Outpatient Neurology

Editors

EVERTON EDMONDSON
DORIS KUNG

NEUROLOGIC CLINICS

www.neurologic.theclinics.com

Consulting Editor
RANDOLPH W. EVANS

February 2023 • Volume 41 • Number 1

ELSEVIER

1600 John F. Kennedy Boulevard • Suite 1800 • Philadelphia, Pennsylvania, 19103-2899

http://www.theclinics.com

NEUROLOGIC CLINICS Volume 41, Number 1
February 2023 ISSN 0733-8619, ISBN-13: 978-0-323-98697-7

Editor: Stacy Eastman
Developmental Editor: Hannah Almira Lopez

Neurologic Clinics (ISSN 0733-8619) is published quarterly by Elsevier Inc., 360 Park Avenue South, New York, NY 10010–1710. Months of issue are February, May, August, and November. Periodicals postage paid at New York, NY, and additional mailing offices. Subscription prices are $353.00 per year for US individuals, $809.00 per year for US institutions, $100.00 per year for US students, $433.00 per year for Canadian individuals, $980.00 per year for Canadian institutions, $489.00 per year for international individuals, $980.00 per year for international institutions, $210.00 for foreign students/residents, and $100.00 for Canadian students/residents. To receive student/resident rate, orders must be accompanied by name of affiliated institution, date of term, and the *signature* of program/residency coordinator on institution letterhead. Orders will be billed at individual rate until proof of status is received. Foreign air speed delivery is included in all *Clinics* subscription prices. All prices are subject to change without notice. **POSTMASTER:** Send address changes to *Neurologic Clinics,* Elsevier Health Sciences Division, Subscription Customer Service, 3251 Riverport Lane, Maryland Heights, MO 63043. **Customer Service: Telephone: 1-800-654-2452 (U.S. and Canada); 314-447-8871 (outside U.S. and Canada). Fax: 314-447-8029. E-mail: journalscustomerservice-usa@elsevier.com (for print support); journalsonlinesupport-usa@elsevier.com (for online support).**

Reprints. For copies of 100 or more of articles in this publication, please contact the Commercial Reprints Department, Elsevier Inc., 360 Park Avenue South, New York, New York, 10010-1710; Tel.: +1-212-633-3874; Fax: +1-212-633-3820, and E-mail: reprints@elsevier.com.

Neurologic Clinics is also published in Spanish by Nueva Editorial Interamericana S.A., Mexico City, Mexico.

Neurologic Clinics is covered in *Current Contents/Clinical Medicine, MEDLINE/PubMed (Index Medicus), EMBASE/Excerpta Medica, and PsycINFO, and ISI/BIOMED.*

Contributors

CONSULTING EDITOR

RANDOLPH W. EVANS, MD
Clinical Professor, Department of Neurology, Baylor College of Medicine, Houston, Texas, USA

EDITORS

EVERTON EDMONDSON, MD
Professor, Neurology, Baylor College of Medicine, Houston, Texas, USA

DORIS KUNG, DO
Associate Professor, Vice Chair of Education, Director of Clinical Sciences, Neurology Department, Baylor College of Medicine, Houston, Texas, USA

AUTHORS

ANTHONY K. ALLAM
School of Medicine, Baylor College of Medicine, Houston, Texas, USA

YAVUZ AYHAN, MD
Atlantic Fellow for Equity in Brain Health Program at GBHI, Department of Neurology, Memory and Aging Center, Weill Institute for Neurosciences, Global Brain Health Institute, University of California, San Francisco (UCSF), San Francisco, California, USA; Trinity College Dublin, Dublin, Ireland; Associate Professor, Department of Psychiatry, Hacettepe University Faculty of Medicine, Ankara, Turkey

FERNANDO X. CUASCUT, MD, MPH
Assistant Professor, Department of Neurology, Maxine Mesinger Multiple Sclerosis Comprehensive Care Center, Houston, Texas, USA

RANDOLPH W. EVANS, MD
Clinical Professor, Department of Neurology, Baylor College of Medicine, Houston, Texas, USA

ERIN FURR STIMMING, MD, FAAN
Director, Neurology Clerkship, Huntington's Disease Society of America (HDSA), Center of Excellence at UTHealth, Professor, Department of Neurology, McGovern Medical School, The University of Texas Health Science Center at Houston (UTHealth), Houston, Texas, USA

RON GADOT, BSc
Department of Neurosurgery, Baylor College of Medicine, Houston, Texas, USA

DAVID GIBBS, BS
Department of Neurologic Surgery, The Ohio State Wexner Medical Center, The Ohio State University College of Medicine, Columbus, Ohio, USA

ALEXANDRA HOVAGUIMIAN, MD
Assistant Professor in Neurology, Beth Israel Deaconess Medical Center, Harvard
Medical School, Boston, Massachusetts, USA

GEORGE J. HUTTON, MD
Professor, Department of Neurology, Maxine Mesinger Multiple Sclerosis Comprehensive
Care Center, Houston, Texas, USA

DORIS KUNG, DO
Associate Professor, Neurology Department, Baylor College of Medicine, Houston,
Texas, USA

SHENG-HAN KUO, MD
Initiative for Columbia Ataxia and Tremor, Columbia University, Department of Neurology,
Columbia University Irving Medical Center, New York, New York, USA

M. BENJAMIN LARKIN, MD, PHARMD
Department of Neurosurgery, Baylor College of Medicine, Houston, Texas, USA

RUPLE S. LAUGHLIN, MD
Associate Professor, EMG Laboratory Director, Department of Neurology, Mayo Clinic,
Rochester, Minnesota, USA

STEPHEN R. MCCAULEY, PhD
Associate Professor, Director of ECCOS, Department of Neurology, Baylor College of
Medicine, H. Ben Taub Department of Physical Medicine and Rehabilitation, Department
of Pediatrics, Baylor College of Medicine, Houston, Texas, USA

BEN G. MCGAHAN, MD
Department of Neurologic Surgery, The Ohio State Wexner Medical Center, Columbus,
Ohio, USA

BRUCE L. MILLER, MD
A.W. and Mary Margaret Clausen Distinguished Professor in Neurology, Director, Memory
and Aging Center, Department of Neurology, Memory and Aging Center, Weill Institute for
Neurosciences, Co-Director, Global Brain Health Institute, University of California, San
Francisco (UCSF), San Francisco, California, USA; Trinity College Dublin, Dublin, Ireland

IRENE PATNIYOT, MD
Section of Neurology and Developmental Neuroscience, Department of Pediatrics, Texas
Children's Hospital Pediatric Headache Clinic, Baylor College of Medicine, Houston,
Texas, USA

CARLOS A. PÉREZ, MD
Assistant Professor, Department of Neurology, Maxine Mesinger Multiple Sclerosis
Comprehensive Care Center, Houston, Texas, USA

KORI A. POROSNICU RODRIGUEZ, MD, MPH
Department of Medicine, Johns Hopkins Bayview Medical Center, Baltimore, Maryland,
USA

MARC PRABLEK, MD
Department of Neurosurgery, Baylor College of Medicine, Houston, Texas, USA

WILLIAM QUBTY, MD
Division of Child Neurology, Minneapolis Clinic of Neurology, Minneapolis, Minnesota, USA

SARA RADMARD, MD
Department of Neurology, Columbia University Irving Medical Center, New York, New York, USA

GAGE RODRIGUEZ, MD
Fellow, Neurology Department, Baylor College of Medicine, Houston, Texas, USA

ALEXANDER E. ROPPER, MD
Department of Neurosurgery, Baylor College of Medicine, Houston, Texas, USA

DEVON I. RUBIN, MD
Professor, EMG Laboratory Director, Department of Neurology, Mayo Clinic, Jacksonville, Florida, USA

RACHEL MARIE E. SALAS, MD, MEd
Assistant Medical Director, Johns Hopkins Center for Sleep and Wellness, Professor of Neurology, Department of Neurology, Johns Hopkins University School of Medicine, Baltimore, Maryland, USA

LOGAN SCHNEIDER, MD
Clinical Lead for Sleep Health, Alphabet, Inc., Clinical Assistant Professor (affiliated) Stanford Sleep Center, Stanford University School of Medicine, Stanford, California, USA

HIMANSHU SHARMA, MD, PhD
Department of Neurosurgery, Baylor College of Medicine, Houston, Texas, USA

MADHU SONI, MD, FAAN
Associate Professor, Director, Clerkship and Advanced Elective Department of Neurological Science, Rush University Medical Center, Chicago, Illinois, USA

ADRIANA M. STRUTT, PhD, ABPP-CN
Professor, Director of BCM Cerebro, Departments of Neurology, Department of Psychiatry and Behavioral Sciences, Baylor College of Medicine, Houston, Texas, USA

ASHLEY A. TAYLOR, MEd
Department of Psychological, Health, and Learning Sciences, Houston, Texas, USA

ASHWIN VISWANATHAN, MD
Department of Neurosurgery, Baylor College of Medicine, Houston, Texas, USA

DAVID S. XU, MD
Department of Neurologic Surgery, The Ohio State Wexner Medical Center, Department of Neurosurgery, The Ohio State University, Columbus, Ohio, USA; Department of Neurologic Surgery, Baylor College of Medicine, Houston, Texas, USA

SELAM A. YOSEPH, MD
Atlantic Fellow for Equity in Brain Health program at GBHI, Department of Neurology, Memory and Aging Center, Weill Institute for Neurosciences, Global Brain Health Institute, University of California, San Francisco (UCSF), San Francisco, California, USA; Trinity College Dublin, Dublin, Ireland; Assistant Professor, Department of Psychiatry, Addis Ababa University, Addis Ababa, Ethiopia

THERESA A. ZESIEWICZ, MD, FAAN
Department of Neurology, University of South Florida (USF), USF Ataxia Research Center, James A Haley Veteran's Hospital, Tampa, Florida, USA

Contents

Chronic insomnia is a clinical diagnosis fulfilled by criteria: (a) difficulty initiating or maintaining sleep, (b) inability to sleep despite having adequate opportunities, (c) having negative daytime effects due to lack of sleep, and (d) sleep difficulty not explained by other disorder—with symptoms at least three times per week during a period of 3 months. Cognitive behavioral therapy is considered a first-line treatment but can be supported with pharmacologic or digital therapeutics. When developing a patient's care plan, we should consider a "personomics" approach in which we personalize care plans as a form of precision sleep medicine.

 Video content accompanies this article at http://www.neurologic. theclinics.com.

Cerebellar ataxia results from damage to the cerebellum and presents as movement incoordination and variability, gait impairment, and slurred speech. Patients with cerebellar ataxia can also have cognitive and mood changes. Although the identification of causes for cerebellar ataxia can be complex, age of presentation, chronicity, family history, and associated movement disorders may provide diagnostic clues. There are many genetic causes for cerebellar ataxia, and the common autosomal dominant and recessive ataxia are due to genetic repeat expansions. Step-by-step approach will lead to the identification of the causes. Symptomatic and potential disease-modifying therapies may benefit patients with cerebellar ataxia.

An electrodiagnostic evaluation is a neurodiagnostic test commonly used to evaluate neuromuscular conditions. A typical electromyography (EMG) report consists of tabular data summarizing findings from nerve conduction studies (NCS) as well as needle EMG (nEMG). A text summary of these findings is also included, followed by a clinical interpretation that evaluates the obtained NCS and nEMG in the context of the clinical presentation. For electrophysiologists and nonelectrophysiologists alike, understanding the elements of EMG report, patterns of findings in common neuromuscular conditions, and potential technical errors that can erroneously influence the clinical interpretation is vital.

> Back pain is a common condition affecting millions of individuals each year. A biopsychosocial approach to back pain provides the best clinical framework. A detailed history and physical examination with a thorough workup are required to exclude emergent or nonoperative etiologies of back pain. The treatment of back pain first uses conventional therapies including lifestyle modifications, nonsteroidal anti-inflammatory drugs, physical therapy, and cognitive behavioral therapy. If these options have been exhausted and pain persists for greater than 6 weeks, imaging and a specialist referral may be indicated.

> Axial neck pain is a common and important problem in the outpatient setting. In isolation, neck pain tends to have a musculoskeletal etiology and responds best to medication and targeted physical therapy. Careful history and physical examination are required to ascertain if there is a neurologic component in addition to the patient's neck pain. For patients needing surgical intervention, there are a variety of approaches and operations that can decompress the appropriate nerve root or the spinal cord itself. These operations are generally well-tolerated and provide significant benefit for appropriately selected patients.

> Multiple sclerosis (MS) is the most prevalent nontraumatic disabling neurologic condition among young adults worldwide. The diagnosis and management of MS is complex. The goal of this review is to provide an updated and practical approach to the diagnosis and treatment approaches in MS, emphasizing current understanding of immunopathogenesis, recent advances, and future directions, for both MS and non-MS clinicians.

> Trigeminal neuralgia is characterized classically by recurrent, evocable, unilateral brief, electric, shocklike pains with an abrupt onset and cessation that affects one or more divisions of the trigeminal nerve. In recent years, the classification of trigeminal neuralgia has been updated based on further understanding. In this manuscript, the authors aim to explain the current understanding of the pathophysiology of trigeminal neuralgia, current diagnosis criteria, and the pharmacologic management and surgical treatments of options currently available.

Dysautonomias are a heterogenous group of disorders that can cause variable symptoms ranging from isolated impairment of one autonomic function to multisystem failure. The causes are also diverse and can be central or peripheral and primary (owing to an intrinsic neurologic cause) or secondary (owing to a disorder that secondarily causes damage to the autonomic nervous system). This review covers common phenotypes of dysautonomias, primary and secondary causes, initial clinical workups, interpretation of common autonomic tests, and first-line treatments. A brief review of autonomic impairment associated with acute and long-COVID is also presented.

Training of students and residents in outpatient settings requires adequate exposure to a broad range of neurologic diseases. A competency-based method has been frequently used to provide a framework for the design and assessment of medical curriculums. However, it is the responsibility of the faculty within a medical school to design the curriculum and ensure its quality. In this article, we review learning objectives, assessment of core competencies, the current status of outpatient neurology education, and the flaws that may affect its quality. We also discuss potential strategies and approaches for the improvement of education and learning process in the outpatient setting, including early clinical exposure of students, cross-disciplinary courses, balancing case mix, near-peer teaching, active learning, electronic and online education, and virtual modules.

NEUROLOGIC CLINICS

ISSUES OF RELATED INTEREST

Neurosurgery Clinics
https://www.neurosurgery.theclinics.com/
Neuroimaging Clinics
https://www.neuroimaging.theclinics.com/
Psychiatric Clinics
https://www.psych.theclinics.com/
Child and Adolescent Psychiatric Clinics
https://www.childpsych.theclinics.com/

THE CLINICS ARE AVAILABLE ONLINE!
Access your subscription at:
www.theclinics.com

Preface

Outpatient Neurology

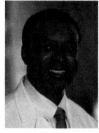

Everton Edmondson, MD   Doris Kung, DO

Editors

Neurologists working in ambulatory clinics encounter a wide variety of neurologic conditions. As new information and treatments emerge, it is often difficult to know sometimes even where to start to diagnose and let alone manage these disorders. We are so fortunate to have an astounding and renowned cadre of neurologists, neurosurgeons, and neurobehavioralists contribute to this issue of *Neurologic Clinics* on Outpatient Neurology. The articles present to the reader rich information with high relevance to the outpatient practice of neurology—from disease entities to differential diagnostic processing and evidence-based therapeutics. Topics illustrate decision processing for the neurologist and provide practical advice and treatment options. The editors of this issue are very honored to have the collaboration of all the authors and appreciate the support of the editorial team and Dr Randolph Evans for his guidance.

Everton Edmondson, MD
Baylor College of Medicine
7200 Cambridge Street, 9th Floor
Houston, TX 77030, USA

Doris Kung, DO
Neurology
Baylor College of Medicine
7200 Cambridge Street, 9th Floor
Houston, TX 77030, USA

E-mail addresses:
everton.edmondson@bcm.edu (E. Edmondson)
kung@bcm.edu (D. Kung)

Neurol Clin 41 (2023) xiii
https://doi.org/10.1016/j.ncl.2022.07.001
0733-8619/23/© 2022 Published by Elsevier Inc.

Insomnia
Personalized Diagnosis and Treatment Options

Kori A. Porosnicu Rodriguez, MD, MPH[a,b],
Rachel Marie E. Salas, MD, MEd[b], Logan Schneider, MD[c,*]

KEYWORDS

- Insomnia • Sleep • Personomics • Somnomics • Cognitive behavioral therapy

KEY POINTS

- Chronic insomnia is a clinical diagnosis made through the International Classification of Sleep Disorders, third edition criteria (ICSD-3): (a) difficulty initiating or maintaining sleep, (b) inability to sleep despite having adequate opportunities for sleep, (c) experiencing negative daytime impacts due to lack of sleep, and (d) sleep difficulty not explained by other sleep/medical disorder—with symptoms occurring at least three nights per week during a period of at least 3 months.
- Cognitive behavioral therapy is the first-line treatment of chronic insomnia.
- Pharmacotherapies are the second-line treatment of insomnia and are only weakly recommended by the American Academy of Sleep Medicine (AASM) guidelines.
- Somnomics is the study of sleep and its relationship to overall patient health from the precision medicine perspective.

INTRODUCTION

The human relationship with sleep has undergone an immense evolution. Our increasing emphasis on productivity and micro-scheduling is no longer limited solely to our work but has permeated our rest. Our ability to closely monitor our sleep habits with a profusion of longitudinally trackable metrics logged on wearable technology and sleep applications has given rise to a wave of emerging "sleep athletes." Concurrently, the prevalence of insomnia continues to rise worldwide, with COVID-19 bringing an onslaught of challenges. The pandemic has augmented the society-wide mental health burden and led to a shift toward telework and virtual social immersion. The blurred line between home and workplace has upended routines and contributed to compromised sleep hygiene and practices,[1] increased insomnia,[2] and poorer sleep quality for some subgroups of sleepers.[3] Now, more than ever, we need to safeguard our sleep for better health and well-being.

[a] Department of Medicine, Johns Hopkins Bayview Medical Center, 4940 Eastern Avenue, Baltimore, MD, USA; [b] Department of Neurology, Johns Hopkins University School of Medicine, 600 North Wolfe Street, Baltimore, MD, USA; [c] Alphabet, Inc., 1600 Amphitheater Parkway, Mountainview, CA 94043, USA
* Corresponding author.
E-mail address: logands@gmail.com
Twitter: @KoriPoRodri (K.A.P.R.); @RachelSalasMD (R.M.E.S.)

Neurol Clin 41 (2023) 1–19
https://doi.org/10.1016/j.ncl.2022.07.004
0733-8619/23/© 2022 Elsevier Inc. All rights reserved.

With the move toward precision medicine, there is an effort to provide personalized high value care. Although the -omics such as proteomics, metabolomics, pharmacogenomics, and so forth are more well known "tools" in the precision medicine toolbox, sleep has also been proposed to be a vital component of precision care. Coined somnomics,[4] the study of sleep, is important across all medical specialties and has been shown to affect several aspects of health. Sleep affects cognition, mood, well-being, metabolism, and immune response and can affect a variety of medical disorders. Further, it is becoming evident that the timing of medication doses may be important for individuals to promote enhanced benefits and reduced side effects, a practice called chronotherapy.[5] Somnomics thus is an area that requires more exploration to achieve high value care.

In this review, we outline the evaluation and management of insomnia while exploring the new frontiers of sleep. We hope to equip clinicians with a clear guide for gold standard management of insomnia and provide a broad overview of the variety of treatment modalities emerging on the market.

BACKGROUND

Epidemiologic studies highlight the elevated prevalence of insomnia disorder sustained over the last decade.[6] More recently in the era of a global crisis, longitudinal studies have shown a 26.7% increase in the incidence of insomnia (symptoms increased from 25.4% to 32.2%, and diagnoses increased from 16.8% to 19%),[2] a phenomenon that has been variously termed "covidsomnia" or "coronasomnia."[7] This is despite—or even possibly because of—the increases in sleep duration that were seen in the general population following COVID-19-related changes in work and social behavioral patterns.[8] Similarly, less enduring disruptions to sleep have demonstrated the consequences of the sociopolitical climate on sleeping patterns,[9] emphasizing that the profusion of the Internet of Things (IoT) can help elucidate the countless sleep disruptors in our daily lives. For example, region-specific bouts of acute insomnia were observed in large-scale smartphone sleep-tracking data sets as a consequence of critical geopolitical events (notably the 2016 U.S. Presidential election and "Brexit"[9]).

The impacts of inadequate sleep on the quality of life are manifold,[10] with some examples being increased cognitive impairment,[11] higher likelihood of mood disorders/chronic pain, elevated risk of suicide, higher rates of prescription sedative/hypnotic use,[12] increased cardiovascular morbidity and mortality, increased accidents, decreased societal productivity, and increased national economic costs.[13] These health impacts and their broad-reaching socioeconomic implications highlight the importance of identifying and addressing insomnia early in our patients.

DEFINITIONS

The International Classification of Sleep Disorders (ICSD) is the primary diagnostic resource for clinicians within sleep medicine. The ICSD-3 delineates three types of insomnia: short-term insomnia disorders, chronic insomnia disorders, and "other" insomnia disorders—which do not fulfill the criteria for the two prior categories. Nearly one in five cases of short-term insomnia develop into chronic insomnia disorders,[14] many of which can persist for years.[6]

PATHOPHYSIOLOGY

Regardless of the duration or characterization (e.g., difficulty initiating or maintaining sleep), a central aspect of insomnia is the concept of hyperarousal. Hyperarousal may be evidenced physiologically in the central and/or peripheral nervous system. Consequently, most patients experience hyperarousal as heightened physiologic (e.g., faster heartbeat and respiration), psychological (e.g., anxiety), or cognitive (e.g., mind racing) activity. This psychophysiological overactivity can interfere with an individual's ability to adequately disengage from the environment for a sound sleep.[15]

The development of insomnia is thought to be the consequence of an individual's predisposition and exposure to a precipitating event, dubbed the "3P Model" of insomnia.[16] In such a diathesis-stress model, individuals with biopsychosocial factors, such as age, sex, and genetic predisposition, may develop insomnia in the face of stressors based on their physical and psychological reactions. The transition to a chronic issue often happens because of maladaptive behaviors and thoughts that serve to perpetuate sleep difficulties. Through repeated associations, individuals reinforce the psychological and/or physiologic hyperarousal through various mechanisms, such as classical conditioning of the bed/bedroom (unconditioned stimulus) with anxiety (conditioned response).

Often accompanying the physiologic sleep associations are cognitive distortions and behavioral adaptations that further reinforce the sleep dysfunctions. For example, many individuals will spend excessive amounts of time worrying about and trying to sleep, often contributing to their insomnia through dilation of the sleep period and "nesting" behaviors that prevent them from straying too far from the bed/bedroom for fear of missing out on the opportunity for sleep.[14] Other cognitive reactions may result in patients developing a "performance anxiety" in response to the approaching sleep period, whereas others have just resigned themselves to the belief that they simply "cannot sleep."[17]

Underpinning the perpetuation of insomnia, as well as the theory behind its treatment, is a disruption of the core physiology of sleep. The two-process model of sleep regulation (**Fig. 1**) explains sleep as a product of the interaction of two components: Process C, a circadian process that is a ~24-h oscillating wakefulness signal, which interacts with and guides Process S, a homeostatic process of sleep debt that gradually accumulates over the course of wake and dissipates over a period of sleep.[18] Factors reducing sleep homeostasis, and thereby, sleep drive, include the caffeine used to combat exhaustion, excessive sleeping (e.g., napping, sleeping longer than the body needs) to make up for perceived sleep inadequacy, and inactivity (e.g., nesting in bed, a generally sedentary lifestyle). Disrupted exposure to typical clock-setting

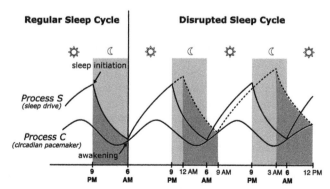

Fig. 1. A representation of the interaction between Process S and Process C and the consequences of delays in sleep onset. The point at which the homeostatic sleep drive (Process S) diminishes to the level where the alerting circadian signal (Process C) is elevated enough to promote awakening takes longer following prolonged wakefulness.

zeitgebers ("time givers"/sleep cues) can cause circadian misalignment with the intended sleep period. From misplaced light exposure at night (instead of at the desired wake time) to mistiming of dietary intake, environmental temperature fluctuations, and even late-night socialization (e.g., the endless stream of social media), the cues necessary for our body to entrain our biological rhythms to our sleep–wake schedule often become desynchronized as individuals with insomnia attempt to orchestrate their lives around their sleep dysfunction.

CLINICAL EVALUATION

Chronic insomnia is primarily a clinical diagnosis. According to the ICSD-3, an insomnia diagnosis necessitates meeting the following criteria:

1. Difficulty with sleep initiation or maintenance.
2. Persisting sleep difficulties despite adequate opportunity for sleep.
3. Negative daytime impacts attributable to lack of sleep, such as fatigue, lack of energy, diminished concentration, emotional lability, and accidents while driving.
4. No other more likely diagnosis.

Chronic insomnia presents as at least 3 months of sleep disturbance and daytime dysfunction at least 3 nights/week, whereas short-term insomnia does not have to last 3 months.[19]

Because insomnia can be either a symptom or a disorder, a thorough sleep history is the first and most important step in evaluating insomnia. The two-process model of sleep regulation and Spielman's 3P behavioral model of insomnia can help inform the history. During the initial visit, one can capture the patient's presleep conditions, difficulty in initiating or maintaining sleep, sleep–wake patterns, sleep-related symptoms, and impact on daytime function. In addition, a sleep environmental scan should be done to search for disruptive factors in the patient's sleep environment from pets and co-sleepers to ambient noises and light pollution. Such questioning can also reveal maladaptive behavior patterns. Moreover, making a distinction between what times in the sleep period are disrupted by insomnia can also be important, as they can have different therapeutic approaches (**Table 1**). Finally, at the initial visit, it will also be important to evaluate for other sleep disorders (e.g., sleep apnea, restless leg syndrome), comorbities, or medications that could be causing the symptom of insomnia.

Questionnaires that can be used as aids in this initial stage include the Pittsburgh Sleep Quality Index, Epworth Sleepiness Scale, and Insomnia Severity Index. These measures provide a validated means of quantifying the severity of a patient's sleep disturbance and daytime impairments at baseline and monitoring the patient's progress during treatment. If additional information is needed, asking the patient to maintain a daily sleep diary can provide a more accurate, real-time account of the patient's sleep. Patients may also be utilizing sleep tracking devices (eg, Sleep Sensing on Nest Hub), which can provide meaningful insights into their sleep patterns and progress. Although commercial sleep trackers provide the benefit of a consistent measure of longitudinal sleep trends within an individual, it must be recognized that these devices often measure and report on metrics that do not yet have a clear, validated role in the clinical management of sleep disorders. In addition, the accuracy of absolute sleep metrics is often poor compared with polysomnography, particularly in clinical populations in which the devices have not been adequately validated.[20,21] Toward this end, consumer wearable companies are attempting to provide transparency regarding their devices and metrics to assist clinicians in using and interpreting patient-generated data (e.g., Fitbit Health Solutions: https://healthsolutions.fitbit.com/providers/).

Table 1
Insomnia issues can affect sleep onset latency, wake after sleep onset, and early morning awakening, each characterized by different criteria and therapeutic approaches

	Sleep Onset Latency Insomnia	Wake After Sleep Onset Insomnia	Early Morning Awakening Insomnia
Definition	Sleep onset latency exceeding 30 min 3 days/wk or more during the last month	Wakefulness exceeding 30 min between periods of sleep 3 days per week or more during the last month	Early morning awakening exceeding 30 min 3 day/wk or more during the last month
Common differential considerations	Medications, anxiety and affective disorders, restless legs syndrome, sleep starts (hypnic jerks), hypnagogic foot tremor, alternating leg muscle activation, sleep-related leg cramps, exploding head syndrome, delayed sleep–wake phase disorder, environmental sleep disturbance	Medications, anxiety and affective disorders, sleep apnea, periodic limb movement disorder, nightmare disorder, narcolepsy, sleep-related leg cramps, environmental sleep disturbance	Medications, anxiety and affective disorders, advanced sleep–wake phase disorder, natural short sleep, nightmare disorder, environmental sleep disturbance
Therapeutic strategies	Limit time in bed before sleep intent. Establish pre-bedtime routines that facilitate preparation for sleep (eg, dimming lights, cooling the environment, tech curfew). Techniques to help quiet the mind (eg, meditation) and calm the body (eg, box breathing). Homeostatic-circadian alignment. Pharmacologic adjunctive therapy with fast onset and relatively short half-life	Stimulus control (eg, leave the sleep space until sleepy). Techniques to help quiet the mind (eg, meditation) and calm the body (eg, box breathing). Homeostatic-circadian alignment. Sleep environment optimization (eg, noise, light, temperature optimization). Pharmacologic adjunctive therapy with either a medium half-life agent at bedtime or a rapid onset, short half-life preparation	Stimulus control (eg, get up and start the morning routine). Homeostatic-circadian alignment. Sleep environment optimization (eg, noise, light, temperature optimization)

At the end of the visit, clinicians can decide whether more in-depth testing is warranted to investigate or validate the experience using in-lab or home polysomnography, actigraphy, or the like. Devices such as the Sleep Profiler can be used for in-home patient-applied polysomnography.[22] However, such diagnostics are often used to elucidate the presence of other primary sleep disorders, such as obstructive sleep apnea, that may be contributory to or causative of insomnia.

MANAGEMENT OF INSOMNIA
Cognitive Behavioral Therapy

As outlined in the Choosing Wisely recommendations,[23] the first-line treatment of chronic insomnia is cognitive behavioral therapy for insomnia (CBT-I). There are various components of CBT-I that can be explored with a patient (**Table 2**). In contrast, only providing patients with general tips on "sleep hygiene" is typically discouraged due to the lack of proven efficacy.[24]

Cognitive interventions involve changing misconceptions that a patient has regarding sleep. These can include negative thoughts around bedtime, such as the fear of not being able to go to sleep, believing that one needs to get more sleep than is necessary or appropriate, or believing that one needs a medication aid to go to sleep. In this vein, education surrounding sleep mechanisms and interactions with daily behaviors is often coupled with an exploration of beliefs that patients have regarding their sleep and impediments thereof. Efforts are made to guide patients to better understand their relationship with sleep, empower them with a sense of control over their ability to get the sleep that they need, and help them set realistic expectations for their sleep and waking function.

Behavioral therapy aims to strengthen the association between the bedroom and sleep with components such as stimulus control and sleep compression. Stimulus control leverages classical conditioning to reestablish the bed and sleep environment as cues to sleep rather than as places where waking activities occur. Establishing a consistent morning rise time and remaining in bed only when sleepy or sleeping leads to the reinforcement of the association between the bedroom and sleep. Sleep compression is another tool that limits "sleep opportunity" to increase sleep efficiency—the proportion of the time in bed spent sleeping—to above 85%.

Although there is efficacy of any individual component of the therapeutic approach to reframing misconceptions or adjusting sleep/wake habits to coordinate sleep drives, the American Academy of Sleep Medicine (AASM)'s 2021 guidelines for the behavioral and psychological treatments for chronic insomnia disorder in adults highlight that a multi-component therapy integrating cognitive and behavioral aspects has the greatest supporting evidence for most insomnia subtypes in various patient populations.[24] Unfortunately, traditional CBT-I is limited in accessibility due to a dearth of qualified behavioral sleep medicine specialists.[25] Consequently, equivalently effective digital CTB-I (dCTB-I) offerings have developed quickly as a means of increasing accessibility and cost-efficacy.[26,27] Although the efficacy of CBT-I in numerous groups has been established, it has been cited that up to 40% of patients do not achieve remission due to heterogeneity within insomnia.[28] As such, groups have sought to use various means—from objective sleep pattern quantification[29] to affective and personality trait characterization[30]—to derive insomnia phenotypes that can provide pathophysiologic insights and identify optimal therapeutic approaches. Interestingly, in one study that identified five stable subtypes of insomnia, therapeutic responses to CBT-I and pharmacotherapies differed between subtypes,[30] suggesting that the potential for a more personalized, data-driven approach to insomnia treatment is on the horizon.

Pharmacotherapy

If CBT-I fails in insomnia remission, pharmacotherapy can be prescribed (**Table 3**). However, it should be noted that every class of agent currently used in the treatment

Table 2
Summary of cognitive behavioral therapy components and targets

Approaches[a]	AASM Strength of Recommendation[b]	What Is This Intervention Trying to Do?	What Does It Involve?	Timeline
CBT-I (multicomponent)	Strong	Address cognitive misperceptions and maladaptive behaviors that are perpetuating sleep difficulties	Cognitive behavioral therapy involving stimulus control and sleep restriction, and mindfulness training involving relaxation promotion	6–10 1-h sessions over a 6–20 wk period
Brief therapy for insomnia (multicomponent)	Conditional recommendation for use	Address cognitive misperceptions and maladaptive behaviors that are perpetuating sleep difficulties	Abbreviated version of CBT-I	4 sessions over 4 wk
Stimulus control therapy (single component)	Conditional recommendation for use	Weaken association between bed/bedroom and wakefulness	Instruct patient to (a) maintain a regular wake time, (b) limit time in bed to only when sleepy, (c) get out of bed if they are unable to sleep, (d) use bedroom for sleep and sex only, and (e) reduce napping in the daytime	Variable
Sleep restriction therapy (single component)	Conditional recommendation for use	Increase sleep drive (pressure for sleep) and sleep efficiency by compressing sleep	Restrict time in bed to patient's average sleep duration (not <5 h), subsequently adjusting time based on sleep efficiency; time in bed is increased by 15–30 min when sleep efficiency is 80%–85% and is decreased by 15–30 min when sleep efficiency is <80%	Variable, but generally weeks (periodic adjustments)
Relaxation therapy (single component)	Conditional recommendation for use	Promote muscle relaxation while reducing cognitive arousal	Exercises to reduce tension such as abdominal breathing, progressive muscle relaxation, and autogenic training; reduced cognitive arousal through guided imagery training and meditation	Variable

(continued on next page)

Table 2
(continued)

Approaches[a]	What Is This Intervention Trying to Do?	What Does It Involve?	AASM Strength of Recommendation[b]	Timeline
Sleep hygiene (single component)	Modify lifestyle and environmental factors to improve sleep conditions	General recommendations about sleep hygiene regarding diet, exercise, substance use, and environmental factors (light, noise, temperature)	Conditional recommendation against use	Variable
Cognitive therapy (single component)	Address potentially harmful beliefs about sleep that may cause increased anxiety and interfere with sleep	Structured psychoeducation, Socratic questioning, thought records, behavioral experiments	No recommendation	Weeks
Biofeedback (single component)	Train physiologic relaxation	Biofeedback device links reduced patient muscle tone (frontalis electromyography) with patient control of auditory tone to train muscle relaxation	No recommendation	4–6 sessions, 30–60 min
Paradoxic intention (single component)	Reduce sleep anxiety by confronting fear	Patient instructed to remain awake as long as possible after staying in bed	No recommendation	Variable
Intensive sleep retraining (single component)	Enhance sleep drive	After 5-h time period in bed, patient undergoes 24-h time period in which they are given opportunities to fall asleep every 30 min; if successful sleep attained, patient is woken up 3 min later, informed of success, and is instructed to remain awake until subsequent 30 min trial	No recommendation	Multiple periods of attempted sleep over a 24-h time period
Mindfulness therapies (multicomponent or single component)	Enhance awareness of one's thoughts and emotions surrounding sleep	Structured exercises to emphasize self-awareness and acceptance conducted either at home or in a group setting	No recommendation	Variable

[a] Multimodal refers to the named therapy offered in conjunction with other CBT components. Single-component therapy is referring to solely the intervention indicated above.
[b] The AASM clinical guidelines provide the recommendation strength for each intervention using the GRADE framework.

of insomnia has been given only a "WEAK" recommendation in the AASM's most recent guidelines.[31] Nonetheless, pharmacotherapies are being prescribed as sleep aids more frequently over the last several decades.[32,33] Commonly used medications with regulatory approval for insomnia include benzodiazepine receptor agonists (BZRAs), nonbenzodiazepine BZRAs ("Z-drugs"), histamine receptor antagonists (e.g., low-dose doxepin), and melatonin receptor agonists (e.g., ramelteon). The first two classes of medications—BZRAs and Z-drugs—both work through activation of the inhibitory γ-aminobutyric acid type A (GABA$_A$) receptor, which results in a global depression of brain function. This rather shotgun approach could be more likened to light anesthesia than physiologic sleep, based on the electroencephalographic changes noted with these agents.[34] It is important to note that benzodiazepines carry a risk of misuse, dependence, tolerance, and withdrawal reactions. Similar risk profiles are seen among the Z-drugs (e.g., zolpidem, eszopiclone, zaleplon), in addition to a risk of parasomnias,such as sleep walking, that prompted the United States Food and Drug Administration (FDA) to issue a black box warning to the entire class of medications.

Antidepressants are also commonly used off-label to treat chronic insomnia; typically trazodone and mirtazapine are used since they have highly selective antihistamine activity at low doses.[35] There is one antidepressant that is FDA-approved for the treatment of insomnia: the low-dose tricyclic antidepressant doxepin that is predominantly antihistaminergic at doses from 3 to 6 mg, and has antiadrenergic, antiserotonergic, and anticholinergic activity typically seen at doses above 75 mg. Toward this end, due to the relative lack of data or regulatory approvals for most antidepressants, such therapies should be reserved for management of a primary psychiatric disorder when comorbid insomnia can be addressed with a single agent.

In 2014, the FDA approved the first dual orexin receptor antagonist for the treatment of insomnia, with subsequent agents (suvorexant, lemborexant) that gained clinical approval demonstrating similar efficacy.[31,36] These agents work to temporarily suppress the activity of the hypocretin system, essentially inducing a state of narcolepsy for the night. Although this is a step toward precision sleep medicine, facilitated by advancements in our understanding of the sleep–wake neurocircuitry, it should be noted that hypocretin is more of a sleep–wake state stabilizer rather than a wake promoting neurotransmitter, per se. As such, individuals with narcolepsy often have sleep instability and disorganized sleep macroarchitecture during the night.[37]

Given that the choice of therapies used in the treatment of insomnia is most strongly predicted by historical prescribing practices (i.e., familiarity),[33] the initiation of more appropriate pharmacotherapies will permeate clinical practice at a relatively glacial pace. However, pharmacogenetics may offer a more patient-centric approach to medication selection that could help tailor treatments to patients while promoting awareness of modern agents that provide a better balance of benefits and risks.[38] Using next-generation sequencing to identify genetic polymorphisms in patients can inform responsiveness and side-effect risks from the array of potential sleep medications, helping clinicians choose an optimal pharmacotherapeutic agent that suits the unique needs of the patient before them.[39]

Complementary Treatments

An important part of precision medicine is personomics[40] which involves respecting the unique belief systems that each patient brings into the clinic. Respecting patients' core beliefs involves focused listening during medical history acquisition and being open to including patient suggestions in an integrated care plan to promote clinician–patient trust, safeguard autonomy, and encourage hope in their clinical

Table 3
Summary of pharmacologic interventions for chronic insomnia

Classes	Medications	AASM Target Recommendation	AASM Strength of Recommendation[a] (Quality of Evidence)	Overdose Side Effects	Withdrawal Side Effects
Dual orexin (hypocretin) receptor antagonists	Suvorexant, Lemborexant, Daridorexant	Sleep maintenance	Weak (low)	Headache, dry mouth, dizziness, dry mouth, abnormal dreams, daytime sleepiness	Typically no withdrawal syndrome
Benzodiazepine receptor agonists	Eszopiclone	Sleep onset and sleep maintenance	Weak (very low)	Headache, dry mouth, nausea, dizziness, tolerance, dependence, bitter/metallic taste Black box: non-rapid eye movement (NREM) parasomnias	Insomnia, irritability, anxiety, tremor, sweating, palpitations, headache, muscular pain and stiffness, perceptual changes
	Zaleplon	Sleep onset	Weak (low)	Drowsiness, dizziness, decreased alertness and concentration, tolerance, dependence Black box: NREM parasomnias	Insomnia, irritability, anxiety, tremor, sweating, palpitations, headache, muscular pain and stiffness, perceptual changes
	Zolpidem	Sleep onset and sleep Maintenance	Weak (very low)	Headache, nausea, diarrhea, daytime sleepiness, tolerance, dependence, Black box:NREM parasomnias	Insomnia, irritability, anxiety, tremor, sweating, palpitations, headache, muscular pain and stiffness, perceptual changes

Class	Drug	Use	Potency (abuse potential)	Side effects	Withdrawal/discontinuation symptoms
Benzodiazepines	Triazolam	Sleep onset	Weak (high)	Dizziness, lightheadedness, coordination difficulties, confusion, headache, tolerance, dependence, respiratory depression	Insomnia, irritability, anxiety, tremor, sweating, palpitations, headache, muscular pain and stiffness, seizure, perceptual changes
	Temazepam	Sleep onset and sleep maintenance	Weak (moderate)	Drowsiness, headache, dizziness, nausea, tiredness, tolerance, dependence, respiratory depression	Insomnia, irritability, anxiety, tremor, sweating, palpitations, headache, muscular pain and stiffness, seizures, perceptual changes
Melatonin receptor agonists	Ramelteon	Sleep onset	Weak (very low)	Dizziness, drowsiness, nausea	Typically no withdrawal syndrome
Heterocyclics	Doxepin	Sleep maintenance	Weak (low)	Drowsiness, dry mouth, constipation, nausea, blurry vision, orthostatic hypotension	Typically minimal: agitation, anxiety, insomnia, dizziness, confusion, headache, irritability, nervousness, depressed mood
	Trazodone	Not recommended	Weak (moderate)	Dry mouth, nausea, headache	Typically minimal: agitation, anxiety, insomnia, dizziness, confusion, headache, irritability, nervousness, depressed mood
Anticonvulsants	Tiagabine	Not recommended	Weak (very low)	Dizziness, memory impairment, headache, diarrhea, asthenia, respiratory depression	Insomnia, irritability, anxiety, tremor, sweating, palpitations, headache, muscular pain and stiffness, seizures, perceptual changes

(continued on next page)

Table 3
(continued)

Classes	Medications	AASM Target Recommendation	AASM Strength of Recommendation[a] (Quality of Evidence)	Overdose Side Effects	Withdrawal Side Effects
OTC preparations	Diphenhydramine	Not recommended	Weak (low)	Dry mouth, urinary retention, pupil dilation, constipation, delirium	Tachycardia, sweating, hypersalivation, mydriasis, hypomimia and hypophonia, dysarthria, eye-movement abnormalities
	Melatonin	Not recommended	Weak (very low)	Headache, dizziness, nausea, drowsiness	Typically no withdrawal syndrome
	L-tryptophan	Not recommended	Weak (high)	Drowsiness, vomiting, diarrhea, headache, blurry vision	Typically no withdrawal syndrome
	Valerian	Not recommended	Weak (low)	Headache, dizziness	Possibly associated with elevated heart rate, unstable blood pressure, tremors, and confusion

[a] The AASM clinical guidelines provide the recommendation strength for each intervention using the GRADE framework.

journey (**Table 4**). Although around 4.5% of patients experiencing insomnia used complementary medicine outside of standard medical care, physicians do not receive sufficient training regarding these treatment modalities.[41]

Many interventions focus on promoting mindfulness within users, a practice that has demonstrated meaningful improvements in measures of insomnia.[42] There has been an explosion of digital offerings such as Headspace and Calm that offer direct-to-consumer options for mindfulness practices and other techniques for winding down for sleep. Somryst, the first and only prescription dCBT-I therapeutic for chronic insomnia, has created lasting improvements in insomnia symptoms. Patients can also explore yoga nidra, massage, acupuncture, meditation, and various forms of sensory stimulation (e.g., tactile, auditory, thermal) to promote relaxation.

Patients often turn to natural supplements to aid in their sleep journey. Some commonly used natural sleep aids include valerian root, lavender, chamomile, passionflower, cannabidiol, and magnesium, most of which have a weak or nonexistent evidence base to support their use.[43] One of the most commonly used over-the-counter sleep aids is melatonin. Although melatonin is better used in physiologic 300 to 500 µg doses for circadian rhythm timing, most individuals typically use 1 to 5 mg due to the slight hypnotic effects. Meta-analyses suggest modest benefits in objective[44,45] and subjective[45] sleep measures; however patients should still be

Table 4
Summary of complementary sleep therapeutics with varying approaches to address sleep difficulties

Approaches	Description	Examples
Digital therapeutics	Prescription digital therapeutics Nonprescription digital therapeutics	Somryst (digital CBT program) Digital CBT programs: SleepHub, Sleepio Meditation apps: Aura, Calm, Headspace
Auditory	Neutral or calming noises	White noise, pink noise, binaural beats, autonomous sensory meridian response
Thermoregulation	Products to maintain comfortable internal temperature or trigger circadian mechanisms	Cooling therapy (eg, Chillow, Chili Cool Mesh Mattress Pad)
Tactile	Intimacy-mimicking compression devices Sensory-stimulating devices or techniques	Sleep Pod, weighted blankets Apollo (vibration therapy), Acupuncture
Visual	Visual cues of sleep-/wake-promoting mechanisms	Light therapy, red light usage
Olfactory	Aromatherapy promoting calming or relaxing effects	Essential oils (lavender, peppermint, chamomile, and so forth)
Relaxation training	Techniques to quiet the mind and calm the body (through parasympathetic tone)	Meditation, yoga Nidra, hypnotherapy, biofeedback, progressive muscle relaxation, guided imagery
Natural Sleep Aids	Various agents with sedating/hypnotic effects	Valerian root, lavender, chamomile, passionflower, cannabidiol, and magnesium

cautious with using supplements since melatonin is unregulated in the United States and studies have demonstrated wide discrepancies between labels and contents (sometimes with no melatonin in the product at all).[46] Although the listed sleep aids often do not produce adverse effects, many of these over-the-counter (OTC) products are unregulated and, like melatonin in the United States, may not contain the ingredient amounts specified.

DISCUSSION

The high and increasing prevalence of insomnia disorders and insomnia symptoms in the general population highlights that the scale of sleep issues in the United States and globally is exceeding the capacity of sleep specialists. Often, individuals turn to their primary care provider or take matters into their own hands. Unfortunately, in such circumstances, many of the best practices in the diagnosis and management of insomnia are often not followed due to a lack of experience or expertise in the management of this common sleep disorder. Nonetheless, front-line clinicians are especially well-poised to make impactful advances in preventing, identifying, and treating insomnia due to their thorough understanding of the various biopsychosocial factors that can promote their patients' sleep health or, when neglected, can result in sleep disorders.. Toward this end, we sought to improve awareness of the state of the field in relation to insomnia to familiarize front-line clinicians, from neurologists to other specialists who may serve as the primary care provider, with the multifaceted nature of the condition and its therapeutic strategies.

First, it is important to understand how insomnia develops and manifests in our current society. Some contend that industrialization transformed our environments and behaviors in ways that are insomniogenic.[47] Prolonged exposure to artificial light and other psychophysiological cues (e.g., social engagement, dietary intake), decreased waking activity levels, [mis]use of readily available psychoactive stimulants (e.g., caffeine) and depressants (e.g., alcohol), and an overemphasis on structured/scheduled efficiency imposed on our sleep schedule are just a few of the potential cognitive and behavioral contributors that have resulted in high rates of sleep dissatisfaction and disordered sleep. Relying on the 3P conceptual framework, we can also see how extrinsic factors may serve to precipitate sleep disruptions that can snowball into long-term sleep issues. However, it is also important to recognize that the breakdown of our usual social rhythms—from the lack of demarcation between professional and social lives to reductions in activity levels—likely compounded the problem.

Given the regular evolution of our society and the challenges it faces, broad prevention of sleep disruption in the face of the next societal stressor is all but impossible. However, individuals and their care partners will need assistance in navigating the complex network of sleep-related factors to prevent acute sleep disruptions from turning into chronic sleep disorders. This often begins with simply discussing sleep health as part of a patient's routine care. The validated RU-SATED paradigm provides a simple mnemonic to aid providers in assessing the many dimensions of sleep health: Routine regularity, Satisftaction, Alertness, Timing (of the sleep period), Efficiency, and Duration.[48] Once issues with sleep have been identified, refining the understanding of an individual's sleep pathology can be accomplished through the involvement of specialized consultations, further diagnostics, and even the incorporation of some of the cutting-edge tools discussed above to create a multifaceted clinical picture of each patient. From discerned patterns in consumer wearable actigraphic data that identify an individual's daily circadian phase,[49] to data-driven sleep phenotypes that predict outcomes[50] as well as response to therapies,[51] to personalized pharmacogenomic profiles that help clinicians choose the optimal treatment regimen by means of identifying the medication with maximal benefit, low side effect profile, and least amount of drug–drug interactions, sleep is at the forefront of integrating various data streams to tailor clinical management to each patient's unique needs.

Despite the promise that the IoT and analytical advances offer to patients and providers alike, we must be careful not to exacerbate the situation through the tools that we use to solve the problem. From the pathology of "orthosomnic" consumers obsessing over impractical sleep goals,[52] which may not be appropriate for them, to a deterministic sense of being "hard wired" for a certain sleep pathology or therapeutic response, the risk of patients getting the wrong message and being led astray by contextless data is high. Particularly as cheap sleep tracking technologies and direct-to-consumer offerings are becoming more ubiquitous, clinicians must become more familiar with the evidence underpinning them to competently assess their limitations and be comfortable interpreting their data in the context of the patient sitting before them.

Beyond the feed-forward model of optimizing insomnia management through precision medicine approaches, we must also consider each patient's unique needs and values. Meeting patients where they are takes a discernment of the biopsychosocial factors that are likely contributing to the perpetuation of their insomnia. Exploring a patient's circumstances through the lens of "personomics" not only provides insights into the misconceptions and maladaptive habits that may be the focus of CBTs, but also serves to offer insight and agency to our patients as part of shared decision-making that helps map out the therapeutic journey together. Without "peeking into the bedroom" to get a glimpse of the sleeping and waking lives of our patients, we cannot truly begin to understand what obstacles are preventing them from sleeping soundly.

SUMMARY

Fundamentally, sleep medicine has always been a forward-looking specialty that embraces big data: distilling hours of physiologic signals into a concerted understanding of someone's night, tracking behavioral patterns of sleep and wake over weeks to discern circadian phase, monitoring therapy adherence from breath to breath in positive airway pressure (PAP) device data downloads. However, simply gathering data will not result in the desired outcomes; engaging patients to provide context to the data and customization to the care is essential to the health care relationship. This therapeutic journey begins by simply asking.

CLINICS CARE POINTS

- Insomnia symptoms and insomnia disorder are highly prevalent in the general population.

- Numerous biopsychosocial factors influence the likelihood of acute onset of insomnia symptoms, including societal stressors such as the COVID-19 pandemic.

- Chronic insomnia is a clinical diagnosis where the following criteria have to be fulfilled: (a) difficulty with sleep initiation/maintenance, (b) inability to sleep despite adequate opportunities for sleep, (c) negative daytime impacts due to lack of sleep, and (d) sleep difficulty is not explained by other sleep/medical disorder. Chronic insomnia involves at least 3 months of sleep disturbances and daytime dysfunction for at least 3 nights/week.

- Spielman's "3P Model" of chronic insomnia can be useful during history taking by allowing the physician to explore (a) predisposing factors, (b) precipitating events, and(c) perpetuating factors for insomnia.
- Assessing sleep health should be done at every clinical visit (as with other vital signs), leveraging simple frameworks that account for its multifaceted nature (e.g., RU-SATED).
- The first-line treatment of insomnia is cognitive behavioral therapy for insomnia (CBT-I); pharmacotherapies should be avoided until a patient has had the opportunity to go through a CBT-I program.
- The second-line treatment of chronic insomnia involves pharmacotherapies, though it is important to note that every class is only weakly recommended by AASM's most recent guidelines.
- The practice of "somnomics" involves the study of sleep and its relationship on overall health and is part of the precision medicine toolbox.

DISCLOSURE

Dr. K.A. Porosnicu Rodriguez has no disclosures. Dr. R.M.E. Salas has the following disclosures: Idorsia, Alliance for Sleep (2022-present); HMP Global, Neurology and Sleep Education Consultant (2021-present); American Medical Association, Health System Science Core Faculty (2021-present); ScholarRX, Editorial Board, Education Consulting (2021-present); UptoDate Chapter-royalty (2016-present). Dr. L. Schneider reports personal fees from Jazz Pharmaceuticals, personal fees from Harmony Biosciences outside the submitted work, and employment at Alphabet, Inc.

REFERENCES

1. Cellini N, Canale N, Mioni G, et al. Changes in sleep pattern, sense of time and digital media use during COVID-19 lockdown in Italy. J Sleep Res 2020;29(4). https://doi.org/10.1111/JSR.13074.
2. Morin CM, Vézina-Im LA, Ivers H, et al. Prevalent, incident, and persistent insomnia in a population-based cohort tested before (2018) and during the first-wave of COVID-19 pandemic (2020). Sleep 2022;45(1). https://doi.org/10.1093/SLEEP/ZSAB258.
3. Kocevska D, Blanken TF, van Someren EJW, et al. Sleep quality during the COVID-19 pandemic: not one size fits all. Sleep Med 2020;76:86.
4. Somnomics: the intersection of sleep medicine and personalized care | Neurodiem. Available at: https://www.neurodiem.com/news/somnomics-the-intersection-of-sleep-medicine-and-personalized-care-BdXnXJdkFGvS94S4ama7Y. Accessed May 10, 2022.
5. Smolensky MH, Hermida RC, Geng YJ. Chronotherapy of cardiac and vascular disease: timing medications to circadian rhythms to optimize treatment effects and outcomes. Curr Opin Pharmacol 2021;57:41–8.
6. Morin CM, Jarrin DC, Ivers H, et al. Incidence, Persistence, and Remission Rates of Insomnia Over 5 Years. JAMA Netw Open 2020;3(11):e2018782.
7. Coronasomnia: Definition, Symptoms, and Solutions | Sleep Foundation. Available at: https://www.sleepfoundation.org/covid-19-and-sleep/coronasomnia. Accessed May 10, 2022.
8. Robbins R, Affouf M, Weaver MD, et al. Estimated Sleep Duration Before and During the COVID-19 Pandemic in Major Metropolitan Areas on Different Continents:

Observational Study of Smartphone App Data. J Med Internet Res 2021;23(2). https://doi.org/10.2196/20546.

9. Anýž J, Bakštein E, Dudysová D, et al. No wink of sleep: Population sleep characteristics in response to the brexit poll and the 2016 U.S. presidential election. Soc Sci Med 2019;222:112–21.

10. Olfson M, Wall M, Liu SM, et al. Insomnia and Impaired Quality of Life in the United States. J Clin Psychiatry 2018;79(5). https://doi.org/10.4088/JCP. 17M12020.

11. Fernandez-Mendoza J, He F, Puzino K, et al. Insomnia with objective short sleep duration is associated with cognitive impairment: a first look at cardiometabolic contributors to brain health. Sleep 2021;44(1). https://doi.org/10.1093/SLEEP/ ZSAA150.

12. Bertisch SM, Herzig SJ, Winkelman JW, et al. National use of prescription medications for insomnia: NHANES 1999-2010. Sleep 2014;37(2):343–9.

13. Streatfeild J, Smith J, Mansfield D, et al. The social and economic cost of sleep disorders. Sleep 2021;44(11). https://doi.org/10.1093/SLEEP/ZSAB132.

14. Perlis ML, Vargas I, Ellis JG, et al. The Natural History of Insomnia: the incidence of acute insomnia and subsequent progression to chronic insomnia or recovery in good sleeper subjects. Sleep 2020;43(6):1–8.

15. Levenson JC, Kay DB, Buysse DJ. The Pathophysiology of Insomnia. Chest 2015; 147(4):1179.

16. Spielman AJ, Caruso LS, Glovinsky PB. A Behavioral Perspective on Insomnia Treatment. Psychiatr Clin North Am 1987;10(4):541–53.

17. Yang CM, Hung CY, Lee HC. Stress-Related Sleep Vulnerability and Maladaptive Sleep Beliefs Predict Insomnia at Long-Term Follow-Up. J Clin Sleep Med 2014; 10(9):997.

18. Borbély AA, Daan S, Wirz-Justice A, et al. The two-process model of sleep regulation: a reappraisal. J Sleep Res 2016;25(2):131–43.

19. Medicine AA of S. International Classification of Sleep Disorders. 3rd ed. Darien, IL: American Academy of Sleep Medicine, 2014. Available at: https://learn.aasm. org/Listing/a1341000002XmRvAAKIt's.

20. Haghayegh S, Khoshnevis S, Smolensky MH, et al. Accuracy of Wristband Fitbit Models in Assessing Sleep: Systematic Review and Meta-Analysis. J Med Internet Res 2019;21(11). https://doi.org/10.2196/16273.

21. Chinoy ED, Cuellar JA, Huwa KE, et al. Performance of seven consumer sleep-tracking devices compared with polysomnography. Sleep 2021;44(5):1–16.

22. Finan PH, Richards JM, Gamaldo CE, et al. Validation of a Wireless, Self-Application, Ambulatory Electroencephalographic Sleep Monitoring Device in Healthy Volunteers. J Clin Sleep Med 2016;12(11):1443.

23. American Academy of Sleep Medicine. Five Things Physicians and Patients Should Question. 2021. Available at: www.aasm.org. Accessed May 10, 2022.

24. Edinger JD, Arnedt JT, Bertisch SM, et al. Behavioral and psychological treatments for chronic insomnia disorder in adults: an American Academy of Sleep Medicine clinical practice guideline. J Clin Sleep Med 2021;17(2):255–62.

25. Thomas A, Grandner M, Nowakowski S, et al. Where are the Behavioral Sleep Medicine Providers and Where are They Needed? A Geographic Assessment. Behav Sleep Med 2016;14(6):687.

26. Darden M, Espie CA, Carl JR, et al. Cost-effectiveness of digital cognitive behavioral therapy (Sleepio) for insomnia: a Markov simulation model in the United States. Sleep 2021;44(4). https://doi.org/10.1093/SLEEP/ZSAA223.

27. Henry AL, Miller CB, Emsley R, et al. Insomnia as a mediating therapeutic target for depressive symptoms: A sub-analysis of participant data from two large randomized controlled trials of a digital sleep intervention. J Sleep Res 2021;30(1): e13140.

28. Galbiati A, Sforza M, Fasiello E, et al. Impact Of Phenotypic Heterogeneity Of Insomnia On The Patients' Response To Cognitive-Behavioral Therapy For Insomnia: Current Perspectives. Nat Sci Sleep 2019;11:367.

29. Foldager J, Peppard PE, Hagen EW, et al. Genetic risk for subjective reports of insomnia associates only weakly with polygraphic measures of insomnia in 2,770 adults. J Clin Sleep Med 2022;18(1):21–9.

30. Blanken TF, Benjamins JS, Borsboom D, et al. Insomnia disorder subtypes derived from life history and traits of affect and personality. Lancet Psychiatry 2019;6(2):151–63.

31. Sateia MJ, Buysse DJ, Krystal AD, et al. Clinical Practice Guideline for the Pharmacologic Treatment of Chronic Insomnia in Adults: An American Academy of Sleep Medicine Clinical Practice Guideline. J Clin Sleep Med 2017;13(2):307–49.

32. America's State of Mind Report | Express Scripts. Available at: https://www.express-scripts.com/corporate/americas-state-of-mind-report. Accessed May 10, 2022.

33. Beam AL, Kartoun U, Pai JK, et al. Predictive Modeling of Physician-Patient Dynamics That Influence Sleep Medication Prescriptions and Clinical Decision-Making. Sci Rep 2017;7(1):1–7.

34. Jang DJ, Lim DK, Kim JK. Polysomnography Analysis of Electroencephalography in Patients Expending Benzodiazepine Drugs. Korean J Clin Lab Sci 2021;53(4): 333–41.

35. Stahl SM. Selective histamine H1 antagonism: novel hypnotic and pharmacologic actions challenge classical notions of antihistamines. CNS Spectr 2008;13(12): 1027–38.

36. Rosenberg R, Citrome L, Drake CL. Advances in the Treatment of Chronic Insomnia: A Narrative Review of New Nonpharmacologic and Pharmacologic Therapies. Neuropsychiatr Dis Treat 2021;17:2549.

37. Roth T, Dauvilliers Y, Mignot E, et al. Disrupted Nighttime Sleep in Narcolepsy. J Clin Sleep Med 2013;9(9):955.

38. Landolt HP, Holst SC, Valomon A. Clinical and Experimental Human Sleep-Wake Pharmacogenetics. Handb Exp Pharmacol 2019;253:207–41.

39. Krystal AD, Prather AA. Sleep Pharmacogenetics: The Promise of Precision Medicine. Sleep Med Clin 2019;14(3):317–31.

40. Ziegelstein RC. Personomics *JAMA Intern Med* 2015;175(6):888–9.

41. Ng JY, Parakh ND. A systematic review and quality assessment of complementary and alternative medicine recommendations in insomnia clinical practice guidelines. BMC Complement Med Therapies 2021;21(1). https://doi.org/10.1186/S12906-021-03223-3.

42. Gong H, Ni CX, Liu YZ, et al. Mindfulness meditation for insomnia: A meta-analysis of randomized controlled trials. J Psychosom Res 2016;89:1–6.

43. Kim J, Lee SL, Kang I, et al. Natural Products from Single Plants as Sleep Aids: A Systematic Review. J Med Food 2018;21(5):433–44.

44. Li T, Jiang S, Han M, et al. Exogenous melatonin as a treatment for secondary sleep disorders: A systematic review and meta-analysis. Front Neuroendocrinol 2019;52:22–8.

45. Fatemeh G, Sajjad M, Niloufar R, et al. Effect of melatonin supplementation on sleep quality: a systematic review and meta-analysis of randomized controlled trials. J Neurol 2022;269(1):205–16.
46. Erland LAE, Saxena PK. Melatonin Natural Health Products and Supplements: Presence of Serotonin and Significant Variability of Melatonin Content. J Clin Sleep Med 2017;13(2):275–81.
47. Ekirch AR. Sleep we have lost: Pre-industrial slumber in the British Isles. Am Hist Rev 2001;106(2):343–85.
48. Buysse DJ. Sleep Health: Can We Define It? Does It Matter? Sleep 2014;37(1):9.
49. Cheng P, Walch O, Huang Y, et al. Predicting circadian misalignment with wearable technology: validation of wrist-worn actigraphy and photometry in night shift workers. Sleep 2021;44(2):1–8.
50. Wallace ML, Lee S, Stone KL, et al. Actigraphy-derived sleep health profiles and mortality in older men and women. Sleep 2022;45(4). https://doi.org/10.1093/SLEEP/ZSAC015.
51. Benjamins JS, Migliorati F, Dekker K, et al. Insomnia heterogeneity: Characteristics to consider for data-driven multivariate subtyping. Sleep Med Rev 2017;36:71–81.
52. Baron KG, Abbott S, Jao N, et al. Orthosomnia: Are Some Patients Taking the Quantified Self Too Far? J Clin Sleep Med 2017;13(2):351.

Evaluation of Cerebellar Ataxic Patients

Sara Radmard, MD[a],*, Theresa A. Zesiewicz, MD[b,c], Sheng-Han Kuo, MD[d,e],*

KEYWORDS

- Cerebellar ataxia • Spinocerebellar ataxia • Multiple system atrophy • Ataxia
- Genetics

KEY POINTS

- Cerebellar ataxia is characterized by movement incoordination and variability.
- The cerebellum plays an important role in scaling precise movements, mood, and cognition.
- The causes of cerebellar ataxia are vast, and once cerebellar ataxia is established based on examination, workup for reversible and genetic causes should be pursued.
- Important diagnostic clues for cerebellar ataxia that guide a diagnostic workup include age of onset, chronicity, and other associated movement disorders.
- Some genetic and acquired causes of cerebellar ataxia have targeted disease-modifying therapies.

Video content accompanies this article at http://www.neurologic.theclinics. com.

INTRODUCTION

Movement precision is critical to voluntary motor execution. Cerebellar ataxia leads to impairment of movement precision, making simple tasks such as eating, dressing, and walking difficult. The causes of cerebellar ataxia can be diverse and thus pose a diagnostic challenge. Therefore, it is important to recognize signs and symptoms, perform a comprehensive workup, and institute a treatment plan for patients with cerebellar ataxia.

---

[a] Department of Neurology, Columbia University Irving Medical Center, 710 West 168th Street, Floor 3, New York, NY 10032, USA; [b] Department of Neurology, University of South Florida (USF), USF Ataxia Research Center, Tampa, FL, USA; [c] James A Haley Veteran's Hospital, Tampa, FL, USA; [d] Initiative for Columbia Ataxia and Tremor, Columbia University, New York, NY, USA; [e] Department of Neurology, Columbia University Irving Medical Center, 650 West 168th Street, Room 305, New York, NY 10032, USA
* Corresponding authors.
E-mail addresses: sr3337@cumc.columbia.edu (S.R.); sk3295@columbia.edu (S.-H.K.)

Neurol Clin 41 (2023) 21–44
https://doi.org/10.1016/j.ncl.2022.05.002
0733-8619/23/© 2022 Elsevier Inc. All rights reserved.

The cerebellum is primarily known for control of voluntary movement coordination, balance maintenance, and eye movements. Cerebellar ataxia is a manifestation of cerebellar damage or degeneration and is typified by specific motor impairments. Clinical manifestations of cerebellar ataxia include speech impairment, limb incoordination, gait instability, and eye movement abnormalities. In addition to motor control, the cerebellum is also involved in cognition.[1–4] Although the cognitive symptoms associated with cerebellar ataxia are not as widely recognized as motor symptoms, they are still disabling to patients and should be evaluated along with the motor impairments.

The causes of cerebellar ataxia are vast. Age of onset, disease course, associated clinical symptoms, as well as laboratory and imaging data provide clues to construct a differential diagnosis, which can include vascular, infectious, inflammatory, paraneoplastic, neoplastic, hereditary, toxic, and degenerative etiologies. Given the diverse causes, diagnostic workup and management can be challenging. This review aims to provide guidance for the diagnosis and management of cerebellar ataxia with a special emphasis on phenomenology, complmented by video clips. The authors highlight the unique features of certain forms of cerebellar ataxia and provide a stepwise diagnostic workup diagram. They also discuss symptomatic and emerging disease-modifying therapies for cerebellar ataxia.

CEREBELLAR ANATOMY

The first step of classic neurology is localization of neurologic deficits. Understanding cerebellar anatomy is critical for assessing ataxia. The cerebellum is composed of the left and right lateral hemispheres connected by the vermis. Outflow fibers from the ipsilateral deep cerebellar nuclei course through the superior cerebellar peduncles to the contralateral thalamus and subsequent contralateral motor cortex. Because the contralateral motor cortex controls ipsilateral limb movements, damages to the ipsilateral cerebellum will result in ipsilateral limb ataxia. The vermis is a midline structure important for truncal control. The flocculonodular lobe receives inputs from vestibular nuclei and regulates posture and eye movements. Discrete lesions in a particular cerebellar area result in ataxia of the corresponding body parts,[4,5] whereas degenerative diseases often involve broad regions of the cerebellum and thus ataxia symptoms are more diffuse.

COGNITION AND MOOD IN CEREBELLAR ATAXIA

The role of the cerebellum in cognition and mood is equally as significant as its role in motor coordination. The cerebellar posterior lobe has extensive neural connections to the limbic and paralimbic areas, prefrontal, temporal, parietal cerebral cortex, and cingulate gyrus.[6–9] Posterior lobe degeneration is linked to cognitive dysfunction in executive and visuospatial domains and personality changes of affect flattening, disinhibition, and impulsivity.[10–12] Depression is common among inherited and degenerative ataxia syndromes and are independent of disease severity.[13,14] Collectively, these impairments are known as cerebellar cognitive affective syndrome.[10] Recognizing and screening cerebellar ataxia patients for these cognitive and psychiatric changes is important for quality of life.

SYMPTOMS OF CEREBELLAR DISEASE

Recognition of the core symptoms and signs is the first step in approaching patients with suspected cerebellar ataxia. The most common and often first presenting symptom of cerebellar ataxia is gait imbalance.[15] Patients may describe unexpected loss of balance, easily tripping or bumping into objects, and finally, progressive falls. Ataxic gait may be described as appearing intoxicated from alcohol. Other ancillary information regarding gait imbalance will further ascertain a diagnosis of cerebellar ataxia. Specifically, gait changes (veering, intoxicated, or shortened cadence), the circumstances surrounding the fall (occurring primarily in the dark or with the eyes closed, foot dragging, sudden balance loss "out of nowhere"), and the progressive nature of falls are important diagnostic clues. Patients with cerebellar ataxia are more likely to have veering or changing gait direction and difficulty turning. Falling with eyes closed or in the dark suggests sensory neuropathy.

Appendicular ataxia manifests as imprecise movements in the hands or legs. Patients complain of "clumsiness," uncoordinated handwriting, or knocking over or dropping objects due to miscalculation of object location or weight. Eye and speech complaints are also common in patients with cerebellar ataxia. Patients may notice "jumpy" eyes or burry vision, corresponding to nystagmus. Double vision is not common in pure cerebellar disease unless late stages of spinocerebellar ataxia (SCA) types 2 and 3 cause partial ophthalmoplegia. Speech may be slurred or reported as more difficult to understand. Lastly, patients may describe vertigo, a sensation the environment or oneself is moving. Oftentimes, patients experience lightheadedness without frank vertigo. Cerebellar vertigo is central in origin and thus typically does not worsen with head movements and is less severe than peripheral vertigo, which is often associated with nausea and vomiting.

EXAMINING PATIENTS WITH CEREBELLAR ATAXIA

Evaluation should begin while observing the patient in the waiting room and walking to the examination room. Observation of speech, eye movements, and abnormal movements continues before direct examination. How much of the history is provided by the patient versus a friend or family member can also help clinicians gauge severity of speech disorder or cognitive and emotional impairment. This spontaneous information provides a valuable glimpse of how ataxia symptoms may affect patients' lives.

Eye Examination

The eye examination should first begin in primary position. Instruct the patient to fixate on a far target, such as a painting on the wall. The examiner is looking for *square wave jerks* (SWJ), which means saccadic intrusions in the horizontal plane that interrupt visual fixation on a target. Some healthy adults may exhibit SWJ; conversely, larger amplitude SWJ are seen in certain cerebellar diseases, such as Friedreich ataxia. SWJ may be observed in atypical parkinsonism with cerebellar involvement, including progressive supranuclear gaze palsy (PSP) and multiple system atrophy (MSA).[16,17]

Next, the patient should gaze at and follow the examiner's finger in vertical and horizontal directions to look for *nystagmus* or bring out *ocular flutter* or *opsoclonus*. Inquire about diplopia during smooth pursuit. *Nystagmus* is involuntary, repetitive eye movements that occur in a to-and-fro manner.[18] Nystagmus of a cerebellar origin involves fast and slow phases and can be directional or multidirectional. Nystagmus is the most common eye finding in cerebellar ataxia. *Ocular flutter* is irregular, oscillatory horizontal/unidirectional bursts of saccadic eye movements, typically induced by blinking or voluntary gaze.[18] *Opsoclonus* is similar to ocular flutter but saccadic oscillations are multidirectional.[18] Both are at a higher frequency than nystagmus and are seen in infectious/parainfectious, immune-mediated, or paraneoplastic cerebellar ataxia.[19]

Lastly, the examiner should test *saccades* to assess speed and accuracy of eye movements. To test saccadic movement, have the patient direct gaze between an examiner's finger then switch gaze quickly to the examiner's nose on command. *Slow saccades* are seen in SCA2 and SCA3[20,21]; however, SCA2 patients particularly have profoundly slow saccades. *Hypometric saccades* occur when eye movements fall short of reaching the intended gaze target. The eyes then make one or more corrective saccades to reach the target. *Hypermetric saccades* occur when eye movements pass the intended gaze target then correct back to the target. Patients with cerebellar ataxia may have co-existence of hypometric and hypermetric saccades with hypometric in one direction and hypermetric saccades in another direction. *Oculomotor apraxia* is a loss of voluntary eye movement control and presents as difficulty initiating a saccade. Eye blinks or head thrust are used to maneuver gaze in a particular direction. Examples of eye findings associated with cerebellar ataxia are shown in Video 1, and eye findings commonly associated with specific cerebellar ataxia syndromes are listed in **Table 1**.

Speech Examination

Speech examination begins while listening to the patient give the history. The most common presenting cerebellar speech impairments are *dysarthria* and *scanning speech*. *Dysarthria* is an abnormal articulation of speech phonemes. *Ataxic dysarthria* is due to uncoordinated, antagonistic muscle movements resulting in imprecise speech. *Scanning speech* has variability in speed, power, syllabic stress, and coordination of muscle movements.[22] It is also described as a *staccato speech* where words or syllables are interrupted by variable pauses. For example, when saying, "Today is a sunny day," a patient may say, "Today is a" pause "sunny day," or "Today is a sun" pause "-ny day." Consonants may be overemphasized or vowels underemphasized or distorted. Another key feature of cerebellar speech is slow speed, possibly a

Table 1	
Specific eye findings seen in cerebellar ataxia syndromes	
Square Wave Jerks	**Friedreich Ataxia**
Slowed saccades	SCA2
	SCA3
	SCA7
Downbeating nystagmus	SCA6
	Multiple system atrophy
Pigmentary retinal macular degeneration	SCA7
Ophthalmoparesis	SCA2
	SCA3
	SCA7
	Kearns-Sayre syndrome
	Miller Fisher syndrome
Oculomotor apraxia	Ataxia with oculomotor ataxia types 1 & 2
	Ataxia telangiectasia
Supranuclear ophthalmoplegia	Niemann-Pick type C
Retinitis pigmentosa	Refsum disease
	Abetalipoproteinemia
	Kearns-Sayre syndrome
	Neuropathy, ataxia, & retinitis pigmentosa

Abbreviation: SCA, spinocerebellar ataxia.

compensatory response to imprecision. Examples of speech impairment in cerebellar ataxia can be listened to in Video 2.

Appendicular Examination

Appendicular ataxia is evaluated by a series of assessments centered around the core clinical feature of appendicular ataxia: dysmetria. *Dysmetria* is inaccurate reaching of a target by the hands, arms, or legs. The ability to predict the accurate distance and speed needed to coordinate muscle movements is the exact function of the cerebellum and is consequently impaired in cerebellar ataxia. Two methods used to assess dysmetria are finger chase and heel-shin slide. Finger chase is performed by the examiner quickly moving his or her finger in a random fashion through space. The patient rapidly mirrors the movements exactly. The degree of dysmetria is estimated by the difference the patient's finger deviates from the examiner's finger. Leg dysmetria is tested by performing heel-shin slide in the lying down position with shoes and socks off and no obstructive clothing below the knee. The patient places a heel onto the contralateral knee and accurately and slowly slides the heel down the shin. The heel is then first rested on the table or bed, then repositioned back to the knee to perform successive movements. Thus, the patient is only instructed to slide down the shin but not up the shin. Grading severity is based on how well the heel maintains contact and the number of times the heel slides off the shin.

Dysdiadochokinesia is irregular and inaccurate rapid alternating synchronous movements. Because one major cerebellar function is control of movement rhythm, cerebellar ataxia manifests as abnormal rapid alternating movements. To perform rapid alternating hand movements, the patient alternates between pronating and supinating the hand as accurately as possible on the ipsilateral thigh. The palmar aspect of the hand will alternate touching the thigh with the dorsal aspect of the hand. To find further subtle cerebellar abnormalities, instruct the patient to perform the movements as fast as possible.

Several types of tremors are present in cerebellar ataxia. *Intention tremor* occurs when tremor amplitude increases as nearing a target and is the most common type of tremor in cerebellar ataxia.[23] Intention tremor is observed in finger-nose-finger testing performed by having the patient extend the index finger and alternate between touching the examiner's finger and the patient's nose or chin (depending on tremor severity). Note the examiner's finger should be fixed during finger-nose-finger testing. Another form of kinetic tremor, *postural tremor*, can also be present.[23,24] Assess postural tremor by observing the patient maintaining their arms in an outstretched or wing-beating position. Lastly, look inside the patient's mouth to assess for palatal tremor seen in progressive ataxia associated with hypertrophic olivary degeneration. The examples of appendicular examinations for cerebellar ataxia can be viewed in Videos 3 and 4.

Sitting Examination

Truncal ataxia manifests as incoordination of the trunk, shoulders, and hips. *Truncal sway* can be observed in the seated position, without back support, and the arms outstretched. In severe cases, patients may not be able to sit unsupported. *Truncal titubation* means increased shaking of the body when standing or sitting, which is common in patients with cerebellar ataxia.

Stance and Gait Examination

Stance is evaluated by observing the patient stand in the natural position, with the feet together and with the feet situated in tandem/heel-to-toe. *Titubation* and *truncal sway* are seen in sitting and standing positions in cerebellar ataxia. Ataxia also manifests as inability to maintain balance, needing to catch oneself by holding onto an object or side-stepping while walking. If ataxia is suspected, the examiner should remain close to the patient to ensure patient safety. *Sensory ataxia*, ataxia due to erroneous sensory inputs, worsens with the eyes closed. Additional examination maneuvers that can bring out subtle ataxic signs include having patients stand on one foot at a time or hop on one foot. Patients with cerebellar ataxia will lose balance.

Gait is evaluated by watching the patient comfortably and safely walking with turns. Turning requires more coordination than natural walking; therefore, patients with cerebellar ataxia may find turning more difficult. Sequentially, tandem walking can further bring out ataxia. Ataxic gait is typically wide based to compensate for imbalance and staggering. Tandem walking forces the patient to walk on a very narrow base, amplifying ataxia. Ataxic patients attempting to walk in tandem may have large amplitude sway or side-stepping to maintain balance. Although wide-based gait is commonly associated with ataxia, the core feature of cerebellar gait is *stride variability*, which is an inability to walk with consistent cadence or direction throughout. The examiner cannot predict where the next step will occur due to variation in stride length, cadence, or speed. Stride variability should still be observed in patients who exhibit wide-based gait. Lastly, some patients may have co-existing spastic gait. *Spastic gait* is a stiff leg walk with foot dragging and circumduction of the leg. A good example is autosomal recessive spastic ataxia of Charlevoix-Saguenay (ARSACS). The examples of ataxic stance and gait can be viewed in Videos 5 and 6.

OTHER MOVEMENT DISORDER EXAMINATION CONSIDERATIONS

Once ataxia is established by cerebellar-specific examination as discussed earlier, looking for other signs of movement disorders is important. These signs include parkinsonism, dystonia, and myoclonus. *Parkinsonism* is defined by bradykinesia, hypokinesia, and rigidity. Parkinsonism is present in MSA, PSP, SCA2, SCA3, and SCA17. Rest tremor is uncommon but may be seen in MSA and SCA2. *Dystonia* is sustained or intermittent muscle contractions that results in abnormal posturing, twisting, or repetitive movements. Facial dystonia and anterocollis (forward neck flexion) are common in MSA. Although dystonia is the prominent feature of Wilson disease, an autosomal recessive disorder caused by excessive copper deposition, some cases can also present with ataxia. Dystonia can be seen in autosomal dominant ataxias, including SCA3 and SCA8, and in autosomal recessive ataxias, including abetalipoproteinemia, ataxia telangiectasia, Niemann-Pick type C (NPC), and polymerase gamma gene-related disorder (POLG) ataxia. *Chorea* is involuntary, random, unsustained, dancelike movements. In the autosomal dominant ataxias, chorea is typically accompanied by dementia in dentatorubral-pallidoluysian atrophy and SCA17. In the autosomal recessive ataxias, chorea is seen in ataxia telangiectasia, abetalipoproteinemia, ataxia with oculomotor apraxia (AOA) types 1 and 2, and POLG ataxia. *Myoclonus* is a fast, involuntary muscle jerk frequently present in mitochondrial disorders and progressive myoclonic epilepsies.

GENERAL NEUROLOGIC EXAMINATION CONSIDERATIONS

Cerebellar disease can affect executive, visuospatial, language, and emotional processing, and these should be screened for in office. The cerebellar cognitive affective/Schmahmann syndrome scale (CCAS-Scale) was devised specifically for patients with cerebellar ataxia.[25] This easy-to-administer scale assesses verbal fluency, executive function, memory, visuospatial, and affect domains.

Additional eye examinations can add to the diagnosis, as delineated in **Table 1**.[21] Fundoscopic examination showing papilledema can suggest optic neuritis due to demyelinating or infectious processes. Relative afferent pupillary defect also suggests a demyelinating process. Pigmentary retinal macular degeneration can be found in SCA7, whereas retinitis pigmentosa is associated with Refsum disease, abetalipopro-teinemia, and Kearns-Sayre syndrome.

Muscle strength examination is not only important for determining cerebellar ataxia cause but also uncovers contributions of weakness to the clinical presentation. Myop-athies typically affect proximal muscles first and are associated with mitochondrial disorders, which often have cerebellar involvement. Distal weakness can be seen in myopathy, neuropathy, or motor neuron disease. Friedreich ataxia is a good example of ataxia associated with distal weakness.

Detailed sensory examination is critical when evaluating a patient for ataxia to distin-guish mainly between cerebellar ataxia and sensory ataxia. Sensory ataxia results from loss of proprioceptive input. Testing vibratory sensation and joint position sense can assess large fiber sensory nerve function. Loss of visual input by closing the eyes can worsen sensory ataxia, whereas it has only minor effects on cerebellar ataxia. Thus, in sensory ataxia, imbalance occurs more at nighttime when it is dark or with the eyes closed; this can be further tested by Romberg sign where the patient stands with feet together and eyes closed. Of course, if the patient falls or steps to the side with the feet together when the eyes are opened, testing with the eyes closed would not yield additional information. Sensory loss associated with polyneuropathy can be seen in many of the autosomal recessive ataxias, mitochondrial neuropathies, and paraneoplastic disorders.

OTHER EXAMINATION CONSIDERATIONS

Examination of the skin and extremities can yield important clinical information. Cholesterol depositions in tendons (ie, xanthomas) are seen in cerebrotendinous xan-thomatosis as subcutaneous nodules or skin papules.[26] Telangiectasias seen in ataxia telangiectasias first appear in the eyes around age 3 to 6 years, then spread to involve the face. Pes cavus and scoliosis are common in Friedreich ataxia. NPC may have hepatosplenomegaly.

CLINICAL RATING SCALES TO TRACK ATAXIA SEVERITY

Clinical ratings scales are important for standardizing evaluation and tracking disease severity; this is particularly important in clinical trials. The scale for the assessment and rating of ataxia (SARA) is a 40-point widely used rating scale for ataxia (**Table 2**).[27] SARA evaluates speech, limb ataxia, tremor, stance, and gait using defined objective measures. SARA is the most widely used ataxia scale and has been validated in the natural history studies for SCAs in both North America[28] and Europe.[29] Eye findings are not included and are better evaluated by the more comprehensive 100-point Inter-national Cooperative Ataxia Rating Scale (ICARS),[30] which evaluates eye movements at rest, with pursuit, for nystagmus and saccadic dysmetria. Alternatively, the brief ataxia rating scale is a more concise ICARS.[31]

EVALUATION OF ATAXIA CAUSE BASED ON PRESENTATION

Once ataxia is established based on examination, the clinician should determine the cause. Chronicity of disease, age of onset, and other notable clinical features can indi-cate differential diagnosis and direct investigatory evaluation.

Table 2
Scale of the Assessment and Rating of Ataxia distribution of score[27]

Assessment	Score Rating
Gait	0–8 0—Normal 1—Slight difficulties seen with tandem only 2—Abnormal gait, cannot perform tandem 3—Staggering gait but walks without support 4—Marked staggering, touching walls intermittently 5—Severe staggering, support of walking stick/cane or light one arm support needed 6—Can walk >10 m but needs walker or person 7—Can walk <10 m with walker or person 8—Cannot walk even with support
Stance	0–6 0—Normal 1—Cannot stand in tandem for >10 s, no sway in other positions 2—Can stand with feet together for >10 s but has sway 3—Can stand in natural position only >10 s 4—Can stand in natural position only >10 s with intermittent support 5—Can stand in natural position only >10 s with constant arm support 6—Cannot stand in natural position >10 s even with constant support
Sitting	0–4 0—Normal 1—Intermittent sway with sitting >10 s 2—Constant sway with sitting >10 s 3—Intermittent support needed with sitting >10 s 4—Unable to sit >10 s without continuous support
Speech disturbance	0–6 0—Normal 1—Slight speech impairment 2—Noticeably impaired speech but easily understood 3—Occasional words difficult to understand 4—Many words difficult to understand 5—Only single words understood 6—Cannot understand speech/anarthria
Finger chase	Right 0–4; Left 0–4 0—Normal 1—Dysmetria <5 cm 2—Dysmetria <15 cm 3—Dysmetria >15 cm 4—Cannot perform 5 consecutive movements
Finger-nose-finger test	Right 0–4; Left 0–4 0—Normal 1—Tremor amplitude <2 cm 2—Tremor amplitude <5 cm 3—Tremor amplitude >5 cm 4—Unable to perform 5 movements

(continued on next page)

Table 2 (continued)	
Assessment	**Score Rating**
Rapid alternating movements	Right 0–4; Left 0–4 0—Normal 1—Slight irregularities, can perform 10 alternations <10 s 2—Clear irregularities, can perform 10 alternations <10 s 3—Many irregularities, interruptions, and undistinguishable movements, performs alterations >10 s 4—Cannot perform 10 alternating movements
Heel-shin slide	Right 0–4; Left 0–4 0—Normal 1—Slightly abnormal, contact with shin maintained 2—Clearly abnormal, can go off shin ≤3 times 3—Severely abnormal, goes off shin ≥4 times 4—Cannot perform
	Total: 40

Appendicular examination, including finger chase, finger-nose-finger, rapid alternating movements, and heel-shin slide, are averaged scores of the left and right sides.

Chronicity

Chronicity of disease can be separated into acute (hours to days), subacute (weeks), chronic (months to years) (**Fig. 1**), or episodic (discrete intervals of worsening) presentations. The ataxia causes of various chronicity are detailed in **Table 3**.[32–34] Acute presentations of ataxia include vascular, demyelinating, and infectious/parainfectious. Varicella is one of the most common causes of acute infectious ataxia, and cerebellar disease is the most frequent neurologic manifestation. As varicella causes a pancerebellar syndrome, it presents with impaired gait, dysarthria, dysmetria, and tremor.[35] Subacute presentations include immune-mediated, paraneoplastic, neoplastic, and some infectious/parainfectious causes. Chronic causes of ataxia include degenerative, hereditary, idiopathic, and structural lesions such as slow-growing neoplasms. Toxic/metabolic causes of cerebellar ataxia span from acute to chronic depending on the dose and exposure.

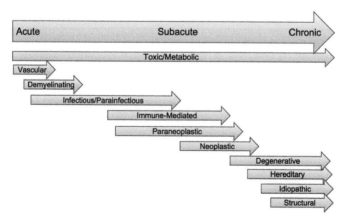

Fig. 1. Causes of cerebellar ataxia and acuity of disease presentation.

Table 3
Disease duration of cerebellar ataxia based on acuity of presentation

Cerebellar Ataxia Causes Based on Disease Duration	

Acute	Vascular
	  Ischemia, hemorrhage, vascular malformation
	Demyelinating
	  Multiple sclerosis, neuromyelitis optica, acute disseminated
	  encephalomyelitis
	Infectious
	  Viral cerebellitis: VZV, EBV, influenza, EV71, parvovirus B19, RSV
	  Bacterial: *Listeria monocytogenes, Mycoplasma pneumoniae, Borrelia*
	  burgdorferi, abscess
	  Fungal: *Aspergillus, Histoplasmosis*
	Parainfectious
	  Bacterial: *Mycoplasma pneumoniae*
	  Viral: measles, mumps, rubella, EBV, pertussis, rotavirus, coxsackie virus
	Toxic/metabolic
	  Antiepileptic drugs, chemotherapy, benzodiazepines, alcohol
	  intoxication, heavy metals, lithium, Wernicke encephalopathy

Subacute	Immune-mediated
	  SLE, Sjögren syndrome, gluten ataxia, thyroid antibody mediated, GAD-65
	  antibody, Miller-Fisher syndrome
	Paraneoplastic
	  Anti-Hu, Yo, Ri, mGluR1, Ma, CRMP, VGKC antibodies
	Neoplastic-posterior fossa tumors
	  Children: medulloblastoma, astrocytomas, ependymoma, brainstem
	  glioma
	  Adults: metastasis, hemangioblastoma, lymphoma
	Infectious
	  HIV, CJD, Whipple disease, JC virus/PML
	Toxic/metabolic
	  Vitamin deficiencies (B1, B12, E), hypothyroidism, hyperparathyroidism

Chronic	Neurodegenerative
	  Multiple system atrophy, progressive supranuclear palsy (less commonly)
	Idiopathic late onset cerebellar ataxia
	Hereditary
	Toxic/metabolic
	  Heavy metals, solvents, phenytoin, alcohol
	Structural/Static
	  Dandy Walker cyst, hydrocephalus, Joubert syndrome, cerebral palsy,
	  Arnold-Chiari malformation, hypoxic ischemic encephalopathy

Abbreviations: CJD, Creutzfeldt-Jakob disease; EBV, Epstein-Barr virus; EV71, enterovirus 71; HIV, human immunodeficiency virus; PML, progressive multifocal leukoencephalopathy; RSV, respiratory syncytial virus; VZV, varicella zoster virus.

Cerebellar ataxia can present episodically with normal examination or milder ataxia between episodes, outlined in **Table 4**. The episodic ataxias can be distinguished clinically based on precipitating factors, duration, and associated clinical phenomenon. Some episodic ataxias are inherited in an autosomal dominant fashion and are associated with mutations in genes encoding ion channels. Episodic ataxia types 1 (EA1) and 2 (EA2) and glucose transporter-1 (GLUT-1) deficiency are the most common types. EA1 attacks are triggered by exercise and startle; EA2 attacks are triggered by stress and alcohol; and GLUT-1 deficiency attacks are triggered by fasting or exercise and is associated with epilepsy.[36] Mitochondrial disorders have notable

Episodic Causes of Ataxia	Features
Table 4	
Episodic causes of cerebellar ataxia	
Genetic	Lasts seconds-minutes
Episodic ataxia type 1	+myokymia between attacks
Episodic ataxia type 2	Lasts hours-days
Episodic ataxia types 3–7	+nystagmus between attacks
Glucose transporter-1 deficiency	Rare
	Recurrent attacks ataxia ± vertigo
	+/− normal examination between attacks
	Paroxysmal exertional dyskinesias
	Ataxia with fasting, exercise, or illness
	Epilepsy
Inborn errors of metabolism	Skin photosensitivity, pellagra-like rash
Hartnup disease	
Mitochondrial disorders	Short stature
MELAS	Hearing and/or vision loss
MERRF	Polyneuropathy, myopathy
NARP	+/−Epilepsy
Demyelinating	Holmes tremor, dysarthria, incoordination
Multiple sclerosis	Cerebellar lesions
Neuromyelitis optica	Can progress to chronic ataxia
	Bulbar dysfunction, diplopia, vertigo, hiccups
	Brainstem, periaqueductal, & peri-third and fourth ventricular lesions
Functional movement disorder	Variability in phenomenology
	Distractable
	Entrainment

Abbreviations: MELAS, mitochondrial encephalomyopathy, lactic acidosis, and stroke-like episodes; MERRF, myoclonus epilepsy with ragged red fibers; NARP, neuropathy, ataxia, and retinitis pigmentosa.

neurologic features, including epilepsy, polyneuropathy, myopathy, and hearing or vision loss. Mitochondrial disorders may present with an episodic onset, then progress into a chronic form of ataxia. Finally, functional movement disorders should be included in the differential diagnosis of episodic ataxia.

Age of Onset

Age of symptom onset can narrow the differential diagnosis. Common causes of cerebellar ataxia in children are toxic ingestion or infectious.[37] Childhood chronic ataxia with a static disease course is consistent with perinatal insults. Childhood progressive ataxias should be evaluated for a genetic or metabolic basis. Children and young adults younger than 25 years should particularly be evaluated for autosomal recessive cerebellar ataxia if family history does not suggest an autosomal dominant inheritance. Adult-onset chronic progressive cerebellar ataxia should be investigated for genetic causes after acquired causes have been largely excluded. Generally, autosomal dominant cerebellar ataxias are more likely to have an age of onset in adulthood. In adults older than 50 years, degenerative causes, including MSA, idiopathic late-onset cerebellar ataxia, and fragile X-associated tremor and ataxia syndrome (FXTAS) should be considered. Regardless of age of onset, reversible causes, including immune-mediated or nutritional, should be investigated.

DIAGNOSTIC INVESTIGATION OF CEREBELLAR ATAXIA

Identifying clinical features of cerebellar ataxia warrants further investigation of the underlying diagnosis of cerebellar dysfunction. Imaging and serum laboratory workup are part of the initial evaluation. Particularly, the clinician should first look for reversible causes. A stepwise approach is outlined in **Fig. 2**.

MRI of the brain is the best initial imaging modality to assess cerebellar atrophy and associated features. A contrasted study should be ordered when there is suspicion for an immune-mediated, neoplastic/paraneoplastic, or infectious processes. Several unique MRI features are associated with specific cerebellar diseases. Cerebellar atrophy is one of the most common imaging features of cerebellar ataxia (**Fig. 3A**). The pattern of cerebellar atrophy can also be helpful; notably, superior vermian atrophy is a hallmark finding in ARSACS (**Fig. 3B**). Pontine atrophy and "hot cross buns sign" can be seen in MSA (**Fig. 3C**) and in some cases of SCA2. Dopamine terminal degeneration in MSA can be evaluated by DaTSCAN (**Fig. 3D**). T2 FLAIR hyperintensities in the cerebellar peduncles are pathognomonic for FXTAS (**Fig. 3E**), and hyperintensities of the deep cerebellar nuclei can be seen in cerebrotendinous xanthomatosis (**Fig. 3F**). In patients with ataxia and palatal tremor, T2 hyperintensity in the inferior olives indicates hypertrophic degeneration (**Fig. 3G**).

Serum laboratory investigation should be performed based on clinical suspicion (see **Fig. 2**). Reversible and acquired causes should be screened for, including vitamin deficiencies, such as vitamin B1, vitamin B12, and vitamin E; immune-mediated causes, including antinuclear antibody, Sjogren antibodies, gluten antibodies, anti-GAD-65 antibodies, and antithyroperoxidase and antithyroglobulin antibodies; and paraneoplastic causes. As the neuropsychological impairments of Wilson disease are treatable, clinicians should screen with serum ceruloplasmin and 24-hour urine copper in patients with ataxia and predominant dystonia.

Cerebrospinal fluid (CSF) analysis is reserved for suspected immune-mediated, paraneoplastic, or infectious processes. For infectious processes, individual viral

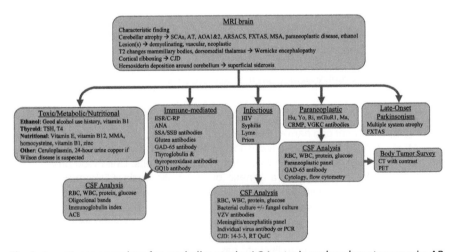

Fig. 2. Investigatory workup for cerebellar ataxia. AOA, ataxia and oculomotor apraxia; ARSACS, autosomal recessive spastic ataxia of Charlevoix-Saguenay; AT, ataxia telangiectasia; CJD, Creutzfeldt-Jakob disease; CSF RT-QuIC, cerebrospinal fluid real-time quaking-induced conversion; TSH, thyroid stimulating hormone; FXTAS, fragile X tremor ataxia syndrome; MMA, methylmalonic acid; MSA, multiple system atrophy; SCA, spinocerebellar ataxia.

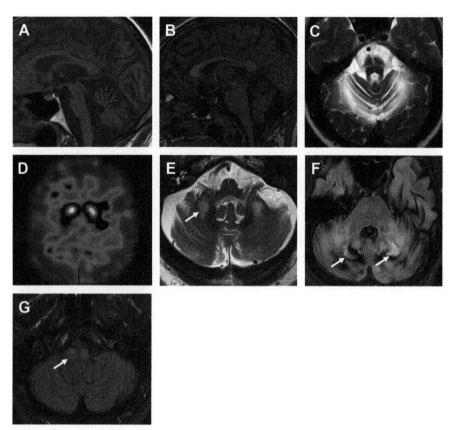

Fig. 3. MRI findings that aid in the diagnosis of a specific ataxia syndrome. (*A*) Cerebellar atrophy in a patient with SCA2. (*B*) Superior cerebellar vermian atrophy in a patient with ARSACS. (*C*) "Hot cross buns" sign in a patient with MSA. (*D*) Asymmetric uptake DaTSCAN in a patient with MSA. (*E*) T2 hyperintensities of middle cerebellar peduncles in a patient with FXTAS (*arrows*). (*F*) T2 hyperintensities of dentate nuclei in a patient with cerebroten-dinous xanthomatosis (*arrows*). (*G*) Inferior olive hypertrophy in a patient with progressive ataxia and palatal tremor (*arrows*). ARSACS, autosomal recessive spastic ataxia of Charlevoix-Saguenay; FXTAS, fragile X tremor ataxia; MSA, multiple system atrophy; SCA, spinocerebellar ataxia.

antibodies and a meningitis/encephalitis panel can identify specific organisms. In cases of suspected Creutzfeldt-Jacob disease, 14-3-3 and real-time quaking-induced conversion (RT-QuIC) should be tested. Elevated oligoclonal bands and immunoglob-ulin index suggest an immune-mediated process. CSF paraneoplastic and anti-GAD65 antibodies sometimes can be found when serum testing is negative.

HEREDITARY CAUSES OF CEREBELLAR ATAXIA

Genetic forms of cerebellar ataxia are categorized based on inheritance pattern: auto-somal dominant, autosomal recessive, X-linked, and mitochondrial inheritance. A detailed family history can reveal an inheritance pattern that directs genetic testing. Notably, autosomal dominant cerebellar ataxia could still be found in 5% of cases without a family history.[38] Determining the underlying genetic diagnosis is prudent for counseling on disease progression, family planning, and/or enrollment in clinical trials for disease-modifying therapies.

Autosomal Dominant Cerebellar Ataxia

Autosomal dominant cerebellar ataxias are labeled SCA nomenclature and numbered by order of discovery. To date, 48 types have been found. The average prevalence is 2.7 (1.5–4.0) per 100,000.[39] Pathologic CAG repeat expansions are the most common genetic mutations found in the SCAs, and SCA1, SCA2, SCA3, SCA6, SCA7, and SCA17 belong to this category. Some SCA trinucleotide repeat expansions result in anticipation or increase in the repeat number with each generation, causing earlier presentation with subsequent generations. SCA3 (also known as Machado-Joseph disease) is the most prevalent and has ethnic predilection in Brazil, Portugal, and China. SCA2 is the second most common autosomal dominant cerebellar ataxia and has ethnic predilection in Spain, Cuba, and Italy.[39,40] Each SCA has different rates of disease progression: SCA1 has the fastest decline followed by SCA3 and SCA2, with SCA6 having the slowest disease progression.[41] Each CAG-repeat SCA has certain unique clinical feature as delineated in **Table 5**. For example, parkinsonism can be seen in SCA2, SCA3, and SCA17[20,42]; chorea can be found in SCA17. SCA2 patients commonly have slowed saccades, hyporeflexia, and tremor, whereas SCA3 patients can have muscle fasciculations, bulging eyes, and restless leg syndrome. SCA6 is a pure cerebellar syndrome associated with downbeating nystagmus.[43] SCA7 causes vision loss due to pigmentary retinal macular degeneration.[44] The second most common type of genetic mutations in SCAs are repeat expansions in noncoding regions, and this category includes SCA8, SCA10, and SCA12. The third category is SCAs with coding sequence alterations, including SCA13, SCA14, SCA15, and SCA35.[45]

Table 5
Notable autosomal dominant cerebellar ataxia syndromes

Genetic Disorder	Mutation	Other Movement Disorder Features	Neurologic Features
SCA1	CAG expansion ATXN1		Early bulbar symptoms Dysarthria, dysphagia Hypermetric saccades
SCA2	CAG expansion ATXN2	Parkinsonism Truncal titubation Postural & rest tremors	Slowed saccades Ophthalmoplegia Hyporeflexia Motor neuron disease
SCA3 (Machado-Joseph disease)	CAG expansion ATXN3	Parkinsonism Dystonia Restless leg syndrome	Fasciculations Bulging eyes Ophthalmoplegia
SCA6	CAG expansion CACN1A	Pure cerebellar syndrome	Downbeating nystagmus
SCA7	CAG expansion ATXN7		Pigmentary retinal macular degeneration Slowed saccades Spasticity
SCA17 (Huntington disease-like)	CAG expansion TBP	Parkinsonism Chorea	Early dysarthria Early dementia Psychiatric disorder

Abbreviation: SCA, spinocerebellar ataxia.

Autosomal Recessive Cerebellar Ataxia

The prevalence of autosomal recessive cerebellar ataxias is 3.3 (1.8–4.9) per 100,000.[39] The most commonly inherited recessive ataxia is Friedreich ataxia followed by AOA and ataxia telangiectasia. Friedreich ataxia and cerebellar ataxia with neuropathy and vestibular areflexia syndrome (CANVAS) are due to repeat expansions, whereas the most of the remaining autosomal recessive cerebellar ataxias are due to sequence alterations.

Peripheral neuropathy is common in the autosomal recessive cerebellar ataxias and can be a defining feature for categorization into 3 types: (1) associated *sensory neuropathy*, which includes Friedreich ataxia and POLG ataxia; (2) associated *sensorimotor neuropathy*, which includes ataxia telangiectasia, cerebrotendinous xanthomatosis, AOA1, AOA2, and ARSACS; and (3) *no neuropathy*, which includes autosomal recessive cerebellar ataxia type 1 and 2 and NPC.

Friedreich ataxia patients often have skeletal abnormalities of pes cavus (**Fig. 4**) and scoliosis. Other systemic issues in Friedreich ataxia are cardiomyopathy and glucose intolerance. Ocular apraxia can be seen in AOA1, AOA2, and ataxia telangiectasia. AOAs are slowly progressive diseases, and ocular apraxia may progress to external ophthalmoplegia. The hallmark of NPC is vertical supranuclear ophthalmoplegia.[46] CANVAS is characterized by cerebellar, vestibular, and sensory neuronopathy degeneration. Oculocephalic reflex produces saccadic eye movements.[47] Selective clinical characteristics in autosomal recessive cerebellar ataxia are listed in **Table 6**.

X-Linked Cerebellar Ataxia

The most notable X-linked inherited ataxia is FXTAS, which is due to a premutation range CGG repeat expansion (55–200 repeats) in the *FMR1* gene. FXTAS usually

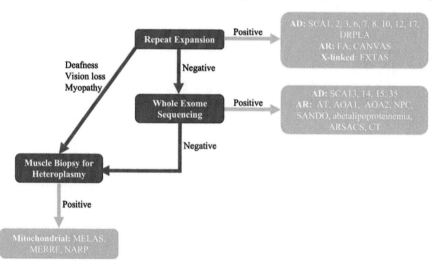

Fig. 4. General examination finding of pes cavus seen in Friedreich ataxia. AD, autosomal dominant; AOA, ataxia with oculomotor apraxia; AR, autosomal recessive; ARSACS, autosomal recessive spastic ataxia of Charlevoix-Saguenay; AT, ataxia telangiectasia; CANVAS, cerebellar ataxia with neuropathy and vestibular areflexia syndrome; CT, cerebrotendinous xanthomatosis; DRPLA, dentatorubral-pallidoluysian atrophy; FA, Friedreich ataxia; FXTAS, fragile X tremor ataxia; MELAS, mitochondrial encephalomyopathy, lactic acidosis, and stroke-like episodes; MERRF, myoclonus epilepsy with ragged red fibers; NARP, neuropathy, ataxia, and retinitis pigmentosa; NPC, Niemann-Pick type C; SANDO, sensory ataxic neuropathy, dysarthria, and ophthalmoparesis; SCA, spinocerebellar ataxia.

Table 6
Notable autosomal recessive cerebellar ataxia features

Genetic Disorder	Mutation	CNS Manifestations	Extra-CNS Manifestations	Further Diagnostics
Friedreich ataxia	GAA repeat *FXN*	Sensory axonal neuropathy Proprioceptive loss, areflexia	Diabetes mellitus Hypertrophic cardiomyopathy Pes cavus, scoliosis	
Ataxia telangiectasia	*ATM*	Dystonia, choreoathetosis Oculomotor apraxia	Recurrent infections (pulmonary) Risk for cancer (lymphoma) Telangiectasias	Elevated CEA and α-fetoprotein
AOA type 1 AOA type 2	*APTX* *SETX*	Mental disability (type 1) Oculomotor apraxia Sensorimotor neuropathy Choreoathetosis		Low albumin Elevated α-fetoprotein
Niemann-Pick type C	*NPC1*	Supranuclear ophthalmoplegia Dystonia Dementia, epilepsy	Hepatosplenomegaly	Elevated oxysterols
CANVAS	*RFC1* repeat	Impaired visually enhanced VOR Sensory neuronopathy		Dorsal vermis and lateral hemispheric atrophy
POLG ataxia/SANDO	*POLG*	Sensory axonal polyneuropathy Epilepsy Chorea, dystonia, myoclonus	Chronic external ophthalmoplegia Bilateral ptosis	
Autosomal recessive cerebellar ataxia type 1	*SYNE1*	Motor neuron disease	Cardiomyopathy Arthrogryposis, pes cavus	
Abetalipoproteinemia	*MTTP*	Retinitis pigmentosa Dystonia, chorea	Steatorrhea, failure to thrive Vitamin E malabsorption	Acanthocytosis Low TG & cholesterol

Disease	Gene			
ARSACS	*SACS*	Sensorimotor neuropathy Loss of vibration sense Spasticity	Distal amyotrophy of feet	Superior cerebellar vermian atrophy, linear T2 pontine hypointensities
Cerebrotendinous xanthomatosis	*CYP27A1*	Cataracts Epilepsy, cognitive impairment	Diarrhea Tendinous xanthomas	Elevated cholestanol Elevated bile alcohols

Abbreviations: AOA, ataxia with oculomotor apraxia; ARSACS, autosomal recessive spastic ataxia of Charlevoix-Saguenay; CANVAS, cerebellar ataxia with neuropathy and vestibular areflexia syndrome; CEA, carcinoembryonic antigen; SANDO, sensory ataxic neuropathy, dysarthria, and ophthalmoparesis; TG, triglycerides; VOR, vestibulo-ocular reflex.

presents as action tremor in men in their 60s. As women have 2 X chromosomes, they are less likely to be affected. Nevertheless, clinicians should investigate family history of premature ovarian insufficiency. FXTAS may present with parkinsonism and ataxia in 20% of cases.[48] Neuropathy and cognitive impairment are also common features.[48] MRI T2 hyperintensities in the middle cerebellar peduncles is a significant clue (see **Fig. 3**E).

Ataxias in Mitochondrial Disorders

Mitochondrial disorders are maternally inherited. Cerebellar ataxia, neuropathy, myopathy, myoclonus, and epilepsy are common neurologic signs. Patients may also have short stature, hearing or vision loss.

Genetic Testing Algorithm

A brief genetic test algorithm is provided in **Fig. 5**. The predominant autosomal dominant, autosomal recessive, and X-linked cerebellar ataxias are repeat expansions and thus are not commonly detected by whole exome sequencing. Thus, the first step of genetic evaluation for cerebellar ataxias is repeat expansion panels, which should include both coding and noncoding repeat expansions. The second step is to pursue either genetic sequence determination of individual ataxia genes or whole exome sequencing to detect sequence alterations and point mutations. If the clinical presentation and inheritance is consistent with mitochondrial disease, muscle biopsy should be performed to detect mitochondrial abnormality.

THERAPEUTIC MANAGEMENT OF CEREBELLAR ATAXIA

Management of ataxia includes a two-pronged approach of medication and physical, occupational, and speech therapies. Physical therapy has been shown to improve balance and mobility in both hereditary and degenerative cerebellar ataxia.[49,50] Patients should be encouraged to perform home exercises, which can improve balance and gait.[51] These evidence-based exercise programs for cerebellar ataxia are demonstrated online and accessible to patients (https://www.ataxia.org/11-exercises-for-ataxia-patients/). In addition, high-intensity exercise improves mobility and balance in cerebellar ataxia[52] and should also be recommended to patients as tolerated.

Pharmacologic therapies for cerebellar ataxia include both symptomatic and potentially disease-modifying therapies. Evidence often comes from clinical trials with small numbers of patients. Selective pharmacologic therapies for cerebellar ataxias are listed in **Table 7**. Immune-mediated cerebellar ataxias and paraneoplastic disorders can be treated with intravenous methylprednisolone or immunoglobulins; plasmapheresis is required in some cases. Certain autosomal recessive ataxias have targeted therapies, including miglustat for NPC, vitamin E for abetalipoproteinemia, and

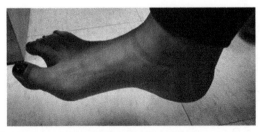

Fig. 5. Algorithm for suspected inherited cerebellar ataxia syndrome.

Table 7
Treatments of cerebellar ataxia

Therapeutic Interventions for Cerebellar Ataxia		
Targeted disease-modifying therapy for acquired disorders	Wernicke encephalopathy & chronic alcohol use	Thiamine, 1500 mg, IV daily x 2 d then 250 mg daily x 5 d
	Immune-mediated	Thiamine, 100 mg, PO daily
	Paraneoplastic	Methylprednisolone, 1000 mg, IV x 3–5 d ± IVIG
	Gluten-associated ataxia	Methylprednisolone, 1000 mg, IV x 5 d + IVIG/plasmapheresis
		Gluten-free diet
Targeted disease-modifying therapy for inherited disorders	Niemann-Pick type C	Miglustat 200 mg TID
	Abetalipoproteinemia	Vitamin E, 150 mg/kg/d
	GLUT-1 deficiency	Ketogenic diet, avoid fasting
	Cerebrotendinous xanthomatosis	Chenodeoxycholic acid, 250 mg, TID
Symptomatic therapy	Cerebellar ataxia	Riluzole, 50 mg, BID
	SCA3	Varenicline, 1 mg, BID
	Episodic ataxia type 1	Carbamazepine
	Episodic ataxia type 2	Acetazolamide, 250–1000 mg/d, 4-aminopyridine, 15 mg/d

Abbreviations: BID, twice daily; d, day(s); GLUT, glucose transporter; IV, intravenous; IVIG, intravenous immunoglobulins; kg, kilograms; mg, milligrams; TID, three times per day.

chenodeoxycholic acid for cerebrotendinous xanthomatosis. Ketogenic diet for GLUT-1 deficiency and gluten-free for gluten-associated ataxias are recommended.

Symptomatic therapies are also available for treating cerebellar ataxia. Riluzole improves gait and speech in a variety of ataxia diseases.[53,54] Valproic acid[55] and varenicline[56] may improve ataxia symptoms in SCA3 patients; however, they both have notable side effects that should be discussed when weighing benefit and risk. Dietary supplementation with coenzyme Q10 (CoQ10) is associated with better outcomes in the natural history study of SCAs; however, randomized clinical trials are lacking.[57] Patients with MSA have reduced cerebellar CoQ10 levels[58,59]; thus further studies are needed to determine supplementation benefits in this population. Carbamazepine decreases attacks in EA1, and both acetazolamide and 4-aminopyridine can decrease attacks in EA2.[60] As SCA6 and EA2 are both caused by mutations in *CACN1A* gene, acetazolamide may mitigate episodic symptoms in SCA6.[61,62] Other therapeutic options, such as amantadine or idebenone, have been reviewed by the American Academy of Neurology and deemed not enough evidence to determine benefit.[63]

Parkinsonism seen in MSA, SCA2, SCA3, SCA8, and SCA17 may be levodopa-responsive, so clinicians can trial levodopa starting 100 mg three times a day to assess the responses. Compared with patients with Parkinson disease, the response tends to be less robust and transient. Higher doses of levodopa up to 1,000-1,200 mg daily may be required to see effects, permitting side effects of sedation, orthostasis, and nausea. Vertigo may respond to benzodiazepines. Nystagmus may improve with symptomatic therapy for memantine, gabapentin,[64] or 4-aminopyridine.[65] Depression should be approached with cognitive behavioral therapy and pharmacologic therapy when indicated.

Active research is ongoing for gene therapy and antisense oligonucleotide targeting of specific genetic forms of cerebellar ataxias.[66] Deep brain stimulation has recently been explored to treat cerebellar ataxias as well.[67,68] Transcranial direct current stimulations and repetitive transcranial magnetic stimulation can have sustained benefits in patients with cerebellar ataxia.[69–71]

CLINICS CARE POINTS

- Once cerebellar ataxia is established based on examination, the etiology should be investigated.
- Each patient should be evaluated for treatable or reversible causes of cerebellar ataxia.
- More investigation is needed for therapeutic medications to treat ataxia symptoms of non-reversible causes of cerebellar ataxia.

SUMMARY

The hallmarks of cerebellar ataxia are incoordination and movement variability. The cerebellum not only controls motor coordination but also plays a role in cognition and mood. After establishing cerebellar ataxia on examination, determining the underlying cause is necessary. The causes of cerebellar ataxia are extensive, and systematic workup includes laboratory studies and imaging. In some cases, genetic testing often leads to a specific cause for cerebellar ataxia. Acquired and reversible causes should be pursued for disease-modifying treatment. Cerebellar ataxia is rapidly expanding, and new therapies are actively being tested, bringing hope for patients with cerebellar ataxia.

FINANCIAL DISCLOSURES/CONFLICTS OF INTEREST

Dr S-H. Kuo has received funding from the National Institutes of Health: NINDS #R01 NS118179 (principal investigator), NINDS #R01 NS104423 (principal investigator), NINDS #R03 NS114871 (principal investigator), the Louis V. Gerstner Jr. Scholar Award, Parkinson's Foundation, National Ataxia Foundation, and International Essential Tremor Foundation. Dr S-H. Kuo served as the Scientific Advisor for Praxis Precision Medicines and Sage Therapeutics. Dr T.A. Zesiewicz has received personal compensation for serving on the advisory boards of Boston Scientific, Reata Pharmaceuticals, and Steminent Biotherapeutics. Dr T.A. Zesiewicz has received personal compensation as senior editor for Neurodegenerative Disease Management and as a consultant for Steminent Biotherapeutics. Dr T.A. Zesiewicz has received royalty payments as co-inventor of varenicline for treating imbalance and nonataxic imbalance. Dr T.A. Zesiewicz has received research grant support as principle investigator for studies from AbbVie, Biogen, Biohaven Pharmaceuticals, Boston Scientific, Bukwang Pharmaceuticals Co, Ltd, Cala Health, Inc, Cavion, Friedreich's Ataxia Research Alliance; Houston Methodist Research Institute, National Institutes of Health, REtrotope Inc; and Takeda Development Center Americas, Inc.

SUPPLEMENTARY DATA

Supplementary data related to this article can be found online at https://doi.org/10.1016/j.ncl.2022.05.002.

REFERENCES

1. Koziol LF, Budding D, Andreasen N, et al. Consensus paper: the cerebellum's role in movement and cognition. Cerebellum 2014;13(1):151–77.

2. Guell X, Gabrieli JDE, Schmahmann JD. Embodied cognition and the cerebellum: Perspectives from the Dysmetria of Thought and the Universal Cerebellar Transform theories. Cortex 2018;100:140–8.
3. Schmahmann JD. The cerebellum and cognition. Neurosci Lett 2019;688:62–75.
4. Roostaei T, Nazeri A, Sahraian MA, et al. The human cerebellum: a review of physiologic neuroanatomy. Neurol Clin 2014;32(4):859–69.
5. Manto M, Bower JM, Conforto AB, et al. Consensus paper: roles of the cerebellum in motor control–the diversity of ideas on cerebellar involvement in movement. Cerebellum 2012;11(2):457–87.
6. Schmahmann JD, Pandya DN. The cerebrocerebellar system. Int Rev Neurobiol 1997;41:31–60.
7. Schmahmann JD, Pandya DN. Projections to the basis pontis from the superior temporal sulcus and superior temporal region in the rhesus monkey. J Comp Neurol 1991;308(2):224–48.
8. Schmahmann JD, Pandya DN. Anatomic organization of the basilar pontine projections from prefrontal cortices in rhesus monkey. J Neurosci 1997;17(1):438–58.
9. Dum RP, Strick PL. An unfolded map of the cerebellar dentate nucleus and its projections to the cerebral cortex. J Neurophysiol 2003;89(1):634–9.
10. Schmahmann JD, Sherman JC. The cerebellar cognitive affective syndrome. Brain 1998;121(Pt 4):561–79.
11. Amokrane N, Viswanathan A, Freedman S, et al. Impulsivity in Cerebellar Ataxias: Testing the Cerebellar Reward Hypothesis in Humans. Mov Disord 2020;35(8):1491–3.
12. Amokrane N, Lin CR, Desai NA, et al. The Impact of Compulsivity and Impulsivity in Cerebellar Ataxia: A Case Series. Tremor Other Hyperkinet Mov (N Y) 2020;10:43.
13. Lo RY, Figueroa KP, Pulst SM, et al. Depression and clinical progression in spinocerebellar ataxias. Parkinsonism Relat Disord 2016;22:87–92.
14. Benrud-Larson LM, Sandroni P, Schrag A, et al. Depressive symptoms and life satisfaction in patients with multiple system atrophy. Mov Disord 2005;20(8):951–7.
15. Luo L, Wang J, Lo RY, et al. The Initial Symptom and Motor Progression in Spinocerebellar Ataxias. Cerebellum 2017;16(3):615–22.
16. Termsarasab P, Thammongkolchai T, Rucker JC, et al. The diagnostic value of saccades in movement disorder patients: a practical guide and review. J Clin Mov Disord 2015;2:14.
17. Rascol O, Sabatini U, Simonetta-Moreau M, et al. Square wave jerks in parkinsonian syndromes. J Neurol Neurosurg Psychiatry 1991;54(7):599–602.
18. Leigh J, Zee DS. The neurology of eye movements. Oxford University Press; 2015.
19. Shaikh AG, Ramat S, Optican LM, et al. Saccadic burst cell membrane dysfunction is responsible for saccadic oscillations. J Neuroophthalmol 2008;28(4):329–36.
20. Kim M, Ahn JH, Mun JK, et al. Extracerebellar Signs and Symptoms in 117 Korean Patients with Early-Stage Spinocerebellar Ataxia. J Clin Neurol 2021;17(2):242–8.
21. Stephen CD, Schmahmann JD. Eye Movement Abnormalities Are Ubiquitous in the Spinocerebellar Ataxias. Cerebellum 2019;18(6):1130–6.
22. Love RJ, Webb WG. The Neuromotor Control of Speech. Neurology for the Speech-Language Pathologist. 2nd edition. Butterworth-Heinemann; 1992:81-111: Chapter 6.

23. Gan SR, Wang J, Figueroa KP, et al. Postural Tremor and Ataxia Progression in Spinocerebellar Ataxias. Tremor Other Hyperkinet Mov (N Y) 2017;7:492.

24. Lai RY, Tomishon D, Figueroa KP, et al. Tremor in the Degenerative Cerebellum: Towards the Understanding of Brain Circuitry for Tremor. Cerebellum 2019; 18(3):519–26.

25. Hoche F, Guell X, Vangel MG, et al. The cerebellar cognitive affective/Schmahmann syndrome scale. Brain 2018;141(1):248–70.

26. Nie S, Chen G, Cao X, et al. Cerebrotendinous xanthomatosis: a comprehensive review of pathogenesis, clinical manifestations, diagnosis, and management. Orphanet J Rare Dis 2014;9:179.

27. Schmitz-Hübsch T, du Montcel ST, Baliko L, et al. Scale for the assessment and rating of ataxia: development of a new clinical scale. Neurology 2006;66(11): 1717–20.

28. Ashizawa T, Figueroa KP, Perlman SL, et al. Clinical characteristics of patients with spinocerebellar ataxias 1, 2, 3 and 6 in the US; a prospective observational study. Orphanet J Rare Dis 2013;8:177.

29. Jacobi H, Bauer P, Giunti P, et al. The natural history of spinocerebellar ataxia type 1, 2, 3, and 6: a 2-year follow-up study. Neurology 2011;77(11):1035–41.

30. Chen ML, Lin CC, Rosenthal LS, et al. Rating scales and biomarkers for CAG-repeat spinocerebellar ataxias: Implications for therapy development. J Neurol Sci 2021;424:117417.

31. Schmahmann JD, Gardner R, MacMore J, et al. Development of a brief ataxia rating scale (BARS) based on a modified form of the ICARS. Mov Disord 2009; 24(12):1820–8.

32. Sawaishi Y, Takada G. Acute cerebellitis. Cerebellum 2002;1(3):223–8.

33. Lancella L, Esposito S, Galli ML, et al. Acute cerebellitis in children: an eleven year retrospective multicentric study in Italy. Ital J Pediatr 2017;43(1):54.

34. Nussinovitch M, Prais D, Volovitz B, et al. Post-infectious acute cerebellar ataxia in children. Clin Pediatr (Phila) 2003;42(7):581–4.

35. Bozzola E, Bozzola M, Tozzi AE, et al. Acute cerebellitis in varicella: a ten year case series and systematic review of the literature. Ital J Pediatr 2014;40:57.

36. Kipfer S, Strupp M. The Clinical Spectrum of Autosomal-Dominant Episodic Ataxias. Mov Disord Clin Pract 2014;1(4):285–90.

37. Pavone P, Praticò AD, Pavone V, et al. Ataxia in children: early recognition and clinical evaluation. Ital J Pediatr 2017;43(1):6.

38. Moseley ML, Benzow KA, Schut LJ, et al. Incidence of dominant spinocerebellar and Friedreich triplet repeats among 361 ataxia families. Neurology 1998;51(6): 1666–71.

39. Ruano L, Melo C, Silva MC, et al. The global epidemiology of hereditary ataxia and spastic paraplegia: a systematic review of prevalence studies. Neuroepidemiology 2014;42(3):174–83.

40. Schöls L, Bauer P, Schmidt T, et al. Autosomal dominant cerebellar ataxias: clinical features, genetics, and pathogenesis. Lancet Neurol 2004;3(5):291–304.

41. Jacobi H, du Montcel ST, Bauer P, et al. Long-term disease progression in spinocerebellar ataxia types 1, 2, 3, and 6: a longitudinal cohort study. Lancet Neurol 2015;14(11):1101–8.

42. Park H, Kim HJ, Jeon BS. Parkinsonism in spinocerebellar ataxia. Biomed Res Int 2015;2015:125273.

43. Yabe I, Sasaki H, Takeichi N, et al. Positional vertigo and macroscopic downbeat positioning nystagmus in spinocerebellar ataxia type 6 (SCA6). J Neurol 2003; 250(4):440–3.

44. Michalik A, Martin JJ, Van Broeckhoven C. Spinocerebellar ataxia type 7 associated with pigmentary retinal dystrophy. Eur J Hum Genet 2004;12(1):2–15.
45. Ashizawa T, Öz G, Paulson HL. Spinocerebellar ataxias: prospects and challenges for therapy development. Nat Rev Neurol 2018;14(10):590–605.
46. Gupta DK, Blanco-Palmero VA, Chung WK, et al. Abnormal Vertical Eye Movements as a Clue for Diagnosis of Niemann-Pick Type C. Tremor Other Hyperkinet Mov (N Y) 2018;8:560.
47. Szmulewicz DJ, Roberts L, McLean CA, et al. Proposed diagnostic criteria for cerebellar ataxia with neuropathy and vestibular areflexia syndrome (CANVAS). Neurol Clin Pract 2016;6(1):61–8.
48. Leehey MA. Fragile X-associated tremor/ataxia syndrome: clinical phenotype, diagnosis, and treatment. J Investig Med 2009;57(8):830–6.
49. Ilg W, Synofzik M, Brötz D, et al. Intensive coordinative training improves motor performance in degenerative cerebellar disease. Neurology 2009;73(22): 1823–30.
50. Miyai I, Ito M, Hattori N, et al. Cerebellar ataxia rehabilitation trial in degenerative cerebellar diseases. Neurorehabil Neural Repair 2012;26(5):515–22.
51. Keller JL, Bastian AJ. A home balance exercise program improves walking in people with cerebellar ataxia. Neurorehabil Neural Repair 2014;28(8):770–8.
52. Synofzik M, Ilg W. Motor training in degenerative spinocerebellar disease: ataxia-specific improvements by intensive physiotherapy and exergames. Biomed Res Int 2014;2014:583507.
53. Ristori G, Romano S, Visconti A, et al. Riluzole in cerebellar ataxia: a randomized, double-blind, placebo-controlled pilot trial. Neurology 2010;74(10):839–45.
54. Romano S, Coarelli G, Marcotulli C, et al. Riluzole in patients with hereditary cerebellar ataxia: a randomised, double-blind, placebo-controlled trial. Lancet Neurol 2015;14(10):985–91.
55. Lei LF, Yang GP, Wang JL, et al. Safety and efficacy of valproic acid treatment in SCA3/MJD patients. Parkinsonism Relat Disord 2016;26:55–61.
56. Zesiewicz TA, Greenstein PE, Sullivan KL, et al. A randomized trial of varenicline (Chantix) for the treatment of spinocerebellar ataxia type 3. Neurology 2012; 78(8):545–50.
57. Lo RY, Figueroa KP, Pulst SM, et al. Coenzyme Q10 and spinocerebellar ataxias. Mov Disord 2015;30(2):214–20.
58. Kuo SH, Quinzii CM. Coenzyme Q10 as a Peripheral Biomarker for Multiple System Atrophy. JAMA Neurol 2016;73(8):917–9.
59. Nakamoto FK, Okamoto S, Mitsui J, et al. The pathogenesis linked to coenzyme Q10 insufficiency in iPSC-derived neurons from patients with multiple-system atrophy. Sci Rep 2018;8(1):14215.
60. Jen JC, Graves TD, Hess EJ, et al. Primary episodic ataxias: diagnosis, pathogenesis and treatment. Brain 2007;130(Pt 10):2484–93.
61. Yabe I, Sasaki H, Yamashita I, et al. Clinical trial of acetazolamide in SCA6, with assessment using the Ataxia Rating Scale and body stabilometry. Acta Neurol Scand 2001;104(1):44–7.
62. Jen JC, Yue Q, Karrim J, et al. Spinocerebellar ataxia type 6 with positional vertigo and acetazolamide responsive episodic ataxia. J Neurol Neurosurg Psychiatry 1998;65(4):565–8.
63. Zesiewicz TA, Wilmot G, Kuo SH, et al. Comprehensive systematic review summary: Treatment of cerebellar motor dysfunction and ataxia: Report of the Guideline Development, Dissemination, and Implementation Subcommittee of the American Academy of Neurology. Neurology 2018;90(10):464–71.

64. Thurtell MJ, Joshi AC, Leone AC, et al. Crossover trial of gabapentin and memantine as treatment for acquired nystagmus. Ann Neurol 2010;67(5):676–80.
65. Tsunemi T, Ishikawa K, Tsukui K, et al. The effect of 3,4-diaminopyridine on the patients with hereditary pure cerebellar ataxia. J Neurol Sci 2010;292(1–2):81–4.
66. Toonen LJ, Schmidt I, Luijsterburg MS, et al. Antisense oligonucleotide-mediated exon skipping as a strategy to reduce proteolytic cleavage of ataxin-3. Sci Rep 2016;6:35200.
67. Cury RG, França C, Duarte KP, et al. Safety and Outcomes of Dentate Nucleus Deep Brain Stimulation for Cerebellar Ataxia. Cerebellum 2021. https://doi.org/10.1007/s12311-021-01326-8.
68. Teixeira MJ, Cury RG, Galhardoni R, et al. Deep brain stimulation of the dentate nucleus improves cerebellar ataxia after cerebellar stroke. Neurology 2015;85(23):2075–6.
69. Chen TX, Yang CY, Willson G, et al. The Efficacy and Safety of Transcranial Direct Current Stimulation for Cerebellar Ataxia: a Systematic Review and Meta-Analysis. Cerebellum 2021;20(1):124–33.
70. Maas RPPW, Toni I, Doorduin J, et al. Cerebellar transcranial direct current stimulation in spinocerebellar ataxia type 3 (SCA3-tDCS): rationale and protocol of a randomized, double-blind, sham-controlled study. BMC Neurol 2019;19(1):149.
71. Manor B, Greenstein PE, Davila-Perez P, et al. Repetitive Transcranial Magnetic Stimulation in Spinocerebellar Ataxia: A Pilot Randomized Controlled Trial. Front Neurol 2019;10:73.

Electrodiagnosis
How to Read Electromyography Reports for the Nonneurophysiologist

Ruple S. Laughlin, MD[a],*, Devon I. Rubin, MD[b]

KEYWORDS

- Electrodiagnosis • Electromyography • EMG • Nerve conduction studies • Needle
- Report interpretation

KEY POINTS

- An electrodiagnostic evaluation (EDX) is a neurodiagnostic study used in the diagnosis and evaluation of neuromuscular disorders, including motor neuron disorders, radiculopathies, mononeuropathies, peripheral neuropathies, neuromuscular junction disorders, and myopathies.
- An EDX study is composed of 2 parts:
  ○ Nerve conduction study, which uses surface electrical stimulation to record motor or sensory nerve responses.
  ○ Needle electromyography, which involves assessment of muscle activity via a needle electrode inserted into muscles.
- Knowledge of the fundamental components of the EDX evaluation allows the nonneurophysiologist to best determine if the study performed was technically reliable as well as sufficient to answer the clinical question posed.

GOALS OF ELECTRODIAGNOSIS

An electrodiagnostic evaluation study should be considered to achieve any of the following goals in a patient with a potential neuromuscular condition:

1. Confirm a diagnosis
2. Exclude alternative diagnosis
3. Define the anatomic extent of involvement
4. Localization of the abnormalities
5. Define severity
6. Determine pathophysiology
7. Follow temporal evolution of a clinical condition or treatment effects.

[a] Department of Neurology, Mayo Clinic Rochester, Mayo E8A, 200 First St SW, Rochester, MN 55905, USA; [b] Department of Neurology, Mayo Clinic Florida, NeurologyFLA — Mangurian Building 4428, 4500 San Pablo Road, Jacksonville, FL 32224, USA
* Corresponding author.
E-mail address: Laughlin.Ruple@mayo.edu

Neurol Clin 41 (2023) 45–60
https://doi.org/10.1016/j.ncl.2022.05.003
0733-8619/23/© 2022 Elsevier Inc. All rights reserved.

INTRODUCTION

An electrodiagnostic evaluation (EDX) is a neurodiagnostic test but also a consultation used in the evaluation of peripheral nervous system disorders. Each study can provide useful information to aid in the diagnosis of common conditions, such as radiculopathies, mononeuropathies, and polyneuropathies, and uncommon disorders, such as myopathies, neuromuscular junction disorders, or motor neuron diseases. EDX can also be used to exclude neuromuscular conditions in patients presenting with vague or nonspecific symptoms, such as numbness or fatigue.

Most nonneuromuscular subspecialist providers, including neurologists, rely on the "clinical interpretation" portion of the report to provide them with the information they need to diagnose and manage their patients. An ideal report interpretation will include all necessary information to assist the referring provider in answering the clinical query posed for the study. Principal elements in the interpretation include localization, chronicity, and severity of a disorder and, in some cases, the specific neuromuscular disease. However, not all EDX findings and interpretations are reported similarly, and the details of the report may be confusing to a provider who does not perform or interpret EDX studies. A basic understanding of the essential components of a report, commonly termed the "EMG report", such as the significance of details within the data tables and what features inform the clinical interpretation, may be helpful to referring providers. Furthermore, because poorly performed EDX studies can lead to inaccurate data and interpretation, understanding the components constituting a reliable study is imperative.

This article will review the basic components of an EDX study and report, highlight general guidelines to understand the reported data, and review key features in reports related to certain diagnoses. A complete review of the methods and interpretations of EDX studies is beyond the scope of this article and can be found elsewhere.[1]

A typical EDX study consists of 2 components: nerve conduction studies (NCS) and needle EMG (nEMG). Because each provides complementary information necessary for an accurate interpretation, nearly every EDX study should include both components; the absence of one part should raise concern about the reliability of the study.

NERVE CONDUCTION STUDIES OVERVIEW

NCS are a technique where an individual nerve is stimulated with sufficient electrical current to depolarize all axons within the nerve.

When studying the integrity of the peripheral *motor* system, the action potentials propagate along the motor axons to the nerve terminal, releasing acetylcholine vesicles that diffuse across the synapse to the muscle endplate, yielding muscle fiber action potentials. The recording electrode is placed over a muscle, and the action potentials from all muscle fibers are recorded, producing a compound muscle action potential (CMAP) (**Fig. 1**). When the *sensory* nerves are studied, a large fiber mixed sensory/motor or pure sensory nerve is stimulated, and the action potentials are recorded at a distal (for antidromic studies) or proximal (for orthodromic studies) site along the nerve, resulting in a sensory nerve action potential (SNAP) (**Fig. 2**). The sensory modalities transmitted by small or unmyelinated sensory nerve fibers (serving pain/temperature or autonomic function) are not assessed with NCS.

NERVE CONDUCTION STUDIES IN AN ELECTROMYOGRAPHY REPORT

The results from each NCS, along with the laboratory reference values, are typically reported in a tabular format in an EMG report. In some laboratories, the NCS

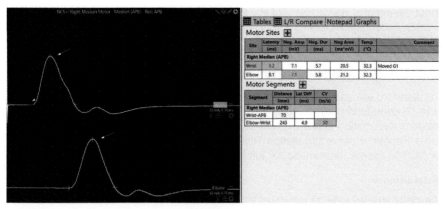

Fig. 1. Compound muscle action potential (CMAP). Typical CMAP recorded from the abductor pollicis brevis with stimulation of the median nerve. Note the waveform consistency in morphology and amplitude (*arrows*) at both sites of stimulation as well as the upward deflection from baseline (*arrowhead*) indicating a well-positioned recording electrode over the muscle endplate site of action potential generation.

waveforms themselves are included in the report. For the EDX specialist who is reviewing an EDX study performed by another provider, reviewing the actual waveforms allows for the assessment of reliability of the study by detecting technical factors that may be present. However, for the nonneurophysiologist, interpreting the waveforms may be difficult. The tabular numerical data provide valuable information

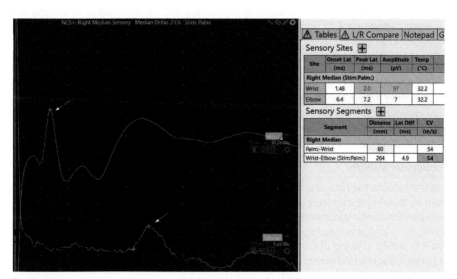

Fig. 2. Sensory nerve action potential (SNAP). Typical antidromic SNAP recorded from the second digit with stimulation of the median mixed nerve at the wrist and elbow. Unlike CMAPs, SNAPs demonstrate temporal dispersion of responses as one stimulates the nerve further from the recording site. The latency is marked at the peak of the response (*arrow*) not the onset. Note the SNAP is recorded at a much smaller sensitivity and therefore more prone to technical errors.

about the integrity and number of axons, as well as the integrity of the neuromuscular junction and muscle fibers for motor NCS. Each of the values reported for a nerve provides different types of information.[2]

REPORTED VALUES DURING MOTOR NERVE CONDUCTION STUDIES

The standard values reported during a motor NCS are (1) distal latency (DL), (2) amplitude, (3) conduction velocity (CV), and in some cases (4) F wave latencies. Each value provides information about the function of different components and sites along the nerve. Repetitive nerve stimulation (RNS) is an advanced technique performed on motor NCS to assess neuromuscular junction integrity (see **Fig. 1**).

Distal Latency

The distal latency reflects the conduction time along the distal segment of the nerve tested (usually distal to the wrist or ankle). Prolonged distal latencies suggest demyelination in the distal segment of the nerve, such as can occur with carpal tunnel syndrome. However, disorders associated with a loss of many fast-conducting large fiber axons may result in a secondary prolongation in the distal latency.

Amplitude

The CMAP amplitude measures the amplitude of the summated action potentials generated directly from the muscle(s) under the recording electrodes after nerve stimulation. Although this value directly reflects the number of muscle fibers, it indirectly reflects the number of motor axons and integrity of the neuromuscular junctions. A reduction in the CMAP amplitude can occur in disorders affecting motor nerves or axons (eg, motor neuron disease, severe mononeuropathy or polyneuropathy, severe radiculopathy), severe myopathies, and some neuromuscular junction disorders. For most motor nerves tested, the nerve is stimulated at 2 or more sites to assess the CV along the segment. In normal nerves, the CMAP amplitude and morphology should be similar at all sites of stimulation as motor axons conduct at similar rates (see **Fig. 1**). Although some EMG reports only report the amplitude at the proximal site of stimulation, others report the amplitude at all sites of stimulation. The latter is helpful to determine the presence of an abnormal drop (usually >20% in most nerves) in amplitude, which could represent focal conduction block or abnormal temporal dispersion, both of which are indicators of focal or multifocal demyelination. A thorough EMG report should also textually describe the presence and site of conduction block or temporal dispersion within the report Summary.

Conduction Velocity

The CV reflects the rate of conduction of action potentials along the nerve. It is calculated by dividing the latency differences at 2 or more stimulation sites by the distances between the sites. Abnormally slowed CV may suggest demyelination along the nerve. However, a process resulting in the loss of many large, fast-conducting axons may result in a mild slowing of CV. Therefore, the diagnosis of demyelinating neuropathies requires a degree of slowing that is disproportionately greater than what would be expected with amplitude reduction.

F Wave Latencies

F waves are late responses that are sometimes performed to assess the proximal segments of nerves. They are performed by stimulating a motor nerve at a distal site and recording the responses that propagate antidromically along the motor axon to the anterior horn cell and then orthodromically back to the muscle. The time that the response takes to course through this pathway is the F wave latency (**Fig. 3**). The F wave latency may be compared with an absolute reference value, although limb length will affect the conduction time. Some laboratories compare the F wave latency to an estimated F wave latency (F estimate) based on the known distal motor CV. Prolongation of the actual F wave latency compared with the F estimate suggests more proximal slowing. Although F waves are insensitive at assessing radiculopathies and many other disorders, they are useful in the evaluation of demyelinating neuropathies or polyradiculopathies (such as chronic inflammatory demyelinating polyradiculopathy).

Repetitive Nerve Stimulation

RNS is an advanced technique in which a motor nerve is stimulated repetitively, usually at (slow) rates of 2 to 5 Hz in a short train (4–6 stimuli) to assess the integrity of neuromuscular transmission. When neuromuscular junctions are intact, the motor (CMAP) amplitude should remain the same with each stimulus. In conditions in which there is an impairment in neuromuscular junctions, there is a drop in amplitude (referred to as *decrement*) with each stimulus. The percent decrement between the first and each subsequent stimulus is calculated, and the maximum decrement between the first and last response is reported. The change in the decrement and CMAP amplitude following brief (10 seconds) or long (60 seconds) exercise is also reported. Some reports include the presence and degree of decrement within the NCS tables, whereas others describe this in a text format within the report Summary.[3]

REPORTED VALUES DURING SENSORY NERVE CONDUCTION STUDIES

As noted above, sensory responses are nerve-to-nerve recordings. Although the main values attained and reported during a sensory NCS are similar to motor NCS and include (1) distal latency (DL), (2) amplitude, and (3) CV, they differ slightly in their neurophysiology (see **Fig. 2**).

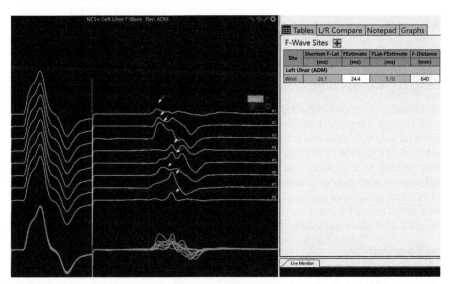

Fig. 3. F waves. F wave responses elicited by distal stimulation of the ulnar nerve. Note the expected variance in F wave latency and morphology with each stimulus (*arrowheads*) but the very uniform CMAP best depicted on the bottom trace (overlay).

Distal Latency

As in motor NCS, the reported distal latency refers to the time that it takes for the action potentials to travel from the stimulation site to the recording electrode. Unlike motor NCS in which the distal latency is marked at the onset of the waveform to assess the fastest fibers, most laboratories report the peak latency of sensory responses, thereby assessing the average speed of the fibers.

Amplitude

The sensory amplitude reflects the number of sensory axons under the recording electrode excited by nerve stimulation at that point. Since sensory axons have a wider variability in diameter and myelination than motor axons, they reach the recording electrode at variable times, resulting in "phase cancellation" and a decrease in the recorded amplitude over longer distance. Given this phenomenon and the fact that amplitudes are small (measured in microvolt rather than millivolt), distal amplitudes are reported and compared with reference values.

Conduction Velocity

CV is obtained in the same manner as in motor NCS, and it uses the onset latencies (measuring the conduction in the fastest fibers) for calculation.

NEEDLE ELECTROMYOGRAPHY OVERVIEW

nEMG is a technique that entails inserting a recording needle electrode into a muscle and recording the electrical signals that are generated directly from muscle fibers at rest and during voluntary contraction. The presence of spontaneous waveforms at rest may indicate certain types of neuromuscular disorders or pathologic conditions. The voluntary motor unit potentials (MUPs) recorded during contraction help to determine the presence and type (neurogenic, myopathic, neuromuscular junction) of neuromuscular disorder as well as the temporal course and severity of the disorder. A detailed review of the types and pathophysiology of changes of different waveforms is beyond the scope of this article and can be found in other sources.[4] However, the significance of each change that is reported in the needle EMG table in the EMG report will be briefly described below.

REPORTED FINDINGS DURING NEEDLE ELECTROMYOGRAPHY

The waveforms recorded during needle EMG are free running waveforms interpreted in real time as the muscle is being examined. Although buffers of EMG activity can be stored for future review, the actual waveforms are not included in an EMG report. The presence or absence of spontaneous waveforms for each muscle is documented and either graded in a table or described in the Summary. Similarly, multiple individual MUPs generated during voluntary contraction within each muscle are graded and the average qualitative grade of abnormality for different MUP parameters is entered into a table. Some laboratories perform quantitative EMG and report the mean numerical value of a given parameter as well.

Insertional Activity

When a needle is moved through a resting muscle, the needle irritates muscle fibers, resulting in brief bursts of action potentials. The bursts should last only while the needle is moved, and the baseline activity should become quiet once needle movement ceases. In disorders in which denervation or irritability of the muscle membranes is present, insertional activity is *increased*, and there is persistent or recurrent firing of the action potentials after needle movement ceases. Increased insertion activity is nonspecific and can be seen in neurogenic or myopathic disorders.

Fibrillation Potentials

Fibrillation potentials are spontaneously firing action potentials of muscle fibers that have lost their innervation (ie, denervated). They are nonspecific and can be seen in neurogenic and some myopathic disorders. Their presence in neurogenic disorders typically occurs when there has been axon loss or degeneration, such as in axonal neuropathies, severe mononeuropathies involving loss of motor fibers, motor neuron diseases, and so forth. Fibrillation potentials occur in myopathies characterized pathologically by fiber necrosis, splitting, or vacuole injury to the fibers.[5] Although the presence of fibrillation potentials often indicates an "active" or ongoing disorder, they can persist in an old or inactive process if the muscle fibers are never fully reinnervated. Fibrillation potentials are graded on a qualitative (1–4+) scale based on the density of fibrillation potentials in the muscle.

Fasciculation Potentials

Fasciculation potentials are spontaneously firing MUPs. These can occur in normal individuals but are also frequently seen in patients with neurogenic disorders. Fasciculation potentials are graded qualitatively based on the number of potentials recorded per minute.

Several rarer spontaneous waveforms may be described in an EMG report. *Complex repetitive discharges* are nonspecific discharges seen in chronic neurogenic or myopathic disorders. *Myotonic discharges* are repetitive discharges that occur at rest or with needle movement because of abnormality of muscle membrane channels. They are nonspecific and can be seen in a variety of myopathies in isolated muscles but when diffusely recorded, suggest a myotonic myopathy or channelopathy. *Myokymic discharges* are grouped discharges, sometimes associated with clinical myokymia, seen in a variety of neurogenic disorders but most classically associated with radiation-induced nerve injury.[6]

Voluntary Motor Unit Potentials

Assessment of voluntary MUPs is necessary to determine the type and timing of a neuromuscular disorder. Each individual MUP is an electrical representation of a portion of the motor unit and extrapolation of the morphology of the MUPs helps to determine the fiber density and distribution of fibers of each motor unit within the muscle. Different MUP parameters are assessed, graded, and reported, and each provides information on the type of disorder, severity, and timing or chronicity of the disorder. Details of the pathophysiology of the parameters and changes can be found elsewhere.[4] A general overview of the significance of each parameter is described here (**Fig. 4**).

- *Recruitment*. Recruitment refers to the number of activated motor units and the firing rates of the motor units relative to the patient's effort of contraction. *Reduced recruitment* occurs when there is loss of motor units (eg, with axonal neurogenic disorders) or block of conduction along axons (eg, with focal demyelination). Reduced recruitment is often associated with clinical weakness. *Rapid (early) recruitment* occurs in myopathies associated with loss of muscle fibers; in this situation, more motor units fire with minimal effort to generate a needed force. *Poor activation* occurs with central (upper motor neuron) disorders or with poor voluntary effort.

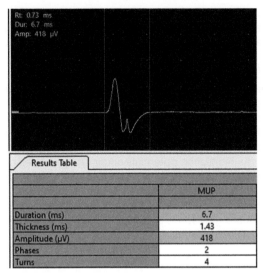

Fig. 4. Motor unit potential (MUP). Example of a voluntary MUP. Top, the waveform of a single MUP (*purple vertical lines* mark the duration). Bottom, value of each parameter of the MUP.

- *Duration and Amplitude.* The duration (baseline to baseline) and amplitude (peak-to-peak) of a MUP are parameters that reflect the overall size of the motor unit, including the density and distribution of fibers in the region around the recording electrode (**Fig. 5**). These are the primary parameters used to help distinguish neurogenic from myopathic disorders. With reinnervation after axon loss, collateral sprouting results in increased fiber density and distribution, thereby resulting in higher amplitude and longer duration MUPs (**Table 1**). Myopathies characterized by loss of muscle fibers are associated with short duration, low amplitude MUPs. However, short duration, low amplitude MUPs can also occur in severe neuromuscular junction disorders and even severe neurogenic disorders where very early reinnervation has just begun (termed "nascent MUPs").
- *Phases and Turns.* Phases and turns refer to the complexity of a MUP and are defined by the number of changes in direction of the MUP (phases cross the baseline and turns do not). Up to 15% of MUPs in a muscle may be polyphasic (>4 phases) or have excess turns. A higher percentage of complex (polyphasic) MUPs suggest less synchronous firing of the muscle fiber action potentials and is seen in early (weeks–months) reinnervation of neurogenic disorders or in myopathies. These parameters may be graded qualitatively or the percent of polyphasic MUPs may be estimated and reported.
- *Stability.* A motor unit with normally functioning neuromuscular junctions is stable; there is no moment-to-moment change in amplitude or morphology as it fires. An unstable MUP indicates impaired neuromuscular transmission and can be seen with neuromuscular junction disorders or with ongoing reinnervation. Stability is not commonly included in the needle EMG table but may be listed in a comment section by each muscle or in the Summary.

Interpreting each of these parameters helps to define the type and chronicity of the underlying process. Although variations occur, the classic findings of several disorders are shown in **Table 1**.

Electromyography
Patient:
MRN:

DOB:	Study Date:	27-Apr-2022 07:15
Sex: F	Location:	Mayo Clinic Hospital in Florida
Staff:	Ordered by:	

** Final Report **

Study Number: 1
Referred for: Bil CTS
Referral Code: 038
Referral Diagnosis: 211

SUMMARY:
Prior to starting the procedure, the patient's identity was verified, pertinent available records were reviewed, the nature of the procedure was explained, the appropriate sites of the exam were confirmed directly with the patient, and a pre-procedure pause was performed for final verification of all of the above.

Nerve conduction studies of both upper limbs revealed an unobtainable right median mixed nerve peak latency. Concentric needle examination of selected right upper limb muscles demonstrated mildly polyphasic motor unit potentials limited to the abductor pollicis brevis muscle.

CLINICAL INTERPRETATION:
Abnormal study. There is electrophysiological evidence of moderate right and mild left median neuropathies at the wrist correlating to a clinical diagnosis of carpal tunnel syndrome. There is no evidence of a right cervical radiculopathy on the current study.

NERVE CONDUCTIONS

Nerve	Type	Record Site	Rep Stim	Side	Amp	Normal Amp	CV	Normal CV	Distal Lat	Normal Lat	F-Wave Lat	F-Wave Est	Temp (°C)
Median	Motor	APB		L	8.1	(>4.0)	51	(>48)	4.3	(<4.5)			31.5
Median	Motor	APB		R	9.5	(>4.0)	50	(>48)	6.1	(<4.5)			30.8
Ulnar	Motor	ADM		R	11.9	(>6.0)	59	(>51)	3.4	(<3.6)			32.0
Median	Sensory	Wrist		L	66	(>50.0)		(>56)	2.3	(<2.3)			31.8
Median	Sensory	Dig II		R	NR	(>15.0)		(>56)	NR	(<3.6)			32.3
Ulnar	Sensory	Wrist		L	27	(>15.0)		(>55)	1.8	(<2.3)			31.9
Ulnar	Sensory	Dig V		R	17	(>10.0)	67	(>54)	3.0	(<3.1)			33.3

NEEDLE EMG

Muscle	Side	Ins Act	Spont Fib	Spont Fasc	MUP Normal	Activ	Recruitment Reduced	Recruitment Rapid	Duration Long	Duration Short	Amplitude High	Amplitude Low	Phases %	Turns
Abductor pollicis brevis	R	NL	0	0	NL								15%	*
First dorsal interosseous	R	NL	0	0	NL									
Pronator teres	R	NL	0	0	NL									
Biceps brachii	R	NL	0	0	NL									
Triceps brachii	R	NL	0	0	NL									

Fig. 5. Standard electromyography (EMG) report example. Sample EMG report from an abnormal study in a patient referred for evaluation of carpal tunnel syndrome. Presented are the key elements of standard EMG report: Summary, interpretation, and tabular presentation of nerve conduction (including temperature reporting), and needle electromyography data.

COMPONENTS OF THE ELECTROMYOGRAPHY REPORT

The EMG report summarizes all the findings of NCS and EMG and provides an overall interpretation of those findings (see **Fig. 5**).[7] Most EMG reports consist of the following sections:

1. Demographics and Referral Indication or Clinical Summary. The report should list or describe the reason for the referral for the EDX study. Some reports will include a brief clinical history and examination findings, whereas others rely on the documentation in the electronic medical record. The EDX consultant should always perform a brief history and examination before the performance of the study.
2. NCS Table. This table lists details for each nerve studied, including the nerve, recording site, and numerical data. Because the studies are performed and data interpreted according to specific reference values and methods, the reference values should always be included in the report.
3. Temperature. Cool limb temperature has a significant impact on nerve conduction time and limbs that are too cold may result in slowed conduction velocities and/or prolonged distal latencies. Cooling will also increase amplitudes and can pseudonormalize neuromuscular junction disorders by facilitating neuromuscular transmission. Therefore, limb temperature should always be measured and maintained above a certain level throughout the study. An appropriate report should include skin temperature.
4. Needle Electromyography Table. This table lists each muscle that was examined and the findings for that muscle. The standard columns include insertional activity, the presence and grade of fibrillation and fasciculation potentials, and each of the voluntary MUP parameters.
5. Summary of Findings. This section summarizes the pertinent abnormalities or absence of abnormalities in a manner that supports the clinical interpretation. This section often includes specific information that may not be captured in the tables, such as the site of focal slowing or conduction block during short segment stimulation or the presence and degree of decrement during RNS.
6. Clinical Interpretation. This is the key part of the report in which the performing electromyographer interprets the EDX findings in the context of the clinical scenario and provides their insight into the patient's condition.

CLUES TO RELIABILITY OF THE ELECTRODIAGNOSTIC EVALUATION STUDY IN THE ELECTROMYOGRAPHY REPORT

Unlike reviewing radiographic images performed at a different location, it is difficult to completely determine reliability of the study simply by review of an EMG report. An EDX study may be fraught with technical situations that can result in data that mimics disease. Furthermore, although NCS waveforms can be included in a report, needle EMG findings are live waveforms that are not included. Thus, reliability of the interpretation depends on the reliability of the performing and interpreting EDX consultant. There are several clues to consider when reviewing the report for reliability.

1. Does the interpreting physician have board certification in clinical neurophysiology or electrodiagnostic medicine? Although subspecialty certification is not an absolute necessity to perform the studies, having sufficient training and successful certification in the field generally reflects a higher level of expertise.
2. Was limb temperature measured and documented in the report? If not, the results may not reliably reflect the integrity of the peripheral nervous system.

Table 1
Characteristics of common disorders noted on electromyography

Condition	Recruitment	Duration/ Amplitude	Phases/Turns	Stability
Acute (days) neurogenic	Reduced	Normal	Normal	Stable
Subacute (weeks) neurogenic	Reduced	Normal	Increased	Unstable
Chronic (months) neurogenic	Reduced	Increased	Increased (may decrease)	Stable
Myopathy	Rapid (early)	Decreased	Normal or increased	Stable
Neuromuscular junction disorder	Normal	Normal (decreased if severe)	Normal	Unstable

3. Were excessive numbers of nerves and muscles examined? The number of nerves and muscles tested varies widely depending on the clinical problem. However, in most uncomplicated studies, approximately 3 to 5 NCS and 5 to 7 muscles are necessary. Studies that include nearly all nerves and muscles in a limb should raise a red flag that the focus of the study was not based on a clinical hypothesis but more on random or algorithmic testing.

DISEASE-SPECIFIC ELECTROMYOGRAPHY REPORT CONSIDERATIONS

The EDX study can assist in making a diagnosis of many types of neuromuscular disorders. Although the final interpretation should indicate the type of disorder and aspects of the findings in each patient, certain specific report findings and considerations may provide additional helpful information.

ELECTROMYOGRAPHY REPORTS IN PERIPHERAL NEUROPATHIES

Peripheral neuropathy (PN) is among the most common indication for EDX testing. The goals of EDX testing in PN are to (1) confirm involvement of large fibers, (2) help elucidate pathophysiology, and (3) define the extent and distribution of abnormalities (length-dependent vs polyradiculoneuropathy). Both NCS and nEMG are necessary to adequately assess PN.[8]

- Most peripheral neuropathies are distal predominant and "length-dependent." In most cases, NCS will begin in the feet but will include the hands if abnormalities are identified in the lower limbs or if the patient is symptomatic in the hands.
- NCS, including F waves, are important in the assessment of PN because they can help to understand the underlying pathophysiology (axonal or demyelinating), which cannot be accomplished with a clinical examination.
  - In axonal neuropathies, the loss of axons results in a reduction of amplitudes. Usually, sensory nerves are affected before the motor nerves. Although this loss of axons can affect the fastest axons yielding slowing of DL and CV, the degree of slowing is mild compared with the degree of axonal loss (**Table 2**).
  - In demyelinating neuropathies, the axons are intact but injury to myelination slows the speed of nerve conduction, resulting in prolongation of DL and slowing of CV disproportionate to the degree of amplitude reduction. It is important that the interpretation of a demyelinating neuropathy incorporates established criteria for demyelination to avoid misdiagnoses (**Table 3**).[9,10]

- Conduction block and dispersion may not be evident in the tabular data in the report but should be summarized in the Summary text.
- Routine NCS are performed on distal limbs (hands and feet). Distal abnormalities can occur with proximal nerve involvement from axonal degeneration. Therefore, NCS alone are insufficient to exclude a process involving proximal nerves or roots, such as polyradiculopathies. A comprehensive EMG includes needle examination of proximal muscles if distal muscles are abnormal. Abnormalities in proximal muscles are unusual in length-dependent neuropathies and may suggest polyradiculopathy or polyradiculoneuropathy.
- Needle abnormalities in distal muscles may be the earliest or first abnormalities on EDX testing in PN because the NCS values are presented as a normal value related to a pooled population. Consequently, although the SNAP amplitude might be within normal range, it may represent a 50% reduction for that patient, which cannot be discerned without a prior comparative study performed in the same manner.
- EDX testing in the EMG laboratory cannot reliably assess for the presence of a small fiber neuropathy and is usually normal.

ELECTROMYOGRAPHY REPORTS IN RADICULOPATHIES

The role of EDX testing in radiculopathies is to (1) identify the presence of injury to one or more nerve roots, (2) localize the process to the specific root(s), (3) exclude other sites of pathologic condition, such as plexus or distal individual nerves, (4) determine whether the process is "active" (ie, ongoing injury to the root), (5) assess the chronicity of the process, and (6) assess the severity of root injury. The combination of NCS and needle EMG can often provide those answers.[11]

- EDX studies primarily assess the motor axons coursing through the root, and the preganglionic sensory roots cannot be reliably tested. Therefore, in root disorders that manifest primarily with pain and/or sensory disturbance or are due to irritation of the roots without axonal degeneration, the study will be normal. Referring physicians should understand that a normal EDX study does not exclude a process involving a root.
- Needle EMG is much more sensitive than NCS in identifying mild injury to the roots. Because abnormalities such as fibrillation potentials may occur even with the loss of only a few axons, changes on needle EMG may be identified when NCS remain normal. An EDX study for radiculopathy that does not include a careful needle examination is an incomplete study.[12,13]
- Fibrillation potentials in all muscles supplied by a specific root imply an "active" process. However, because fibrillation potentials take 2 to 3 weeks to develop,

Table 2
Nerve conduction studies in axonal peripheral neuropathy

CMAP Amplitude	Conduction Velocity	Distal Latency	Conduction Block or Temporal Dispersion
70%–99% normal	Normal to >70%	Normal	No
50%–70% normal	>70% normal	<130% normal	No
<50% normal	>50%	Any (indeterminate)	No

the EDX study should be performed at least 3 weeks after symptom onset to adequately assess for a recent onset radiculopathy.

- Although fibrillation potentials imply an active process, they can persist for months or years in an old, severe process with incomplete reinnervation. Therefore, the presence of fibrillation potentials, particularly in distal but not proximal muscles supplied by a root, may be the residua of an old process.

ELECTROMYOGRAPHY REPORTS IN MONONEUROPATHIES

EDX studies are often used to (1) confirm the presence of a mononeuropathy, (2) localize the focal areas of entrapment if possible, and (3) exclude alternative diagnoses (ie, cervical radiculopathy vs median neuropathy). The most common mononeuropathies (median nerve at the wrist, ulnar nerve at the elbow, and fibular nerve at the knee) are readily assessed by EDX testing but many other individual nerves can be assessed. The EDX evaluation of a mononeuropathy includes NCS and nEMG in most cases. For some nerves (eg, suprascapular, axillary, anterior interosseous, phrenic), there is not a sensory component to test but NCS can often be helpful to exclude a more diffuse process in suspected mononeuropathies (plexopathies, mononeuritis multiplex, and so forth).[14]

- Sensory NCS are typically affected first in compressive mononeuropathies that have motor and sensory axons.
- In compression mononeuropathies, NCS typically show slowing of latencies/CV before amplitude, implying that focal demyelination occurs first. With ongoing compression, axonal loss follows. Demyelination without axonal loss supports a better prognosis.
- In some nerves (ulnar neuropathy at the elbow, fibular neuropathy at knee), short segment stimulation can be helpful to precisely localize the area of focal conduction block or slowing. These stimulation sites are not typically presented in the tabular data but should be summarized in the report.

ELECTROMYOGRAPHY REPORTS IN MYOPATHIES

The goals of EDX studies in suspected myopathies are to (1) confirm the localization of a disorder to the muscle, (2) exclude other mimicking disorders (eg, neuromuscular junction disorders or motor neuron diseases), (3) identify the distribution of muscle involvement and subclinical muscle involvement, (4) provide clues to the underlying pathologic condition, and (5) help guide selection of muscle for potential biopsy.[15]

- Nerve conduction studies are usually normal in most myopathies, unless severe, because most myopathies are proximal in nature. Needle EMG is the most sensitive test to identify myopathy.
- The pattern of nEMG findings helps to define the differential diagnosis for causes of myopathy.
  - Fibrillation potentials are typically seen in myopathies characterized by muscle fiber necrosis, splitting, or vacuolar injury. These include inflammatory myopathies, muscular dystrophies, and toxic myopathies.[5]
  - Diffuse myotonic discharges are seen in myotonic dystrophies and muscle channelopathies (eg, myotonia congenita, hyperkalemic periodic paralysis).
- EDX testing may be normal in certain types of myopathies, including steroid-induced myopathy, metabolic myopathies, and some congenital myopathies.

Table 3			
Nerve conduction studies in demyelinating peripheral neuropathy			
CMAP Amplitude	Conduction Velocity	Distal Latency	Conduction Block/ Temporal Dispersion
Normal	<70% normal	>150% normal	
50%–99% normal	<50% normal	>150% normal	Yes, acquired*
<50% normal	If amplitude <50%, indeterminate		Yes, acquired*

* Some uncommon hereditary neuropathies can demonstrate conduction block (i.e. hereditary neuropathy with liability to pressure palsy)

ELECTROMYOGRAPHY REPORTS IN NEUROMUSCULAR JUNCTION DISORDERS

The goals of EDX studies in neuromuscular junction (NMJ) disorders are to (1) confirm a disorder of the NMJ, (2) determine whether the disorder involves the postsynaptic junction (eg, myasthenia gravis) or presynaptic junction (eg, Lambert Eaton myasthenic syndrome), (3) define severity, and (4) assess response to treatment.[3]

- RNS is a key component of the EDX study used to assess the NMJ integrity. The report should document which nerve–muscle combinations were studied, as well as the rate of stimulation and maximum degree of decrement or increment.
- Many technical factors during RNS can result in unreliable responses or falsely appearing decrement, which is difficult to discern when only reading a report. If the data are shown, 3 sets of RNS at rest should be performed, and the degree of decrement should be similar among each set. Wide variations in the degree of decrement should raise the suspicion for a technical problem. If the waveforms or percent decrement for each stimulus is included, the largest degree of decrement should always be between the first and second stimulus.
- RNS of proximal muscles are more often abnormal than distal muscles in myasthenia gravis and should be performed if there is a high clinical suspicion of disease.
- The only needle EMG feature indicates an NMJ disorders is MUP instability, which can easily be overlooked and not universally present on routine nEMG. An optimal study should comment on the presence or absence of MUP instability.
- The study should be performed with patients withholding their pyridostigmine (Mestinon) for at least 8 hours, and when the effects of other therapies (intravenous immunoglobulin, plasma exchange) are at their least impact to reduce false negative findings.

ANOMALOUS ANATOMY IN THE ELECTROMYOGRAPHY REPORT

There are several normal anatomic variants that may be reported in EMG reports. These have no clinical significance but can be misinterpreted as pathologic condition.

- Martin-Gruber anastomosis (or median-to-ulnar crossover). This is an anatomic variant in the forearm in which some ulnar innervated muscles are supplied by fibers that course with the median nerve in the upper arm but crossover to the ulnar nerve in the forearm. If not identified by the electromyographer, this could potentially mimic an ulnar neuropathy in the forearm.

- Riche-Cannieu anastomosis (or "all ulnar hand"). This is a rare anatomic variant by which the thenar muscles are supplied by the deep branch of the ulnar nerve such that all hand muscles are supplied by the ulnar nerve. This can produce an apparent low median motor amplitude on NCS.
- Accessory fibular (peroneal) nerve. An anatomic variant in the leg by which a portion of the extensor digitorum muscle is supplied by the superficial fibular (rather than deep fibular) branch. This finding does not mimic any disease.

SUMMARY

An EDX study provides depth to the evaluation in the neuromuscular patient beyond the clinical evaluation. Understanding the key components of an EMG report, including components of NCS and nEMG and common pitfalls and technical factors that can influence results is imperative for electromyographers. This knowledge is important for nonneurophysiologists who are ordering and using the EDX test to complement their history and examination.

DISCLOSURE

Dr R.S. Laughlin has no disclosures. Dr D.I. Rubin receives royalties on sale of education products from AANEM, Demos publishing and Wolters Kluwer publishing.

REFERENCES

1. Rubin DI. Practical Concepts in Electromyography. Neurol Clin 2021;39(4):ix–x.
2. O'Bryan R, Kincaid J. Nerve Conduction Studies: Basic Concepts and Patterns of Abnormalities. Neurol Clin 2021;39(4):897–917.
3. Katzberg HD, Abraham A. Electrodiagnostic Assessment of Neuromuscular Junction Disorders. Neurol Clin 2021;39(4):1051–70.
4. Rubin DI. Needle Electromyography Waveforms During Needle Electromyography. Neurol Clin 2021;39(4):919–38.
5. Sener U, Martinez-Thompson J, Laughlin RS, et al. Needle electromyography and histopathologic correlation in myopathies. Muscle Nerve 2019;59(3):315–20.
6. Oishi T, Ryan CS, Vazquez Do Campo R, et al. Quantitative analysis of myokymic discharges in radiation versus nonradiation cases. Muscle Nerve 2021;63(6): 861–7.
7. Jablecki CK, Busis NA, Brandstater MA, et al. Reporting the results of needle EMG and nerve conduction studies: an educational report. Muscle Nerve 2005; 32(5):682–5.
8. Vazquez Do Campo R. Electrodiagnostic Assessment of Polyneuropathy. Neurol Clin 2021;39(4):1015–34.
9. Shaibani A, Al Sultani H. Refractory Chronic Immune-mediated Demyelinating Polyneuropathy. Neurol Clin 2020;38(3):591–605.
10. Allen JA. The Misdiagnosis of CIDP: A Review. Neurol Ther 2020;9(1):43–54.
11. Cho SC, Ferrante MA, Levin KH, et al. Utility of electrodiagnostic testing in evaluating patients with lumbosacral radiculopathy: An evidence-based review. Muscle Nerve 2010;42(2):276–82.
12. Dillingham TR, Annaswamy TM, Plastaras CT. Evaluation of persons with suspected lumbosacral and cervical radiculopathy: Electrodiagnostic assessment and implications for treatment and outcomes (Part II). Muscle Nerve 2020; 62(4):474–84.

13. Dillingham TR, Annaswamy TM, Plastaras CT. Evaluation of persons with suspected lumbosacral and cervical radiculopathy: Electrodiagnostic assessment and implications for treatment and outcomes (Part I). Muscle Nerve 2020;62(4): 462–73.
14. Patel K, Horak HA. Electrodiagnosis of Common Mononeuropathies: Median, Ulnar, and Fibular (Peroneal) Neuropathies. Neurol Clin 2021;39(4):939–55.
15. Martinez-Thompson JM. Electrodiagnostic Assessment of Myopathy. Neurol Clin 2021;39(4):1035–49.

Back Pain
Differential Diagnosis and Management

David Gibbs, BS[a,b], Ben G. McGahan, MD[a],
Alexander E. Ropper, MD[c], David S. Xu, MD[a,c],*

KEYWORDS

- Back pain • Outpatient • Diagnosis • Management

KEY POINTS

- Back pain is common.
- Therapy requires a biopsychosocial approach.
- Surgery is effective in reducing pain and improving quality of life.
- A thorough workup is required to exclude nonoperative etiologies of back pain.

INTRODUCTION

Back pain is currently the most common musculoskeletal complaint affecting millions of individuals every year.[1–3] Back pain significantly contributes to patient morbidity and health care costs[4–6] and is the leading cause of activity limitations and work absenteeism.[7–9] The earliest reports of back pain date back to 1500 BC where the Edwin Smith papyrus documented backache and vertebral column ailments.[10] Before the nineteenth century, back pain had often been considered an incurable rheumatologic disease without a clear pathophysiological mechanism.[11] Although the treatment of back pain remains a pertinent clinical challenge, numerous advances in imaging and medical knowledge have advanced the care that can be provided to patients suffering with back pain.

Back pain is a multifactorial condition that is best approached from a biopsychosocial cognitive framework.[12] A biopsychosocial approach seeks to incorporate the numerous factors that may contribute to a patient's chronic pain and has demonstrated remarkable clinical efficacy when applied in the context of chronic low back pain. Although there are surgically amendable etiologies of back pain, the

[a] Department of Neurological Surgery, The Ohio State Wexner Medical Center, 410 West 10th Street, Columbus, OH 43210, USA; [b] The Ohio State University College of Medicine, 370 West 9th street, Columbus, OH 43210, USA; [c] Department of Neurological Surgery, Baylor College of Medicine, 1 Baylor Plaza, Houston, TX 77030, USA
* Corresponding author. Department of Neurological Surgery, The Ohio State Wexner Medical Center, 410 West 10th Street, Columbus, OH 43210.
E-mail address: David.xu@osumc.edu

Neurol Clin 41 (2023) 61–76
https://doi.org/10.1016/j.ncl.2022.07.002   neurologic.theclinics.com
0733-8619/23/© 2022 Elsevier Inc. All rights reserved.

effective treatment of nonoperative back pain is of paramount clinical utility. Estimates state that surgical intervention is only indicated for approximately half of patients presenting with chronic back pain.[13] Determining which patients would benefit from surgery and working to develop effective treatments among both operative and nonoperative cohorts of back pain are of significant clinical utility and relevance. In the United States, as high as 8.0% of a primary care physician's patient population may present with back pain.[14] Throughout this article, the authors discuss the current literature and guidelines surrounding the assessment, diagnosis, and treatment of back pain for nonsurgical providers.

Differential Diagnosis

The differential diagnosis for back pain is multifactorial with many diagnoses sharing similar presenting signs and symptoms. A general understanding of spinal and paraspinal anatomy is foundational to assist in categorizing etiologies of back pain. Moving from cranial to caudal, the spine is divided into cervical, thoracic, and lumbosacral regions that often present with distinct clinical signs and symptoms. When assessing a patient with back pain, it is essential to confidently rule out "red flag" causes of acute or chronic back pain. Oftentimes, clinical scenarios are unique, but generally, red flags include new onset or progressive motor or sensory loss, urinary or bowel incontinence, history of cancer or recent surgical spinal procedure, and trauma.[15] To better guide clinical decision-making, the differential diagnoses for back pain can be broadly categorized into infectious, neoplastic, inflammatory, degenerative, deformative, traumatic, or inherited/metabolic etiologies.

Infectious

The infectious etiologies of back pain are typically related to immunocompromised states or high-risk behaviors such as IV drug use. Spinal and paraspinal infections often present as back pain with fever and limited range of motion in the affected region. Physical examination may demonstrate erythema or evidence of deep tissue infection. In the appropriate clinical context, granulomatous diseases may also affect the spine. The dissemination of *Mycobacterium tuberculosis* to the spine is often referred to as Pott's disease.[16] In addition, IV drug use is an independent risk factor for infection of the vertebral body, disc space, and epidural space.[17]

Neoplastic

Vertebral column metastasis is the most common site of any bony metastasis and often requires surgical decompression and radiation therapy.[18,19] Patients with metastatic spine lesions may present with mechanical or neurogenic back pain due to spinal cord compression. Further, systemic symptoms may or may not be present. Given the increasing age of the population and the increased incidence of spinal metastasis, a high clinical suspicion for malignancy should be exercised until proven otherwise in elderly patients and those with a past medical history of cancer.[20]

Inflammatory

There are a variety of inflammatory spondyloarthropathies that may affect the spine and lead to back pain.[21] Often referred to as the seronegative spondyloarthropathies, conditions such as reactive arthritis, ankylosing spondylitis, and rheumatoid arthritis may all have varied effects on the spine. In addition, Langerhans cell histiocytosis may present with vertebra plana causing back pain. A thorough past medical history and review of symptoms are essential in elucidating these inflammatory/autoimmune etiologies of back pain.

Degenerative

Osteoarthritis of the spine is the most common cause of adult back pain.[22] Degenerative disc disease (DDD) refers to the gradual collapse of the intervertebral disc resulting in a loss of disc height and the subsequent development of neurologic sequelae. DDD often occurs in the lumbosacral spine and progresses until symptoms of lower extremity radiculopathy require surgical intervention.[23,24] Patients often present with chronic, non-emergent low back pain, and physical examination may be demonstrate a positive straight leg raise test and limited range of motion.

Deformative

Similar to DDD, deformity in the spine may be a significant contributor to back pain. Adult spinal deformity patients often present with postural instability and gait imbalances. Further, a limited range of motion and abnormal imaging often confirms this diagnosis.

Traumatic

Traumatic etiologies of back pain often present with signs and symptoms concerning for vertebral column fracture, spinal instability, or neurologic injury. A timely history and physical examination are essential when surgical emergencies such as ensure cauda equina syndrome or traumatic spinal cord injury are suspected. Normal imaging in the context of traumatic back pain often suggests musculoskeletal etiologies including muscle strains or torsional sprains.

Inherited and/or Metabolic

There is an extensive differential of inherited or metabolic conditions that may affect the spine leading to back pain. Conditions that affect bone quality or pain receptors in the back may include osteogenesis imperfecta, osteomalacia/rickets, Paget's disease of bone, and diabetic neuropathy, among many others. A family history and evaluation of bone quality may help to elucidate these diagnoses.

Red Flags

Before an extended workup and nonoperative therapy, urgent conditions presenting with back pain such as cauda equina syndrome, pancreatitis, and abdominal aortic aneurysm must be ruled out. A detailed history and careful physical examination are essential elements involved in the diagnosis and assessment of a patient with back pain. A clinical presentation with "red flags" warranting urgent evaluation and intervention may include a history of cancer, unexplained weight loss, fever, intravenous drug use, trauma, bowel/bladder incontinence, urinary retention, saddle anesthesia, and/or neurologic symptoms present longer than 1 month and worsening.

ASSESSMENT AND DIAGNOSIS

The initial diagnosis and assessment of back pain seeks to characterize the severity, etiology, and associated symptoms and to evaluate if further testing and intervention is indicated. Estimates claim that up to 60% of all patients presenting to a primary care physician will complain of back pain.[25] Given its prevalence, providers are tasked with efficiently differentiating who will benefit from further testing and specialist care.

When assessing a patient with back pain, it is important to obtain a broad medical history to determine the duration, intensity, and characterization of pain, the alleviating and exacerbating factors, and the presence of constitutional symptoms (fever, night sweats, weight loss, substance use, depression, and so forth). When conducting a physical examination, following inspection for asymmetries, palpation for localizing pain, and assessment of neurologic function (strength, reflexes, and sensation), the straight leg raise test and evaluation of Waddell's nonorganic signs may be used. The straight leg raise test, also referred to as the Lasegue test, is performed by having the patient lie supine and then gently flexing at the hip with their knee extended. A positive test occurs when flexion less than 45° elicits the patient's pain, in the appropriate dermatomal distribution. Dorsiflexion of the foot during this maneuver increases the sensitivity of Lasegue's test and is referred to as Bragard's sign.[26,27] Waddell's nonorganic signs are notable examination characteristics that signify pain may be psychogenic in nature rather than anatomic.[28] Waddell's signs include tenderness, simulation, distraction, regional disturbances, and overreaction. Eliciting pain within the first 30° of rotation or witnessing a discrepancy in testing when a patient is distracted are both examples of positive inorganic (Waddell) signs.[28,29]

The most common etiologies of surgically treatable back pain can be grouped as axial (mechanical), radicular (neuropathic), or referred, defined by the characteristics of pain produced.[30,31] Although these categories provide a useful framework, it should be noted that etiologies may produce multiple types of back pain and that each patient may present differently, requiring nuanced clinical judgment.

Axial/Mechanical Back Pain

Axial, or mechanical, pain is characterized by deformity and/or degeneration of the mechanical integrity of the axial skeleton and paraspinal musculature. Mechanical pain can vary in its presentation ranging from a nonspecific, dull ache to a sharp, stabbing pain. Patients may complain of mechanical "catching" or "popping" sensations in their spine with flexion and extension and often exhibit weakness and a limited range of motion. Muscle strain is a common cause of axial pain. Axial back pain is frequently degenerative and can be thought of as osteoarthritis of the spine, with pain improving with rest and worsening with activity.

Radicular/Neuropathic Back Pain

Radicular, or neuropathic, pain is characterized by compression and damage of nerves. Radiculopathy refers to the compression of a nerve root as it exits the spine. Neuropathy refers to damage of a nerve outside the central nervous system. Neuropathic pain is often caused by compressive conditions including a herniated disc, spinal stenosis, or spondylolisthesis. This type of back pain is often described as deep, burning, shooting pain and may be localized to a dermatomal distribution. Neuropathic pain can be very severe and is often accompanied by numbness or weakness in the dermatome/myotome of the compressed nerve or nerve root. The straight leg raise test will likely be positive among this cohort.

REFERRED PAIN AND NONSPECIFIC BACK PAIN

Referred pain may be caused by numerous etiologies. This type of back pain is often described as dull or achy and frequently changes location. DDD is a common cause of referred pain to the pelvic girdle. Finally, there is a subset of patients that complain of persistent back pain despite absence of any identifiable anatomic abnormalities.[32] These patients typically present with varied clinical symptoms with pain affecting their quality of life. Although surgical intervention is not recommended among this cohort, individualized medical and behavioral therapy may provide some relief. The determination of Waddell's signs may be beneficial within this cohort.[28]

IMAGING AND ADDITIONAL TESTING

Following a thorough history and physical examination, further assessment of persistent back pain commonly uses medical imaging. Standard imaging is not indicated until symptoms have persisted for greater than 6 weeks, unless there are any red flag symptoms, in which prompt imaging is indicated.[3,33–35] Various studies have identified minimal benefit for early imaging of non-emergent back pain, unless there is significant patient anxiety.[35,36] If there is concern for cauda equina syndrome, urgent referral and MRI are indicated. There is currently insufficient evidence in the literature to recommend specific imaging sequences, and thus this determination may be best suited for a specialist. Laboratory testing is often not required before referral, but if there is concern for osteopenia/osteoporosis or metabolic conditions, relevant studies may be pursued (DEXA scans of the hip and spine, electromyography [EMG], hemoglobin A1c [HbA1C], alkaline phosphatase [ALP]).

MEDICAL AND PSYCHOLOGICAL TREATMENT OPTIONS
Pharmacology

When treating back pain, a biopsychosocial approach provides the most appropriate framework for improving a patient's quality of life and functional status.[37] Biologically, back pain is treated with nonselective, nonsteroidal anti-inflammatory drugs (NSAIDs). Multiple studies have sought to identify novel therapeutic strategies for the medical management of back pain. Recent data suggesting that antidepressants and steroids are ineffective in treating back pain.[38–40] Further, there is insufficient evidence in the literature to suggest the use of anticonvulsants, vitamin D, selective NSAIDs, and topical lidocaine.[41,42] Opioid use for back pain is a highly contested topic with evidence recommending opioids only in limited cases of severe pain with their use restricted to the shortest duration due to their potential for abuse.[43] Finally, topical capsicum cream has been shown to effectively reduce back pain and is recommended for short-term treatment with use up to 3 months.[44,45] In summary, current data regarding pharmacologic options for back pain support the use of nonselective NSAIDs, topical capsicum cream, and opioids in very rare circumstances. Data concerning the efficacy of anticonvulsants, vitamin D, topical lidocaine, and other medications remain inconclusive.

Psychotherapy

When seeking to address the psychosocial aspects of back pain, cognitive behavioral therapy (CBT) and physical therapy (PT) are mainstays of treatment. When compared with PT alone for back pain, CBT with PT significantly improves pain scores and functional outcomes such as time until return to work.[46,47] Psychological illness is prevalent among patients with back pain, yet there is limited conclusive data to support the treatment of anxiety or depression as a means of specifically improving a patient's back pain.[48] The role of CBT for patients with surgically treated back pain remains unclear.[49] Education plays a significant role in the care of patients with chronic conditions. Despite the burden and typical chronology of back pain, educational instruction has not been clearly associated with improved compliance to treatment protocols or to improved pain or functional outcomes.[50–52] Kinesiophobia, defined as "an excessive, irrational, and debilitating fear of physical movement and activity resulting from a feeling of vulnerability due to painful injury or reinjury," has been identified as a psychosocial factor predictive of a poor response to low back pain treatment.[53–55] There is no doubt that lifestyle modification and weight loss have profound effects on a patient comorbidities and overall level of health.[56]

Using a biopsychosocial approach, the treatment of back pain first uses conventional therapies including lifestyle modifications, NSAIDs, PT, and CBT. If these options have been exhausted and pain persists for greater than 6 weeks, imaging and a specialist referral may be indicated. Further, if pharmacologic and psychosocial therapies have failed to improve symptoms or if symptoms are worsening, surgical treatment may be indicated. The clinical decision to pursue surgery for non-emergent back pain varies with each patient but is often considered for patients who have failed conservative treatment and remain in pain greater than 3 months. Current medical and psychological therapies for back pain remain a popular topic of study, and improved therapies will likely continue to develop throughout the coming years.

PHYSICAL MEDICINE AND REHABILITATION

The mainstay treatment of back pain is conservative care and rehabilitation encompassing multiple specialties including PT, physical medicine and rehabilitation, and other alternative therapies. The treatments included in this category are patient education and special programs such as back school, physical agents such as heat and cold, ultrasound, electrical stimulation, laser stimulation, dry needling and acupuncture, braces, spinal manipulation, different exercise programs, and yoga. This section will go over these treatments and briefly discuss the evidence for or against each. As with healthy patients, one of the best treatments for patients with back pain is physical activity.

Patient education regarding back pain has many forms including in office teaching, patient handouts, and specialty programs like back school. Back school refers to several different programs that teach patients about back pain and how to avoid it. For example, one program will have four 1-hour classes over 2 weeks to teach anatomy and causes of low back pain, function of the muscles, ergonomics, and advice for physical activity. In a randomized controlled trial, back school and exercise for chronic low back pain was found to improve pain and function at 6 months compared with exercise alone.[57] Home-based education and exercise can also be successful in reducing low back pain and improving function.[58,59]

A common at home treatment of low back pain has been the local application of heat or cold. Several randomized controlled trials have concluded that the addition of heat to either NSAIDs or exercise can improve pain and disability.[60–64] One study also showed that the application of cold can be helpful to treat pain, although potentially less helpful than heat.[65]

Ultrasound therapy has been investigated for help in treatment of patients with low back pain. Ultrasound therapy uses sound vibrations to deliver heat to deep tissues of the back. Two randomized controlled trials demonstrated that the addition of ultrasound therapy did not add any additional benefit to conservative care.[66,67] Similarly, randomized controlled trials demonstrated that the use of lasers for cutaneous stimulation did not have any benefit in the treatment of low back pain.[68,69]

Transcutaneous electrical nerve stimulation (TENS) provides low-voltage electrical impulses through a battery-powered device on the surface of the skin. TENS is thought to help alleviate pain by disrupting transmission of pain signals. Evidence for TENS efficacy is mixed. In a randomized controlled trial comparing TENS and a sham TENS with and without the addition of exercise, TENS demonstrated no improvement in pain for patients with chronic back pain.[70] Although other randomized controlled trials concluded immediate improved pain and function for patients with chronic low back pain, the affect seems to be beneficial for only a short period of time.[71,72]

Dry needling is the use of thin needles to stimulate myofascial trigger points. There is a lack of solid evidence for the use of dry needling to treat back pain. A randomized controlled trial demonstrated that the addition of dry needling to PT improved back pain more than PT alone. The study did have flaws of a small sample size and poorly defined outcomes.[73] Acupuncture is similar to dry needling with the use of thin needles to provide stimulation although the targets are not myofascial trigger points but traditional Chinese medicine meridian theory targets. When acupuncture is compared with sham acupuncture, the results are conflicting whether it helps with low back pain.[74–78] When acupuncture is studied by comparing standard PT or PT with the addition of acupuncture, then randomized controlled trials do demonstrate significant improvement in pain and function with the addition of acupuncture to standard therapy.[79–81]

Lumbar belts, braces, and corsets have been used to provide musculoskeletal support and alleviate back pain. The evidence is conflicting on the efficacy of this as a treatment of back pain. One randomized controlled trial investigated the use of an elastic lumbar belt and found improvement in pain and functions in patients with subacute lumbar back pain.[82] However, when this study was controlled for differences between the groups, there was no longer significance. Another randomized controlled trial demonstrated no difference in pain or disability when adding a back brace to education, although patients with the brace did have a lower chance of recurrent back pain.[83]

Spinal manipulative therapy (SMT) is performed by chiropractors with their hands to apply controlled thrusts to the spine. SMT is an option for both acute and chronic back pain. However, the evidence is more robust for chronic back pain.[84–86]

Several difference exercise programs are used to treat back pain. The evidence seems to suggest that at least some activity is better than none, although specific exercise programs may be no better than standard PT. There is some evidence to support in addition to PT the use of active stabilization programs,[87,88] McKenzie method exercises for centralization,[89,90] yoga,[91,92] and work hardening.[93,94]

INTERVENTIONAL TREATMENT

More invasive treatments than PT, physical medicine, rehabilitation, and alternative treatments that fall short of surgical treatment are referred to as interventional treatments. These interventional treatments are often performed by pain anesthesiologists in the clinic. These procedures include epidural steroid injections, facet injections, facet nerve blocks and neurotomies, trigger point injections, and sacroiliac join injections. More invasive procedures than these injections, often done by neurosurgeons, include spinal cord stimulation and intrathecal drug delivery via pump.

Epidural steroid injections can be done either caudally through the sacral hiatus or between the lamina at any spinal level. There is not strong evidence for or against the use of epidural steroid injections for treatment of low back pain.[95] In one study of patients undergoing caudal epidural steroid injections, only 20% of patients had at least 50% reduction in pain.[96] Interlaminar injections have a slightly higher rate of success with 40% of patients having a 50% reduction in their pain at 6 months.[97]

A common location for the source of low back pain is the facet joints that wear and tear with time and use. The facet joints have become popular targets for interventional therapy. Injections of local anesthetic into the lumbar facet joints have been used for both diagnostic localization of the patient's source of back pain as well as to treat the pain itself. The use of these blocks to predict the facet joint as the pain generator only has a positive predictive value of 16% and is therefore not useful.[98] In patients who have 50% reduction in pain after facet joint injections, further injections with steroids do not provide clinically meaningful improvement at 6 months.[99] Alcohol, such as phenol, has been injected around facets for a similar purpose of ablating facet joint pain. Although the short-term outcomes at 1 month are 62% of patients report good outcome, only 36% at 6 months.[100] Another similar interventional treatment of facet joint pain is radiofrequency and thermal denervation of the facet joint. Patients have some initial improvement in their pain but at 6 months have no significant improvement.[101] With stringent patient selection, the use of thermal ablation of the medial branches of the dorsal rami that innervate the facet can provide significant improvement to pain and function at 12 months.[102] The stringent patient selection was age greater than 17 years, with continuous low back with focal tenderness over the facet joints, pain on hyperextension, absence of neurologic defect, unresponsiveness to conservative treatment, no radicular syndrome, and no indication for low back surgery.

For patient with pain at the sacroiliac joint, intra-articular steroid injections may be considered for pain relief.[103–105] Trigger point injections, or myofascial injections of local anesthetic or botulinum toxin, at locations of low back pain were not found effective in a randomized control trial.[106]

Spinal cord stimulation is the placement of electrodes dorsal to the spinal cord in the epidural space. The stimulating electrodes are thought to work in decreasing pain by stimulating the dorsal columns of the spinal cord and blocking transmission of pain signals via the gate-control theory. Typically, percutaneous trial leads are placed by a neurosurgeon in a same day surgery under light sedation, and the leads are attached to an external battery. If the patient has success with the trial, usually a 50% reduction in their pain, then they are recommended to have permanent implantation of leads and an implantable pulse generator. Spinal cord stimulators lead to a significant decrease in pain and around 70% decrease in the use of opioids at 12 months.[107]

SURGICAL TREATMENTS

Surgery can be helpful for low back pain when a specific surgical pathology can be addressed, such as a herniated disc causing nerve compression, slippage of one vertebral body of the one below (spondylolisthesis), an unstable fracture, spinal canal stenosis causing compression of neural structures, tumors, and so forth. However, there is, in general, a lack of evidence to support the use of surgery for the treatment of back pain alone.

If a patient has DDD without spondylolisthesis or herniated disc causing severe disabling chronic (>2 years) low back pain and they have failed other conservative treatments, then a fusion across that level can be recommended for treatment of their pain.[108] In the largest prospective randomized study of 339 patients with chronic back pain, half were randomized to lumbar fusion and the other half randomized to intensive rehab. Those who underwent surgery had a small but significant improvement in their disability scores compared with those that underwent an intensive rehab program.[109] The clinical significance of this small improvement is debated and must be weighed against the risk of complications of undergoing lumbar fusion. In a large systematic review of nearly 1500 publications, lumbar fusion was found to be equivalent to intensive rehabilitative programs, and there were moderate benefits to surgery compared with nonoperative treatment.[110]

There are many considerations when deciding if surgery is appropriate for a patient with chronic low back pain. Chief among them is the patient's comorbidities. Patients with other medical issues are at significantly higher risk of postoperative complications. Most commonly obesity and diabetes can lead to wound complications, infections, and failure to fuse. Smoking can prevent fusion and cause wound complications and must be stopped before surgery. Elderly patients, especially females, are typically screened for osteoporosis and treated if needed before surgery for fusion.

Spinal fusion can be done through several different approaches and techniques. The approach can be anterior, lateral, or posterior. Some techniques can be more minimally invasive and can be done with outpatient surgery or an overnight stay in the hospital. Other techniques require a hospital stay of 3 to 5 days and weeks of PT and rehabilitation. Complications from spinal fusion are not rare. In the prospective randomized study of 339 patients, 19 of the 176 surgical patients (11%) had complications, 11 (6%) needed a reoperation.[109] The most common complications were dural tears and problems with implanted hardware.

DISCUSSION

In this article, the authors have summarized some of the most useful information regarding workup and treatment of back pain. Back pain affects millions of people every year and is the most common musculoskeletal complaint and the leading cause of disability.[1–37] As such, there is a vast amount of literature regarding the cause, workup, and treatment of back pain. Controversies continue to exist within back pain literature and further research is needed to clarify the best course of treatment of patient with back pain. A good reference for further reading is the North American Spine Society's guidelines for back pain.[95] Their latest guideline is from 2020 and is endorsed by the major national societies of neurosurgeons, physical medicine, and rehabilitation and has contributions from societies of family medicine, orthopedics, pain specialists, anesthesiology, and PT.

The differential diagnosis for back pain is long and diverse. Categorizing the possible cause into infectious, neoplastic, inflammatory, degenerative, deformative, traumatic, or inherited/metabolic can helpful when initially encountering a patient for back pain. Identifying red flag symptoms of new neurologic deficits, bowel or bladder incontinence, history of trauma, or cancer are important to prompt further workup and treatment. Imaging is not indicated unless pain has been ongoing for 6 weeks or there are red flag symptoms.

Most people with acute back pain will go on to have resolution of symptoms within a few weeks. The goal of treating chronic back pain is not the complete relief of symptoms, but to achieve resumption of activities of daily living. As such, most likely any kind of regular movement and exercise is probably beneficial. The standard of care is NSAIDs to treat pain followed by PT for strengthening core muscles. Adjuvants that may provide some additional benefit are back school, heat or cold application, acupuncture, SMT, and exercises such as stabilization, centralization, hardening, and yoga. All of the treatments discussed need to be weighed against the potential of complications from that treatment, especially surgery. In some cases, surgery of a fusion may be beneficial even weighing the risks of a surgical operation.

Future directions in the workup and treatment of back pain will likely be pioneered by the assistance of artificial intelligence. Digitalized health care data will soon be analyzed to customize treatment to specific patients and their unique pathology. This may lead the way in which back pain patient may benefit best from certain treatments.

In conclusion, back pain is something nearly every medical doctor will encounter. It is important is rule out red flags and to work with patients toward the goal of getting them back to their activities of daily living. This is accomplished by exercise and adjuvants to improve movement.

CLINICS CARE POINTS

- Back pain is very common and typically is benign and self limited.
- Treatment relies not only on medical and pharmacologic therapy, but also psychosocial engagement.
- Persistent back pain longer than 6 weeks warrants additional imaging and labratory analysis.
- Structural causes of persistent back pain respond to surgical intervention.

DISCLOSURE

The authors have nothing to disclose.

REFERENCES

1. Hoy D, Bain C, Williams G, et al. A systematic review of the global prevalence of low back pain. Arthritis Rheum 2012;64(6):2028–37.
2. Hoy D, Brooks P, Blyth F, et al. The Epidemiology of low back pain. Best Pract Res Clin Rheumatol 2010;24(6):769–81.
3. Maher C, Underwood M, Buchbinder R. Non-specific low back pain. Lancet 2017;389(10070):736–47.
4. Buchbinder R, van Tulder M, Öberg B, et al. Low back pain: a call for action. Lancet 2018;391(10137):2384–8.
5. Hoy D, March L, Brooks P, et al. The global burden of low back pain: estimates from the Global Burden of Disease 2010 study. Ann Rheum Dis 2014;73(6): 968–74.
6. Erdem MN, Erken HY, Aydogan M. The effectiveness of non-surgical treatments, re-discectomy and minimally invasive transforaminal lumbar interbody fusion in post-discectomy pain syndrome. J Spine Surg 2018;4(2):414–22.
7. Driscoll T, Jacklyn G, Orchard J, et al. The global burden of occupationally related low back pain: estimates from the Global Burden of Disease 2010 study. Ann Rheum Dis 2014;73(6):975–81.
8. Global, regional, and national incidence, prevalence, and years lived with disability for 354 diseases and injuries for 195 countries and territories, 1990-2017: a systematic analysis for the Global Burden of Disease Study 2017. Lancet 2018;392(10159):1789–858.
9. Lee H, Hübscher M, Moseley GL, et al. How does pain lead to disability? A systematic review and meta-analysis of mediation studies in people with back and neck pain. Pain 2015;156(6):988–97.
10. van Middendorp JJ, Sanchez GM, Burridge AL. The Edwin Smith papyrus: a clinical reappraisal of the oldest known document on spinal injuries. Eur Spine J 2010;19(11):1815–23.
11. Allan DB, Waddell G. An historical perspective on low back pain and disability. Acta Orthop Scand Suppl 1989;234:1–23.
12. Kamper SJ, Apeldoorn AT, Chiarotto A, et al. Multidisciplinary biopsychosocial rehabilitation for chronic low back pain. Cochrane Database Syst Rev 2014;(9):Cd000963.
13. Feuerstein M, Marcus SC, Huang GD. National trends in nonoperative care for nonspecific back pain. Spine J 2004;4(1):56–63.

14. Kent PM, Keating JL. The epidemiology of low back pain in primary care. Chiropr Osteopat 2005;13:13.

15. Will JS, Bury DC, Miller JA. Mechanical Low Back Pain. Am Fam Physician 2018; 98(7):421–8.

16. Turgut M. Pott's disease. *J Neurosurg* Jul 1997;87(1):136–8.

17. Lener S, Hartmann S, Barbagallo GMV, et al. Management of spinal infection: a review of the literature. Acta Neurochir (Wien) 2018;160(3):487–96.

18. Patchell RA, Tibbs PA, Regine WF, et al. Direct decompressive surgical resection in the treatment of spinal cord compression caused by metastatic cancer: a randomised trial. Lancet 2005;366(9486):643–8.

19. Maccauro G, Spinelli MS, Mauro S, et al. Physiopathology of spine metastasis. Int J Surg Oncol 2011;2011:107969.

20. Beaufort Q, Terrier LM, Dubory A, et al. Spine Metastasis in Elderly: Encouraging Results for Better Survival. Spine (Phila Pa 1976) 2021;46(11):751–9.

21. Dougados M, Baeten D. Spondyloarthritis. Lancet 2011;377(9783):2127–37.

22. Goode AP, Carey TS, Jordan JM. Low back pain and lumbar spine osteoarthritis: how are they related? Curr Rheumatol Rep 2013;15(2):305.

23. Battié MC, Joshi AB, Gibbons LE. Degenerative Disc Disease: What is in a Name? Spine (Phila Pa 1976) 2019;44(21):1523–9.

24. Battié MC, Videman T. Lumbar disc degeneration: epidemiology and genetics. J Bone Joint Surg Am 2006;88(Suppl 2):3–9.

25. Atlas SJ, Deyo RA. Evaluating and managing acute low back pain in the primary care setting. J Gen Intern Med 2001;16(2):120–31.

26. Camino Willhuber GO, Piuzzi NS. Straight leg raise test. StatPearls. StatPearls Publishing. StatPearls Publishing LLC.; 2021. Copyright © 2021.

27. Vroomen PC, de Krom MC, Knottnerus JA. Consistency of history taking and physical examination in patients with suspected lumbar nerve root involvement. Spine (Phila Pa 1976) 2000;25(1):91–6 [discussion: 97].

28. D'Souza RS, Dowling TJ, Law L, et al. StatPearls. StatPearls Publishing. StatPearls Publishing LLC; 2021. Copyright © 2021.

29. Yoo JU, McIver TC, Hiratzka J, et al. The presence of Waddell signs depends on age and gender, not diagnosis. Bone Joint J 2018;100-b(2):219–25.

30. Urits I, Burshtein A, Sharma M, et al. Low Back Pain, a Comprehensive Review: Pathophysiology, Diagnosis, and Treatment. Curr Pain Headache Rep 2019; 23(3):23.

31. Hooten WM, Cohen SP. Evaluation and Treatment of Low Back Pain: A Clinically Focused Review for Primary Care Specialists. Mayo Clin Proc 2015;90(12): 1699–718.

32. Popkirov S, Enax-Krumova EK, Mainka T, et al. Functional pain disorders - more than nociplastic pain. NeuroRehabilitation 2020;47(3):343–53.

33. Foster A, Croot L, Brazier J, et al. The facilitators and barriers to implementing patient reported outcome measures in organisations delivering health related services: a systematic review of reviews. J Patient Rep Outcomes 2018;2:46.

34. Oliveira CB, Maher CG, Pinto RZ, et al. Clinical practice guidelines for the management of non-specific low back pain in primary care: an updated overview. Eur Spine J 2018;27(11):2791–803.

35. Kerry S, Hilton S, Dundas D, et al. Radiography for low back pain: a randomised controlled trial and observational study in primary care. Br J Gen Pract 2002; 52(479):469–74.

36. Lemmers GPG, van Lankveld W, Westert GP, et al. Imaging versus no imaging for low back pain: a systematic review, measuring costs, healthcare utilization and absence from work. Eur Spine J 2019;28(5):937–50.

37. Schiltenwolf M, Buchner M, Heindl B, et al. Comparison of a biopsychosocial therapy (BT) with a conventional biomedical therapy (MT) of subacute low back pain in the first episode of sick leave: a randomized controlled trial. Eur Spine J 2006;15(7):1083–92.

38. Muehlbacher M, Nickel MK, Kettler C, et al. Topiramate in treatment of patients with chronic low back pain: a randomized, double-blind, placebo-controlled study. Clin J Pain 2006;22(6):526–31.

39. Atkinson JH, Slater MA, Wahlgren DR, et al. Effects of noradrenergic and serotonergic antidepressants on chronic low back pain intensity. Pain 1999;83(2): 137–45.

40. Eskin B, Shih RD, Fiesseler FW, et al. Prednisone for emergency department low back pain: a randomized controlled trial. J Emerg Med 2014;47(1):65–70.

41. Gimbel J, Linn R, Hale M, et al. Lidocaine patch treatment in patients with low back pain: results of an open-label, nonrandomized pilot study. Am J Ther 2005;12(4):311–9.

42. Sandoughi M, Zakeri Z, Mirhosainee Z, et al. The effect of vitamin D on nonspecific low back pain. Int J Rheum Dis 2015;18(8):854–8.

43. Ruoff GE, Rosenthal N, Jordan D, et al. Tramadol/acetaminophen combination tablets for the treatment of chronic lower back pain: a multicenter, randomized, double-blind, placebo-controlled outpatient study. Clin Ther 2003;25(4): 1123–41.

44. Frerick H, Keitel W, Kuhn U, et al. Topical treatment of chronic low back pain with a capsicum plaster. Pain 2003;106(1–2):59–64.

45. Keitel W, Frerick H, Kuhn U, et al. Capsicum pain plaster in chronic non-specific low back pain. Arzneimittelforschung 2001;51(11):896–903.

46. Turner JA, Jensen MP. Efficacy of cognitive therapy for chronic low back pain. Pain 1993;52(2):169–77.

47. Dufour N, Thamsborg G, Oefeldt A, et al. Treatment of chronic low back pain: a randomized, clinical trial comparing group-based multidisciplinary biopsychosocial rehabilitation and intensive individual therapist-assisted back muscle strengthening exercises. Spine (Phila Pa 1976) 2010;35(5):469–76.

48. Hampel P, Tlach L. Cognitive-behavioral management training of depressive symptoms among inpatient orthopedic patients with chronic low back pain and depressive symptoms: A 2-year longitudinal study. J Back Musculoskelet Rehabil 2015;28(1):49–60.

49. Rolving N, Sogaard R, Nielsen CV, et al. Preoperative Cognitive-Behavioral Patient Education Versus Standard Care for Lumbar Spinal Fusion Patients: Economic Evaluation Alongside a Randomized Controlled Trial. Spine (Phila Pa 1976) 2016;41(1):18–25.

50. Basler HD, Bertalanffy H, Quint S, et al. TTM-based counselling in physiotherapy does not contribute to an increase of adherence to activity recommendations in older adults with chronic low back pain–a randomised controlled trial. Eur J Pain 2007;11(1):31–7.

51. Johnson RE, Jones GT, Wiles NJ, et al. Active exercise, education, and cognitive behavioral therapy for persistent disabling low back pain: a randomized controlled trial. Spine (Phila Pa 1976) 2007;32(15):1578–85.

52. Zhang Y, Wan L, Wang X. The effect of health education in patients with chronic low back pain. J Int Med Res 2014;42(3):815–20.

53. Monticone M, Ferrante S, Rocca B, et al. Effect of a long-lasting multidisciplinary program on disability and fear-avoidance behaviors in patients with chronic low back pain: results of a randomized controlled trial. Clin J Pain 2013;29(11): 929–38.

54. Woods MP, Asmundson GJG. Evaluating the efficacy of graded in vivo exposure for the treatment of fear in patients with chronic back pain: a randomized controlled clinical trial. Pain 2008;136(3):271–80.

55. Larsson C, Ekvall Hansson E, Sundquist K, et al. Kinesiophobia and its relation to pain characteristics and cognitive affective variables in older adults with chronic pain. BMC Geriatr 2016;16:128.

56. Keeley P, Creed F, Tomenson B, et al. Psychosocial predictors of health-related quality of life and health service utilisation in people with chronic low back pain. Pain 2008;135(1–2):142–50.

57. Durmus D, Unal M, Kuru O. How effective is a modified exercise program on its own or with back school in chronic low back pain? A randomized-controlled clinical trial. J Back Musculoskelet Rehabil 2014;27(4):553–61.

58. Kuukkanen T, Mälkiä E, Kautiainen H, et al. Effectiveness of a home exercise programme in low back pain: a randomized five-year follow-up study. Physiother Res Int 2007;12(4):213–24.

59. Shirado O, Doi T, Akai M, et al. Multicenter randomized controlled trial to evaluate the effect of home-based exercise on patients with chronic low back pain: the Japan low back pain exercise therapy study. Spine (Phila Pa 1976) 2010;35(17):E811–9.

60. Kettenmann B, Wille C, Lurie-Luke E, et al. Impact of continuous low level heatwrap therapy in acute low back pain patients: subjective and objective measurements. Clin J Pain 2007;23(8):663–8.

61. Mayer JM, Ralph L, Look M, et al. Treating acute low back pain with continuous low-level heat wrap therapy and/or exercise: a randomized controlled trial. Spine J 2005;5(4):395–403.

62. Nadler SF, Steiner DJ, Erasala GN, et al. Continuous low-level heatwrap therapy for treating acute nonspecific low back pain. Arch Phys Med Rehabil 2003; 84(3):329–34.

63. Nadler SF, Steiner DJ, Petty SR, et al. Overnight use of continuous low-level heatwrap therapy for relief of low back pain. Arch Phys Med Rehabil 2003; 84(3):335–42.

64. Tao XG, Bernacki EJ. A randomized clinical trial of continuous low-level heat therapy for acute muscular low back pain in the workplace. J Occup Environ Med 2005;47(12):1298–306.

65. Dehghan M, Farahbod F. The efficacy of thermotherapy and cryotherapy on pain relief in patients with acute low back pain, a clinical trial study. J Clin Diagn Res 2014;8(9):Lc01–4.

66. Ebadi S, Ansari NN, Naghdi S, et al. The effect of continuous ultrasound on chronic non-specific low back pain: a single blind placebo-controlled randomized trial. BMC Musculoskelet Disord 2012;13:192.

67. Durmus D, Alayli G, Goktepe AS, et al. Is phonophoresis effective in the treatment of chronic low back pain? A single-blind randomized controlled trial. Rheumatol Int 2013;33(7):1737–44.

68. Glazov G, Schattner P, Lopez D, et al. Laser acupuncture for chronic non-specific low back pain: a controlled clinical trial. Acupunct Med 2009;27(3): 94–100.

69. Glazov G, Yelland M, Emery J. Low-dose laser acupuncture for non-specific chronic low back pain: a double-blind randomised controlled trial. Acupunct Med 2014;32(2):116–23.

70. Deyo RA, Walsh NE, Martin DC, et al. A controlled trial of transcutaneous electrical nerve stimulation (TENS) and exercise for chronic low back pain. N Engl J Med 1990;322(23):1627–34.

71. Thompson JW, Bower S, Tyrer SP. A double blind randomised controlled clinical trial on the effect of transcutaneous spinal electroanalgesia (TSE) on low back pain. Eur J Pain 2008;12(3):371–7.

72. Jarzem PFHE, Arcaro N, Kaczorowski J. Transcutaneous Electrical Nerve Stimulation [TENS] for Short-Term Treatment of Low Back Pain–Randomized Double Blind Crossover Study of Sham versus Conventional TENS. J Musculoskelet Pain 2005;13(2).

73. Gunn CC, Milbrandt WE, Little AS, et al. Dry needling of muscle motor points for chronic low-back pain: a randomized clinical trial with long-term follow-up. Spine (Phila Pa 1976) 1980;5(3):279–91.

74. Cherkin DC, Sherman KJ, Avins AL, et al. A randomized trial comparing acupuncture, simulated acupuncture, and usual care for chronic low back pain. Arch Intern Med 2009;169(9):858–66.

75. Cho YJ, Song YK, Cha YY, et al. Acupuncture for chronic low back pain: a multi-center, randomized, patient-assessor blind, sham-controlled clinical trial. Spine (Phila Pa 1976) 2013;38(7):549–57.

76. Vas J, Aranda JM, Modesto M, et al. Acupuncture in patients with acute low back pain: a multicentre randomised controlled clinical trial. Pain 2012;153(9):1883–9.

77. Carlsson CP, Sjölund BH. Acupuncture for chronic low back pain: a randomized placebo-controlled study with long-term follow-up. Clin J Pain 2001;17(4):296–305.

78. Kerr DP, Walsh DM, Baxter D. Acupuncture in the management of chronic low back pain: a blinded randomized controlled trial. Clin J Pain 2003;19(6):364–70.

79. Haake M, Müller HH, Schade-Brittinger C, et al. German Acupuncture Trials (GERAC) for chronic low back pain: randomized, multicenter, blinded, parallel-group trial with 3 groups. Arch Intern Med 2007;167(17):1892–8.

80. Witt CM, Jena S, Selim D, et al. Pragmatic randomized trial evaluating the clinical and economic effectiveness of acupuncture for chronic low back pain. Am J Epidemiol 2006;164(5):487–96.

81. Yeung CK, Leung MC, Chow DH. The use of electro-acupuncture in conjunction with exercise for the treatment of chronic low-back pain. J Altern Complement Med 2003;9(4):479–90.

82. Calmels P, Queneau P, Hamonet C, et al. Effectiveness of a lumbar belt in sub-acute low back pain: an open, multicentric, and randomized clinical study. Spine (Phila Pa 1976) 2009;34(3):215–20.

83. Oleske DM, Lavender SA, Andersson GB, et al. Are back supports plus education more effective than education alone in promoting recovery from low back pain?: Results from a randomized clinical trial. Spine (Phila Pa 1976) 2007;32(19):2050–7.

84. Haas M, Vavrek D, Peterson D, et al. Dose-response and efficacy of spinal manipulation for care of chronic low back pain: a randomized controlled trial. Spine J 2014;14(7):1106–16.

85. Hancock MJ, Maher CG, Latimer J, et al. Assessment of diclofenac or spinal manipulative therapy, or both, in addition to recommended first-line treatment

for acute low back pain: a randomised controlled trial. Lancet 2007;370(9599): 1638–43.

86. Dougherty PE, Karuza J, Dunn AS, et al. Spinal Manipulative Therapy for Chronic Lower Back Pain in Older Veterans: A Prospective, Randomized, Placebo-Controlled Trial. Geriatr Orthop Surg Rehabil 2014;5(4):154–64.

87. Lomond KV, Henry SM, Hitt JR, et al. Altered postural responses persist following physical therapy of general versus specific trunk exercises in people with low back pain. Man Ther 2014;19(5):425–32.

88. Ganesh GS, Chhabra D, Pattnaik M, et al. Effect of trunk muscles training using a star excursion balance test grid on strength, endurance and disability in persons with chronic low back pain. J Back Musculoskelet Rehabil 2015;28(3): 521–30.

89. Garcia AN, Costa Lda C, da Silva TM, et al. Effectiveness of back school versus McKenzie exercises in patients with chronic nonspecific low back pain: a randomized controlled trial. Phys Ther 2013;93(6):729–47.

90. Petersen T, Kryger P, Ekdahl C, et al. The effect of McKenzie therapy as compared with that of intensive strengthening training for the treatment of patients with subacute or chronic low back pain: A randomized controlled trial. Spine (Phila Pa 1976) 2002;27(16):1702–9.

91. Aboagye E, Karlsson ML, Hagberg J, et al. Cost-effectiveness of early interventions for non-specific low back pain: a randomized controlled study investigating medical yoga, exercise therapy and self-care advice. J Rehabil Med 2015;47(2):167–73.

92. Tilbrook HE, Cox H, Hewitt CE, et al. Yoga for chronic low back pain: a randomized trial. Ann Intern Med 2011;155(9):569–78.

93. Sang LS, Ying Eria LP. Outcome evaluation of work hardening program for manual workers with work-related back injury. Work 2005;25(4):297–305.

94. Bendix T, Bendix A, Labriola M, et al. Functional restoration versus outpatient physical training in chronic low back pain: a randomized comparative study. Spine (Phila Pa 1976) 2000;25(19):2494–500.

95. Scott Kreiner PM, Resnick Daniel, Norman Chutkan. North American Spine Society. Evidence-Based Clinical Guidelines for Multidisciplinary Spine Care: Diagnosis & Treatment of Low Back Pain. Clin Guideline 2020;217.

96. Southern D, Lutz GE, Cooper G, et al. Are fluoroscopic caudal epidural steroid injections effective for managing chronic low back pain? Pain Physician 2003; 6(2):167–72.

97. Lee JW, Shin HI, Park SY, et al. Therapeutic trial of fluoroscopic interlaminar epidural steroid injection for axial low back pain: effectiveness and outcome predictors. AJNR Am J Neuroradiol 2010;31(10):1817–23.

98. Schwarzer AC, Derby R, Aprill CN, et al. The value of the provocation response in lumbar zygapophyseal joint injections. Clin J Pain 1994;10(4):309–13.

99. Carette S, Marcoux S, Truchon R, et al. A controlled trial of corticosteroid injections into facet joints for chronic low back pain. N Engl J Med 1991;325(14): 1002–7.

100. Schulte TL, Pietilä TA, Heidenreich J, et al. Injection therapy of lumbar facet syndrome: a prospective study. Acta Neurochir (Wien) 2006;148(11):1165–72 [discussion: 1172].

101. Lakemeier S, Lind M, Schultz W, et al. A comparison of intraarticular lumbar facet joint steroid injections and lumbar facet joint radiofrequency denervation in the treatment of low back pain: a randomized, controlled, double-blind trial. Anesth Analg 2013;117(1):228–35.

102. Tekin I, Mirzai H, Ok G, et al. A comparison of conventional and pulsed radiofrequency denervation in the treatment of chronic facet joint pain. Clin J Pain 2007; 23(6):524–9.
103. Chakraverty R, Dias R. Audit of conservative management of chronic low back pain in a secondary care setting–part I: facet joint and sacroiliac joint interventions. Acupunct Med 2004;22(4):207–13.
104. Cusi M, Saunders J, Hungerford B, et al. The use of prolotherapy in the sacroiliac joint. Br J Sports Med 2010;44(2):100–4.
105. Slipman CW, Lipetz JS, Plastaras CT, et al. Fluoroscopically guided therapeutic sacroiliac joint injections for sacroiliac joint syndrome. Am J Phys Med Rehabil 2001;80(6):425–32.
106. De Andrés J, Adsuara VM, Palmisani S, et al. A double-blind, controlled, randomized trial to evaluate the efficacy of botulinum toxin for the treatment of lumbar myofascial pain in humans. Reg Anesth Pain Med 2010;35(3):255–60.
107. Vallejo R, Zevallos LM, Lowe J, et al. Is spinal cord stimulation an effective treatment option for discogenic pain? Pain Pract 2012;12(3):194–201.
108. Eck JC, Sharan A, Ghogawala Z, et al. Guideline update for the performance of fusion procedures for degenerative disease of the lumbar spine. Part 7: lumbar fusion for intractable low-back pain without stenosis or spondylolisthesis. J Neurosurg Spine 2014;21(1):42–7.
109. Fairbank J, Frost H, Wilson-MacDonald J, et al. Randomised controlled trial to compare surgical stabilisation of the lumbar spine with an intensive rehabilitation programme for patients with chronic low back pain: the MRC spine stabilisation trial. Bmj 2005;330(7502):1233.
110. Chou R, Baisden J, Carragee EJ, et al. Surgery for low back pain: a review of the evidence for an American Pain Society Clinical Practice Guideline. Spine (Phila Pa 1976) 2009;34(10):1094–109.

Neck Pain
Differential Diagnosis and Management

Marc Prablek, MD[a], Ron Gadot, BSc[a], David S. Xu, MD[b],
Alexander E. Ropper, MD[a],*

KEYWORDS

• Neck pain • Cervical myelopathy • Cervical radiculopathy • Cervical spondylosis

KEY POINTS

• Neck pain is a frequent patient complaint in the outpatient neurology setting and is commonly the result of musculoskeletal strain.
• Careful clinical history and examination are required to diagnose cervical radiculopathy or cervical myelopathy in the setting of neck pain.
• Red flag symptoms that may indicate underlying cervical spinal cord or nerve root compression include radiating arm pain, hand numbness, loss of dexterity, and gait imbalance.

INTRODUCTION

Neck pain is a common complaint across outpatient medicine, especially in primary care, neurology, and neurosurgery clinics. Recent epidemiological studies show that neck pain has a global prevalence of 3551 people and 352 years lived with disability per 100,000 people.[1] This pain can be debilitating and can negatively affect a patient's quality of life and functional status. In most cases, neck pain responds well to nonoperative treatment including physical therapy and pain medication.[2] Nevertheless, there are particular patients for whom surgery is appropriate. Determining which patients might benefit from surgical evaluation is a vital skill in the outpatient setting to avoid delays in care and to start patients on the most expedient route to recovery. This determination is largely dependent on a patient's symptoms, physical examination findings, and relevant neck imaging findings. Broadly speaking, patients with symptoms of cervical radiculopathy (CR) or cervical spondylotic myelopathy (CSM), which

---

Disclosures/Conflicts of Interest: Dr M. Prablek, Mr R. Gadot, and Dr D.S. Xu have nothing to disclose. Dr A.E. Ropper receives consulting fees from Globus Medical, Stryker, and Mizuho OSI. None of these have a bearing on this article.
[a] Department of Neurosurgery, Baylor College of Medicine, 7200 Cambridge St. Suite 9A, Houston, TX. 77030, USA; [b] Department of Neurosurgery, Ohio State College of Medicine, 370 W. 9th Avenue, Columbus, OH 43210, USA
* Corresponding author.
E-mail address: Alexander.Ropper@bcm.edu

can be attributed to a structural cause for these pathologies on imaging, would likely benefit most from surgery or more urgent intervention. Therefore, the clinical encounter in patients with neck pain should focus on ruling these disorders in or out. A summary of important syndromes with neck pain that may be amenable to surgical treatment is provided in **Table 1**.

Muscle strain is likely the most common cause of neck pain. This is usually self-resolving and can be treated with home exercise, physical therapy, and nonsteroidal anti-inflammatories. Much of the diagnostic encounter for patients with neck pain tends to focus on inquiring about red flag symptoms and examining for concerning clinical signs. Although cervical nerve root or spinal cord compression may not themselves result in neck pain, the cause of the diseases, degenerated facets and cervical intervertebral discs, may result in neck pain. Clinicians generally focus on ensuring the lack of these red flag symptoms and signs to be able to reassure patients about the self-resolving nature of neck pain, and safe recommendations of conservative care.

DIAGNOSTIC WORKUP

A thorough history and physical examination are critical in making the proper diagnosis of patients with neck pain. Important historical factors in the evaluation of cervicalgia, CR, or cervical myelopathy include a history of trauma, neurologic injury, infection, or malignancy. Patients with recent trauma may present with muscle strain; however, failure of this to resolve may necessitate the need for imaging to ensure there is no fracture or spondylolisthesis. Patients with infection may present with neck pain due to discitis or osteomyelitis. This type of mechanical neck pain with movement can sometimes be differentiated from the classic signs of meningitis. Furthermore, patients with CR classically report a lancinating, electrical pain that radiates from the neck into specific dermatomal distributions. Patients with CSM may report difficulty with gait, hand dexterity, or with bowel or bladder incontinence. The presence of any of these factors in a patient's history might suggest a need for further imaging to assess compression of the spinal cord or cervical nerve roots. In rare cases, vascular pathology, such as arterial dissection, or other compressive pathologies, such as thoracic outlet syndrome, may be included in the differential diagnosis.

It is important to assess for any weakness, especially in the upper extremity myotomes. Traditionally, the C5 myotome involves the deltoid and shoulder flexion, the C6 myotome involves the bicep and arm flexion, the C7 myotome involves the triceps and arm and wrist extension, and the C8 and T1 myotomes involve the intrinsic muscles of the hand. Diminished reflexes in the triceps and biceps may also suggest a cervical root compression. Any weakness in these myotomes, especially with corresponding dermatomal pain, suggests a severe CR and may warrant further imaging and/or surgical referral. In CSM, patients may or may not have dermatomal/myotomal distribution of symptoms, but patients with advanced disease frequently exhibit hyperreflexia and/or ankle clonus. These patients may also report diminished sensation in the hands. Many patients with CR and CSM do not report neck pain.

MRI is the generally preferred method for identifying surgical pathology of the neck. MRI provides excellent visualization of the spinal cord and nerve roots, as well as the vertebrae, intervertebral discs, and spinal ligaments. Although computed tomography (CT) does provide excellent visualization of bony elements and has a role in surgical planning, it is inferior to MRI in visualizing the important soft tissue and neural structures of the spine. Contrasted imaging of the spine (whether CT or MRI) is of limited benefit unless there is suspicion for malignancy or abscess as the etiology of symptoms. In

Table 1
Summary of neck pain and associated syndromes

Condition	Typical Symptoms	Physical Examination Findings	Imaging Findings	Initial Treatment Modality	When to Seek Surgical Treatment
Axial neck pain (cervicalgia)	Midline pain, pain with movement of neck	No neurologic deficits	Variable, frequently without structural pathology	Physical therapy, exercise, massage	Limited cases that do not respond to conservative management
Cervical radiculopathy	Pain radiating from neck to shoulder or arms	Dermatomal pain, numbness, or weakness, Spurling sign	Compression of affected nerve root	Physical therapy, exercise, massage, traction	Neurologic deficit or no response to conservative management
Cervical myelopathy	Pain, hand numbness, gait disturbance, fine motor skill loss	Hand grip weakness, hyperreflexia, gait instability	Focal or multilevel cervical spinal cord compression	Certain symptoms may respond to physical therapy, generally requires surgical evaluation	Patients with symptoms of myelopathy and spinal cord compression on imaging

patients who cannot undergo MRI, CT myelography, in which contrast is infused into the intrathecal space via lumbar puncture, is the imaging modality of choice.

Degenerative findings on MRI are very common even in the absence of symptoms.[2] The challenge for clinicians is to correlate the patient's symptoms with any reported imaging findings. Even in patients with clear symptoms of radiculopathy, MRI findings may suggest compression at a different nerve root level or not at all.[3] Worrisome MRI features such as severe spinal cord edema, presence of tumor, or syringomyelia may prompt more urgent surgical referral.

Electromyography (EMG) and nerve conduction studies (NCS) can also be helpful in correlating imaging findings and symptoms to a single nerve root level, which may aid in diagnosis. If severe radiculopathy is present, Wallerian degeneration can occur leading to spontaneous muscle fiber firing, which can be detected by EMG in the form of fibrillation potentials and positive sharp waves. EMG/NCS can also identify peripheral nerve syndromes such as carpal or cubital tunnel syndrome, which may masquerade as CR. In addition, selective nerve root block can also be used as a diagnostic tool.[4] If a patient exhibits relief of symptoms following a particular nerve root block, it may be implicated as the cause of the patient's symptoms.

CERVICAL RADICULOPATHY

CR is a common syndrome in adults and is generally characterized by lancinating radiating pain from the neck to the shoulder or upper extremities.[5] When severe, radiculopathy can be accompanied by weakness in the myotome corresponding to the affected nerve root. Clinical examination remains the mainstay of diagnosis, and imaging findings alone are an insufficient justification for surgery in most cases. Musculoskeletal shoulder pain or postural pain can mimic high CR, and disorders of peripheral nerves, such as carpal tunnel and cubital tunnel can mimic lower nerve root pathology as well.

Typically, pain produced by compression of a cervical nerve root will be temporarily relieved by gentle traction of the cervical spine.[2] This temporarily expands the cervical neural foramina and can provide some relief throughout the duration of the maneuver. Another useful maneuver that functions via a similar mechanism is the shoulder abduction maneuver,[2] in which the patient places his or her hand ipsilateral to the pain behind their head, which may help relieve pain. In addition, downward pressure on the head while turned toward the side of the pain may provoke the pain (Spurling sign).[2] The presence of any of these signs may point toward a radicular etiology of pain rather than a musculoskeletal one. As previously mentioned, EMG and NCS may be helpful in situations in which the etiology of neck and arm pain may be unclear. These studies may also help distinguish between cervical radicular dysfunction and peripheral nerve entrapment syndromes, (e.g., carpal and cubital tunnel syndromes).

In addition, most CR can be managed conservatively. Physical therapy is frequently helpful in alleviating the symptoms of pain and can also aid in functional recovery.[6–9] Patients failing physical therapy may also be candidates for interventional pain treatments such as nerve blocks or epidural steroid injections. Surgery may be indicated for patients who have failed nonoperative management measures, or patients with focal weakness that might be relieved by alleviating cervical nerve root compression.

Surgical options for the treatment of CR are well-described and effective in properly selected patients. Broadly speaking, these options can be divided into anterior approaches and posterior approaches. Anterior approaches are commonly used when a cervical nerve root is compressed by an intervertebral disc or osteophyte associated with the vertebral body. These approaches include anterior foraminotomy, anterior cervical discectomy with fusion (ACDF), and cervical disc arthroplasty (cervical total disc replacement), among others. Each of these approaches seeks to remove the offending disc fragment or osteophyte causing nerve root compression. They take advantage of well-defined deep investing fascial planes between the sternocleido-mastoid, carotid sheath, and the strap muscles to approach the spine while avoiding major structures of the neck, including the esophagus, trachea, internal jugular vein, carotid artery, and vagus nerve. Following decompression of the disc or osteophyte through this anterior approach, hardware may be placed: an artificial disc in the case of disc arthroplasty, and a disc spacer with a plate and screws in the case of ACDF. Some studies report that cervical disc arthroplasty may be more cost-effective than ACDF based on long-term outcomes; however, further study is required to adequately draw conclusions across an increasingly heterogeneous patient population with cervical degenerative disc disease.[10] Anterior approaches tend to be well-tolerated by patients with relatively little postsurgical pain, as muscles are not transgressed. Nevertheless, patients do frequently complain of dysphagia and sometimes dysphonia following surgery, which are typically self-limited.[11] Rarer complications include injury to the esophagus, trachea, recurrent laryngeal nerve, or postoperative hematoma.

Posterior approaches for cervical nerve root decompression are also commonly performed and are especially useful to address issues such as hypertrophy of facet joints or ligamentum flavum, which might be causing nerve root compression. Most commonly, compression of a single nerve root will be addressed posteriorly with a for-aminotomy. Typically, a midline incision is made at the level of pathology, and the posterior cervical musculature is dissected away from the spinous process and lamina. A laminotomy is then made and medial facetectomy performed to decompress the posterior aspect of the neural foramen. Minimally invasive approaches also can be used, in which an incision is made directly over the facet joint and tubular retractors are used to provide a corridor through the cervical musculature directly to the lateral lamina and facet joint. Although manipulation and dissection of the posterior cervical musculature generally provokes more postoperative pain than in anterior approaches, these operations are generally well-tolerated without prolonged hospital stays.

Overall, there is significant equipoise between surgical options for CR, as all options provide similar pain benefit to patients.[12-14] The selection of approach is largely individualized to the patient's particular pathology, as well as surgeon preference.

CERVICAL MYELOPATHY

CSM is a relatively common and important spinal pathology that is frequently managed with surgery. Typical symptoms include neck pain, gait disturbance, hand numbness, and difficulty with fine motor coordination, such as buttoning buttons or tying shoelaces.[2,15-17] Physical examination may reveal upper extremity weakness, hand numbness, and diffuse hyperreflexia, as well as the presence of pathologic reflexes such as Babinski or Hoffman. Gait examination may reveal wide-based, unsteady gait with positive Romberg sign.

Imaging typically reveals compression of the spinal cord in the cervical spine. Cases of severe or longstanding pathology may demonstrate T2 signal change within the spinal cord or syringomyelia on MRI. Although some cases of CSM are due to focal compression or pathology, frequently CSM is caused by multilevel pathology in the cervical spine and may be accompanied by cervical deformity. Imaging is helpful in distinguishing extrinsic myelopathy as seen with CSM from intrinsic myelopathies, such as those caused by inflammatory diseases or intramedullary spinal cord tumors.

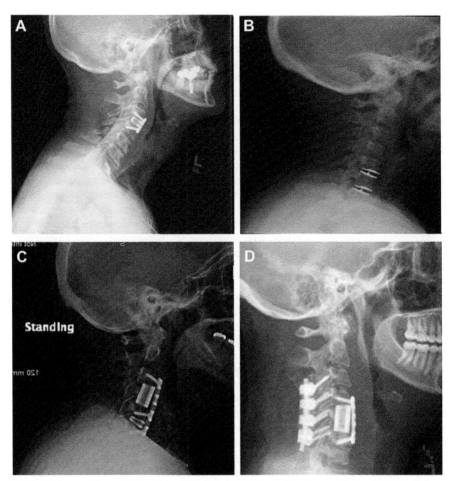

Fig. 1. Postoperative radiographs of the cervical spine following cervical spine decompressions and reconstructions. (*A*) Postoperative lateral radiograph following an anterior cervical discectomy and plating (ACDF) at C3-4. A small titanium spacer is used to reconstruct the disc space followed by placement of a small plate and screws to fixate the construct. (*B*) Postoperative lateral radiograph following placement of cervical arthroplasty (total disc replacement) devices at C5-6 and C6-7. Standard anterior discectomies were performed at these levels to decompress the spinal cord and nerve roots in a patient with multilevel radiculopathies from disc herniations. This was followed by placement of the artificial discs, which allow normal physiologic motion of the cervical spine following surgery. (*C*) Postoperative radiograph of a patient who had a large extruded C3-4 disc herniation that migrated behind the C4 vertebral body as well as central C5-6 disc herniation resulting in cervical spondylotic myelopathy. Anterior decompression and reconstruction were accomplished with a C4 corpectomy and C5-6 ACDF with anterior fixation from C3-6. (*D*) Postoperative radiograph of a patient with severe myelopathy from both ventral and dorsal spinal cord compression. The patient was treated with a C5 corpectomy for anterior decompression and a posterior decompression with a laminectomy and instrumented fusion from C3-6. The posterior lateral mass screws and rods are seen spanning from C3-6 posteriorly.

Patients with signs, symptoms, physical examination, and imaging findings consistent with CSM should prompt surgical referral, as they rarely improve without surgical decompression. In contrast with CR, the threshold for surgical intervention is lower in symptomatic patients with imaging findings of CSM. Patients who decline surgery or cannot tolerate surgery may benefit from occupational therapy or physical therapy for gait training and hand function, but generally the natural history of CSM is progressive. It should be noted that even with timely surgical decompression, patients with severe chronic spinal cord damage may not recover significant neurologic function postoperatively, and the goal of surgery rather is to halt further decline. Patients must be counseled appropriately to endure adequate understanding of the goals of surgery and to have grounded expectations of postoperative function.

As with CR, CSM may be addressed surgically via an anterior approach or posterior approach, and some patients may require multiple approaches. The technical goal of the operation is to achieve central decompression of the cervical spinal cord. Anterior approaches to treat CSM are generally similar to those used for radiculopathy, but the presence of multilevel pathology may favor multilevel ACDF or arthroplasty depending on the patient's particular pathology. Multi- and single-level anterior approaches are still well-tolerated and have similar complication profiles.[18] In cases in which there is ventral spinal cord compression beyond the level of disc space, a complete vertebral corpectomy may be required followed by anterior spinal column reconstruction.

Posterior approaches for multilevel cervical pathology generally involve multilevel laminectomies, with or without fusion. Fusion is generally accomplished with bilateral rod and screw constructs around which new bone growth occurs, converting the segmented mobile spine into a solid, fused unit (**Fig. 1**). This is typically performed to prevent post-laminectomy kyphotic deformities, which can be very debilitating and difficult to treat; nevertheless, large studies have shown similar pain and functional outcomes for patients with or without fusion.[19] Laminoplasty, where the cervical lamina are hinged open and secured to the lateral masses, accomplishes canal decompression but retains segmental motion. These posterior surgeries typically result in significant postoperative pain from larger-scale dissection of the posterior cervical musculature, as well as musculoskeletal discomfort associated with a newly nonmobile spine.[20] Generally, multilevel anterior and posterior cervical surgeries both achieve the goal of spinal cord decompression, but have different complication profiles that may be tailored according to the patient's needs.[21]

Combined approaches using both anterior and posterior instrumentation techniques are generally reserved for more severe cases of CSM or patients with compression as a result of cervical deformity. The ability to reconstruct both the anterior and posterior elements of the spine can be a powerful tool in restoring the normal cervical lordosis and centering the weight of the head over the middle of the shoulders. This, coupled with decompression of the spinal cord, makes a combined approach an attractive surgical option for select patients.

SUMMARY

Axial neck pain is a common and important problem in the outpatient setting. In isolation, neck pain tends to have a musculoskeletal etiology and responds best to medication and targeted physical therapy. Careful history and physical examination are required to ascertain if there is a neurologic component in addition to the patient's neck pain. In particular, CR and CSM are conditions that commonly present with neck pain that might benefit from surgical evaluation and treatment in select patients. Patients with acute neurologic decline warrant urgent evaluation and may even necessitate transfer to an emergent care center. For patients needing surgical intervention, there are a variety of approaches and operations that can decompress the appropriate nerve root or the spinal cord itself. These operations are generally well-tolerated and provide significant benefit for appropriately selected patients.

CLINICS CARE POINTS

- Neck pain is most commonly the result of musculoskeletal strain.
- Most cases of cervical radiculaopthy will improve or resolve with non-surgical measures.
- The natural history of cervical spondylotic myelopathy is slowly progressive.

REFERENCES

1. Safiri S, Kolahi A-A, Hoy D, et al. Global, regional, and national burden of neck pain in the general population, 1990-2017: systematic analysis of the Global Burden of Disease Study. BMJ 2017;2020:m791.
2. Theodore N. Degenerative cervical spondylosis. New Engl J Med 2020;383(2): 159–68.
3. Redebrandt HN, Brandt C, Hawran S, et al. Clinical evaluation versus magnetic resonance imaging findings in patients with radicular arm pain—a pragmatic study. Health Sci Rep 2022;5(3):1–10.
4. Yang D, Xu L, Hu Y, et al. Diagnosis and treatment of cervical spondylotic radiculopathy using selective nerve root block (SNRB): where are we now? Pain Ther 2022;11(2):341–57.
5. Luyao H, Xiaoxiao Y, Tianxiao F, et al. Management of cervical spondylotic radiculopathy: a systematic review. Glob Spine J 2022. 219256822210752.
6. Mańko G, Jekiełek M, Ambroży T, et al. Physiotherapeutic methods in the treatment of cervical discopathy and degenerative cervical myelopathy: a prospective study. Life 2022;12(4):513.
7. Alshami AM, Bamhair DA. Effect of manual therapy with exercise in patients with chronic cervical radiculopathy: a randomized clinical trial. Trials 2021; 22(716):1–12.
8. Senol D, Kizilay F, Toy S, et al. Evaluation of visual and auditory reaction time, pain, and hand grip strength performance before and after conventional physiotherapy in patients with herniated cervical intervertebral disc with radiculopathy. North Clin Istanb 2021;8(6):581–7.
9. Thoomes E, Thoomes-de Graaf M, Cleland JA, et al. Timing of evidence-based nonsurgical interventions as part of multimodal treatment guidelines for the management of cervical radiculopathy: a Delphi study. Phys Ther 2022;102(5):1–9.
10. Schuermans VNE, Smeets AYJM, Boselie AFM, et al. Cost-effectiveness of anterior surgical decompression surgery for cervical degenerative disk disease: a systematic review of economic evaluations. Eur Spine J 2022;31(5):1206–18.
11. Yi Y-Y, Chen H, Xu H-W, et al. Changes in intervertebral distraction: a possible factor for predicting dysphagia after anterior cervical spinal surgery. J Clin Neurosci 2022;100:82–8.
12. Padhye K, Shultz P, Alcala C, et al. Surgical treatment of single level cervical radiculopathy: a comparison of anterior cervical decompression and fusion (ACDF) versus cervical disk arthroplasty (CDA) versus posterior cervical foraminotomy (PCF). Clin Spine Surg 2022;35(4):149–54.

13. Divi SN, Goyal DKC, Woods BI, et al. How do patients with predominant neck pain improve after anterior cervical discectomy and fusion for cervical radiculopathy? Int J Spine Surg 2022;16(2):240–6.
14. Shahi P, Vaishnav AS, Lee R, et al. Outcomes of cervical disc replacement in patients with neck pain greater than arm pain. Spine J 2022;22(9):1481–9.
15. Inose H, Hirai T, Yoshii T, et al. Factors contributing to neck pain in patients with degenerative cervical myelopathy: a prospective multicenter study. J Orthop Surg 2022;30(1). 102255362210918.
16. Chen S, Wang Y, Wu X, et al. Degeneration of the sensorimotor tract in degenerative cervical myelopathy and compensatory structural changes in the brain. Front Aging Neurosci 2022;14:784263.
17. Choy WJ, Chen L, Quel De Oliveira C, et al. Gait assessment tools for degenerative cervical myelopathy: a systematic review. J Spine Surg 2022;8(1):149–62.
18. Luo C-A, Lim AS, Lu M-L, et al. The surgical outcome of multilevel anterior cervical discectomy and fusion in myelopathic elderly and younger patients. Scientific Rep 2022;12(4495):1–9.
19. Revesz DF, Charalampidis A, Gerdhem P. Effectiveness of laminectomy with fusion and laminectomy alone in degenerative cervical myelopathy. Eur Spine J 2022;31(5):1300–8.
20. Nunna RS, Khalid S, Chiu RG, et al. Anterior vs posterior approach in multilevel cervical spondylotic myelopathy: a nationwide propensity-matched analysis of complications, outcomes, and narcotic use. Int J Spine Surg 2022;16(1):88–94.
21. Joo PY, Jayaram RH, McLaughlin WM, et al. Four-level anterior versus posterior cervical fusions: perioperative outcomes and five-year reoperation rates. North Am Spine Soc J (NASSJ) 2022;10:100115.

Immunopathogenesis, Diagnosis, and Treatment of Multiple Sclerosis: A Clinical Update

Carlos A. Pérez, MD*, Fernando X. Cuascut, MD, MPH,
George J. Hutton, MD

KEYWORDS

- Multiple sclerosis • Central nervous system • Demyelination • Diagnosis
- Treatment

KEY POINTS

- Multiple sclerosis (MS) is the most common acquired demyelinating disorder of the central nervous system with various phenotypic presentations and patterns of disease expression.
- The multidimensional construct of phenotypic differences in clinical expression and long-term outcomes across racial groups can be explained by a complex interaction between social, environmental, and genetic factors.
- Recent advances in basic immunology have contributed to an improved understanding of the fundamental principles of MS immunopathogenesis.
- New approaches to MS therapy and goals of care are driven by the rapidly evolving treatment armamentarium and expanding knowledge of disease pathophysiology.

INTRODUCTION

The clinical and phenotypic spectrum of the immune-mediated central nervous system (CNS) demyelinating disorders is broad.[1] Multiple sclerosis (MS) is the most common inflammatory disorder of the CNS and serves as a prototype to inform the diagnosis and treatment of related demyelinating disorders.[2] Although certain clinical features are characteristic of MS, its phenotypic manifestations are highly variable.[3,4] Despite the rapid evolution of the therapeutic landscape, treatment options for the progressive disease are currently limited.[5,6] This review discusses the diagnostic approach, clinical features, and treatment approaches in MS, emphasizing current understanding of immunopathogenesis, recent advances, and future directions.

Department of Neurology, Maxine Mesinger Multiple Sclerosis Comprehensive Care Center, 7200 Cambridge Street, Suite 9A, Houston, TX, USA
* Corresponding author.
E-mail address: Carlos.Perez@bcm.edu

Neurol Clin 41 (2023) 87–106
https://doi.org/10.1016/j.ncl.2022.05.004
0733-8619/23/© 2022 Elsevier Inc. All rights reserved.
neurologic.theclinics.com

BACKGROUND

MS is a chronic neurodegenerative disease with a complex etiopathogenesis characterized by CNS inflammation and demyelination.[1,2] It typically presents in young adults aged 20 to 30 years with unilateral optic neuritis, transverse myelitis, sensory disturbances, or brainstem syndromes developing over several days.[7] It more commonly affects women (female-to-male sex ratio of approximately 3:1).[8] Its overall worldwide prevalence ranges from 5 to 300 per 100,000 people and increases at higher latitudes.[9,10] In a recent study, an estimated one million adults lived with MS in the United States in 2017.[11]

The diagnosis is made based on a combination of signs and symptoms, radiographic findings (eg, MRI T2 lesions), and laboratory findings (eg, cerebrospinal fluid [CSF]–specific oligoclonal bands), which are components of the 2017 McDonald diagnostic criteria[12] (**Table 1**). Specific MRI requirements for the spatial and temporal dissemination of demyelinating plaques in time and space are also defined (**Box 1**). Integrating the clinical history, neurologic examination, brain, and spinal cord MRI findings and laboratory evidence to rule out other conditions remains fundamental in making a reliable diagnosis of MS or an alternative diagnosis.[3] Several studies have suggested that a poor prognosis is related to several risk factors, including male gender, late age of onset; motor, cerebellar, and sphincter involvement at onset; a progressive course at onset, shorter interattack intervals, a high number of early attacks, and early residual disability.[13–15]

PATHOPHYSIOLOGY

A combination of genetic, epigenetic, and environmental factors contributes to the overall risk of developing MS in susceptible individuals.[16] Among the latter, the Epstein-Barr virus (EBV) is a putative culprit.[17] Most people infected with this common virus do not develop MS. Yet, a recent study using data from millions of US military recruits monitored during 20 years determined that EBV infection preceded the development of disease and significantly increased the risk of developing MS.[18] These observations support a causal role of EBV infection in MS etiopathogenesis. Although mechanisms such as molecular mimicry between viral proteins and CNS antigens could represent a mechanistic basis in at least a subset of patients, the possible role of EBV as an active driver of disease progression[18,19] suggests that targeted elimination of EBV-infected cells without suppressing the broader immune system could represent a potential therapeutic target in MS.

Similarly, intestinal commensal microbiota may serve as potential environmental factors implicated in MS pathogenesis. Initial studies of intestinal microbiome have identified multisystem alterations in the gut microbiota of MS patients compared with healthy controls, providing evidence of reduced diversity in the normal flora of patients with active MS.[9,16,20–22] Additionally, a recent study addressed the differential gut microbiota profile in patients with primary progressive multiple sclerosis (PPMS) relative to controls.[23] Recently, several oral disease-modifying treatments (DMTs) were shown to inhibit the growth of *Clostridium* in vitro.[24] This feature has been proposed to contribute to overall anti-inflammatory mechanism of action of these drugs, including treatment efficacy and response, suggesting that gut microbiota modulation may be a promising interventional approach to MS therapy.

RACIAL AND ETHNIC DISPARITIES

The incidence, prevalence, and severity of MS differ by race and ethnicity. There is burgeoning evidence that Hispanics and African Americans with MS present at a

Table 1
2017 McDonald criteria for diagnosis of multiple sclerosis

Clinical Presentation	Additional Data Needed for a Diagnosis of MS
Two or more attacks and objective clinical evidence of 2 ore more lesions Two or more attacks and objective clinical evidence of 1 lesion with historical evidence of prior attack involving a lesion in a different location	None. Dissemination in space (DIS) and dissemination in time (DIT) criteria have been met
Two or more attacks and objective clinical evidence of 1 lesion	One of these criteria: • DIS: additional clinical attack implicating different CNS site. • DIS: ≥1 symptomatic or asymptomatic MS-typical T2 lesions in 2 or more areas of the CNS: periventricular, cortical/juxtacortical, infratentorial or spinal cord
1 attack and objective clinical evidence of 2 or more lesions	One of these criteria: • DIT: additional clinical attack • DIT: simultaneous presence of both enhancing and nonenhancing symptomatic or asymptomatic MRI-typical MRI lesions • DIT: new T2 or enhancing MRI lesion compared with baseline lesion scan (without regard to timing of baseline scan) • Cerebrospinal fluid-specific oligoclonal bands (not present in serum)
1 attack and objective clinical evidence of 1 lesion	One of these criteria: • DIS: additional clinical attack implicating different CNS site • DIS: ≥1 symptomatic or asymptomatic MS-typical T2 lesions in 2 or more areas of the CNS: periventricular, cortical/juxtacortical, infratentorial, or spinal cord AND one of these criteria: • DIT: additional clinical attack • DIT: simultaneous presence of both enhancing and nonenhancing symptomatic or asymptomatic MRI-typical MRI lesions • DIT: new T2 or enhancing MRI lesion compared with baseline lesion scan (without regard to timing of baseline scan)

Abbreviation: CNS, central nervous system.

younger age and demonstrate faster disability accumulation compared with their Caucasian counterparts of European ancestry.[25-27] This multidimensional construct of phenotypic differences and patterns of disease expression across racial and ethnic groups can be explained by a complex interaction between socioeconomic, environmental, and genetic factors.[28,29]

Epidemiologic data in MS suggest that socioeconomic disparities and barriers to health-care access may account, at least in part, for the differences in clinical outcomes across racial groups.[25,30] However, data from small matched cohort studies

---

Box 1
2017 McDonald criteria definitions for demonstration of dissemination in space and time

Dissemination in space
- One or more T2-hyperintense lesion(s) in 2 or more areas of the CNS: periventricular, cortical or juxtacortical, infratentorial, and spinal cord.

Dissemination in time
- Simultaneous presence of gadolinium-enhancing and nonenhancing lesions at any time or by a new T2-hyperintense or gadolinium-enhancing lesion on follow-up MRI, irrespective of the timing of the baseline MRI.
  OR
- Presence of CSF oligoclonal bands.

Abbreviations: CNS, central nervous system; CSF, cerebrospinal fluid.

---

have shown that differences in MS outcome can persist despite a lack of significant socioeconomic disparities or patterns of DMT use between racial groups.[26,31] Additionally, significant cross-sectional differences in baseline regional MRI volume measures and MRI-based volumetric correlates of MS-related disability among racial groups have been reported.[26,32] These observations raise important questions regarding the complex interaction between genetic predisposition and environmental factors in determining long-term prognosis across racial and ethnic MS groups.[33]

Despite recent advances in DMT options, clinically significant health disparities remain between racial/ethnic groups. There is growing concern about a differential response to DMTs among minority groups.[29,31,33–35] Nevertheless, minority population enrollment in phase 3 studies has remained less than 10% since the 1990s,[36–40] which limits the generalizability of evidence-based approaches to therapy. In addition, MS-specific mortality trends demonstrate distinctive disparities by race/ethnicity and age, suggesting an unequal burden of disease, which creates an unmet need to identify tailored, multifaceted approaches to therapy selection, and access to care in MS.

CLINICAL FEATURES

Most commonly, the pattern and clinical course of MS is categorized into several phenotypic subtypes. The overall disease course in relapsing-remitting multiple sclerosis (RRMS) is characterized by an asymptomatic, preclinical phase (radiologically isolated syndrome [RIS]), a subclinical, clinical phase (clinically isolated syndrome [CIS]), RRMS, and a progressive phase (secondary progressive multiple sclerosis [SPMS]).[1] PPMS is the least common clinical MS phenotype characterized by progressive neurologic deterioration and disability accumulation from the onset of symptoms without any relapses, plateaus, or temporary improvements.[41]

Relapsing-Remitting Phase

Approximately 60% to 70% of patients with a first clinical episode do not fulfill 2017 McDonald diagnostic criteria for MS.[42] A *CIS* is defined as the first episode of acute or subacute onset of neurological symptoms caused by inflammatory demyelination, lasting more than 24 hours and occurring in the absence of fever, infection, or encephalopathy.[16] Up to one-third of CIS patients experience a monophasic illness with no further clinical or subclinical demyelinating activity.[43] If a patient has a normal brain MRI, the risk of future development of MS is reduced to about 10% to 30%.[43] However, approximately 80% of subjects with CIS experience a second clinical demyelinating event and are diagnosed with clinically definite MS within 20 years.[44]

RRMS is defined as the presence of clinically distinct neurological events affecting different parts of the CNS separated in time (arbitrarily defined as at least one month apart) and in space.[45,46] Current diagnostic criteria are based on this core rule.[47] Between attacks, the symptoms may disappear altogether but permanent neurologic deficits often remain as the disease advances.[48] Moreover, one must see typical lesions in location, orientation, and shape on MRI. Other diagnostic possibilities should be entertained in the absence of these typical lesions.

Progressive Phase

The progressive phase of MS is established after 1 year of clinical progression.[47] During this phase, patients can continue to have active disease with symptomatic relapses or asymptomatic MRI activity.[49] This phase is classified into subgroups based on the presence or absence of preceding clinical relapses. *SPMS* refers to relapsing-remitting MS followed by the progressive phase.[47,49] *PPMS* is characterized by disease progression from the onset in the absence of symptomatic relapses.[47] Of note, the differences between the progressive MS subtypes do not seem to be because of different progression mechanisms but rather due to subclinical disease activity in some individuals.[50]

Radiologically Isolated Syndrome

The term *RIS* refers to the incidental detection of radiological findings highly suggestive of MS in the absence of clinical signs and symptoms of CNS demyelination.[51,52] Risk factors for a first clinical event include age (<37 years), sex (male), the presence of spinal cord lesions, high cerebral lesion load, gadolinium-enhancing lesions, positive CSF oligoclonal bands, and abnormal visual evoked potentials.[47,53,54] In a retrospective study of 451 patients with RIS, clinical events were identified in 34% of subjects within 5 years from their initial brain MRI. Of those who developed symptoms, 9.6% fulfilled criteria for PPMS. Additional follow-up data in 277 of the initial 451 patients showed that the cumulative probability of a first clinical event at 10 years was 51.2%, suggesting that approximately half of all individuals with RIS experienced a first clinical event within 10 years of the index MRI. Active monitoring of RIS patients with periodic clinical and radiological follow-up every 6 to 12 months is recommended.[51,55]

Multiple Sclerosis Phenotypes as a Continuum

As our understanding of MS expands in light of new insights into clinical relapse rate and imaging data, the concept of MS phenotypes as a continuum, rather than discreet phenotypic subtypes, has been proposed (**Fig. 1**).[50] This concept is primarily based on the premise that the lack of genetic, pathologic, and immunologic evidence does not justify the stratification of relapsing-remitting and progressive forms as 2 separate entities. It argues that MS progresses along a continuum from relapsing to progressive forms, with differing levels of neurologic reserve accounting for known clinical and phenotypic differences.[50] In addition, it provides the scientific rationale for early intervention with highly effective DMTs and promotes adaptation of healthy lifestyles to build a neurologic reserve and improve neurologic function over time.

DIAGNOSTIC EVALUATION

A diagnosis of MS is made through a combination of clinical history, neurologic examination, MRI, and exclusion of other diagnostic possibilities.[56,57] Ancillary tests, such as CSF studies, evoked potentials, and ocular coherence tomography, may be helpful but are not always necessary.[12]

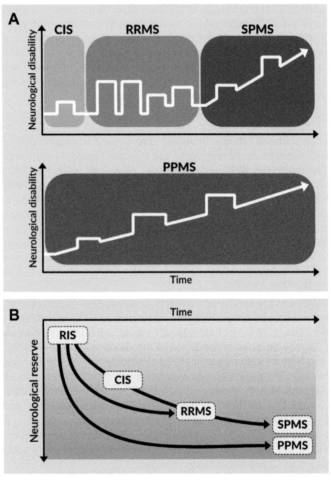

Fig. 1. Multiple sclerosis classifications. (*A*) As phenotypes primarily determined by neurologic disability, and (*B*) as a continuum primarily driven by loss of neurologic reserve. CIS, clinically isolated syndrome; PPMS, primary progressive multiple sclerosis; RIS, radiologically isolated syndrome; RRMS, relapsing-remitting multiple sclerosis; SPMS, secondary progressive multiple sclerosis. (*From* Vollmer TL, Nair K V., Williams IM, et al. Multiple Sclerosis Phenotypes as a Continuum. Neurol Clin Pract 2021; 11: 342–351; with permission.)

Neuroimaging

MRI has become an integral part of the diagnostic process owing to its ability to sensitively and noninvasively demonstrate the spatial and temporal dissemination of demyelinating plaques in the brain and spinal cord.[58] In addition to its fundamental diagnostic role, MRI is used for prognostic evaluations and to monitor subclinical disease activity and DMT effects.[59]

Ancillary Tests

In a change from previous revisions, the 2017 McDonald criteria recommend that demonstration of 2 or more CSF oligoclonal bands may substitute for the demonstration of clinical or MRI dissemination in time.[47] This notable revision enables earlier diagnosis of MS in a patient with objective evidence of a single clinical attack typical for MS with an MRI that only demonstrates dissemination in space.

Multiple Sclerosis Mimics

Antibody testing for aquaporin 4 (AQP4) and myelin oligodendrocyte glycoprotein (MOG) antibodies is usually performed to exclude similar demyelinating conditions, often with overlapping clinical and radiographic features.[60] Autoimmune encephalitis and paraneoplastic antibody panels also may be helpful, especially when a patient presents with encephalopathy or has a known history of malignancy.[61] Visual-evoked potentials (VEPs), brainstem auditory, evoked potentials, and somatosensory potentials may be helpful to provide objective evidence of past injury, particularly when a diagnosis of MS cannot be established based on current diagnostic criteria.[16,62]

OTHER CENTRAL NERVOUS SYSTEM DEMYELINATING DISEASES
Neuromyelitis Optica Spectrum Disorder

Neuromyelitis optica spectrum disorder (NMOSD) is a relapsing, demyelinating CNS disorder with 6 core clinical characteristics: optic neuritis, myelitis, area postrema syndrome, acute brainstem syndrome, diencephalic syndrome, and cerebral syndrome.[63] The presence of anti-AQP4 antibodies is highly specific for NMOSD.[64] The AQP4 protein, which is highly expressed within astrocyte foot processes, is critical for the formation and overall integrity of the blood–brain barrier (BBB).[65] Binding of anti-AQP4 antibodies leads to astrocytic dysfunction and a series of inflammatory cascades that promote demyelination and necrosis.[66] Excluding NMOSD as a potential MS mimic is essential given its distinct pathogenesis. In addition, individuals with NMOSD may worsen when treated with some MS therapies, including interferon-beta, natalizumab, and fingolimod.[67] Unlike MS, NMOSD typically presents with longitudinally extensive transverse myelitis when there is spinal cord involvement.[64] An estimated 10% to 30% of patients with NMOSD can be AQP4 antibody-negative.[65] Among them, approximately half are MOG-IgG seropositive.[68] **Fig. 2** illustrates an exemplary MRI scan that shows a typical demyelinating lesion with involvement of the area postrema.

Myelin Oligodendrocyte Glycoprotein-Associated Disease

More recently, antibodies against the MOG were found in NMOSD patients who tested negative for the AQP4 antibody. Myelin oligodendrocyte glycoprotein-associated disease (MOGAD) is an inflammatory, immune-mediated demyelinating disorder of the CNS.[69] MOG is a protein expressed on the outer myelin membrane of oligodendrocytes, and MOG antibodies are increasingly identified in patients with an acute demyelinating syndrome.[70] The clinical phenotype associated with the presence of MOG antibodies ranges from acute disseminated encephalomyelitis (ADEM)-like presentations in children to a more optico-spinal presentation in adults.[71] Approximately 50% of patients with MOG antibodies follow a relapsing course, with relapses typically occurring within a few months or up to 10 years or more after the initial attack.[69] Usually, the prognosis is satisfactory, with either complete or partial recovery after immunotherapy.[71]

Acute Disseminated Encephalomyelitis

ADEM is a monophasic, immune-mediated demyelinating CNS disorder that typically follows a febrile infection or vaccination.[72] Although it is commonly recognized in

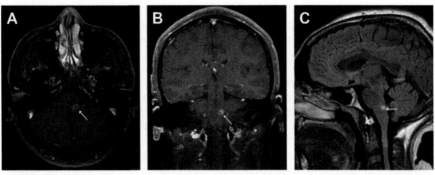

Fig. 2. Postgadolinium axial (*A*) and coronal (*B*) T1-weighted, and sagittal T2-weighted (*C*) images showing a 7 mm peripherally enhancing lesion in the left dorsal medulla with involvement of the area postrema in a patient with neuromyelitis optica spectrum disorder (yellow arrow).

children, it can also occur in adults, typically between the age of 30 and 50 years, and with equal gender preponderance.[73] Acute symptom progression is generally rapid.[72] In childhood ADEM, long-lasting fever, and headaches occur more frequently but motor and sensory deficits predominate in adults.[72] Radiologically, ADEM presents as large, poorly demarcated T2 hyperintense white matter lesions that may affect both hemispheres and often involve the thalamus and the basal ganglia.[73] Typically, ADEM is a monophasic event with no new disease activity after 3 months of disease onset. However, multiphasic ADEM does occur and is defined as a second ADEM event more than 3 months after the initial event.[64]

TREATMENT
Acute Management

The mainstay for the treatment of acute MS relapses is high-dose corticosteroids, which has class I and II evidence for accelerating functional recovery following an acute attack in adult MS populations.[1] For relapses that do not respond sufficiently to steroids, one may consider concurrent or consecutive treatment with therapeutic plasma exchange.[74]

Disease-Modifying Therapies

Treatment strategies for MS have undergone a profound change within the last few years owing to an ongoing expansion of the therapeutic armamentarium. There are many treatment options available (**Table 2**) with variable mechanisms of action (**Fig. 3**). The effect of these drugs seems to be more significant when the treatment is initiated soon after the onset of symptoms.[75]

INJECTABLE THERAPIES

Interferon-beta (IFNβ) was the first DMT available to treat MS in the 1990s.[76] Four different types of IFNβ are currently approved. The exact mechanism of action is unknown but may include stabilization of the BBB, antiproliferative mechanisms, and promotion of a shift from a proinflammatory to an anti-inflammatory milieu.[77,78] Interferons have a well-known and favorable safety profile with established long-term efficacy. Possible side effects may include flu-like symptoms, depression, hepatotoxicity, lymphopenia, and injection-site reactions, including necrosis.[79] Shortly after their

Table 2
Currently approved disease-modifying treatments for multiple sclerosis

Injectable	Oral	Infused
Interferons	Teriflunomide (Aubagio®)	Natalizumab (Tysabri®)
• IFNβ-1a	Fumarates	Alemtuzumab (Lemtrada®)
○ Avonex®	• Dimethyl fumarate	Ocrelizumab (Ocrevus®)
○ Rebif®	(Tecfidera®)	
• IFNβ-1b	• Diroximel fumarate	
○ Betaseron®	(Vumerity®)	
○ Extavia®	• Monomethyl fumarate	
• Peg IFNβ-1a	(Bafiertam®)	
○ Plegridy®	Sphingosine-1-phosphate	
Glatiramer acetate	inhibitors	
• Copaxone®	• Fingolimod (Gilenya®)	
• Glatopa®	• Siponimod (Mayzent®)	
• Glatiramer acetate injection	• Ozanimod (Zeposia®)	
Ofatumumab (Kesimpta®)	• Ponesimod (Ponvory®)	
	Cladribine (Mavenclad®)	

approval, glatiramer acetate was approved with similar efficacy.[80] Its mechanism of action is unclear but it is thought to promote the upregulation of T-regulatory cells, inducing an anti-inflammatory milieu.[81] Although it is known to have an excellent long-term profile, it has no proven effect on disability progression.[82] In the current landscape, the use of IFNβ and glatiramer acetate has diminished due to the development of alternative DMTs with improved tolerability and higher efficacy.[46,77,82] The most recently approved injectable, ofatumumab, is a subcutaneous fully human

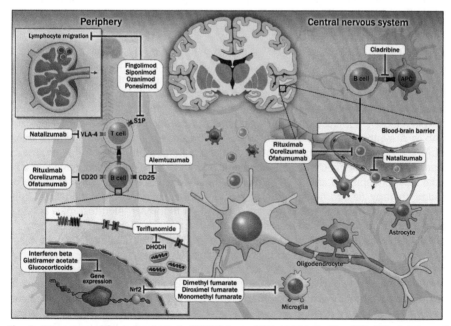

Fig. 3. Disease-modifying treatments (DMTs) in multiple sclerosis. Simplified illustration of various cell types and DMT sites of action in the periphery and within the central nervous system.

anti-CD20 monoclonal antibody that selectively depletes B-cells.[83] It provides higher therapeutic efficacy in reducing clinical relapse risk compared with IFNβ and glatiramer acetate and is similar in efficacy to the infusion therapies.[84]

ORAL THERAPIES

The oral medications are newer additions to the therapeutic armamentarium for MS that trade the convenience of an oral formulation for the long-term safety profile of IFNβ and glatiramer acetate. Teriflunomide is an inhibitor of dihydroorotate dehydrogenase, an enzyme involved in pyrimidine synthesis, that is thought to act by reducing the proliferation of proinflammatory lymphocytes.[85] Common safety concerns include hepatotoxicity and infection.[75] The fumarates (dimethyl, diroximel, and monomethyl fumarate) are a class of oral medications that may exert their anti-inflammatory and neuroprotective effects based on their effects on the nuclear factor-kappa B and nuclear factor erythroid 2-related factor 2 pathways, respectively.[85,86] Commonly reported side effects to include flushing, gastrointestinal upset, and lymphopenia.[87] Sphingosine-1-phosphate receptor modulators (fingolimod, siponimod, ozanimod, and ponesimod) are thought to act by retaining lymphocytes (including autoreactive lymphocytes) within peripheral lymph nodes.[5,77] Due to the possibility of first-dose bradycardia from interaction with receptors on cardiac myocytes, all patients started on fingolimod require first-dose observation.[88] Conversely, only patients with a cardiac history or abnormal electrocardiogram are suggested to undergo a first-dose observation with siponimod and ponesimod. There is no first-dose observation recommendation for ozanimod. Notably, among currently used DMTs, only siponimod has data for efficacy in patients with SPMS.[87] Finally, cladribine is a synthetic adenosine analog that suppresses the immune system by disrupting DNA synthesis and repair, and inducing apoptosis in lymphocytes.[89] Overall, the oral medications are more efficacious than IFNβ and glatiramer acetate, except for teriflunomide, and cladribine has the highest efficacy within the oral group.

INFUSION THERAPIES

Monoclonal antibody infusions (natalizumab, ocrelizumab, alemtuzumab) have higher efficacy than IFNβ, glatiramer acetate, and the oral DMTs. All of these medications can cause infusion reactions (headache, nausea, urticaria, pruritus, and so forth) that can be mitigated by administering antihistamines, antipyretics, and steroids.[89] Natalizumab is a synthetic monoclonal antibody that selectively inhibits very late antigen (VLA)-4 integrins, preventing leukocyte migration across the BBB.[77,90] It has been associated with latent JC virus infection activation known to cause progressive multifocal leukoencephalopathy.[91] Cessation of natalizumab treatment in the absence of bridge therapy (ie, corticosteroids) or the introduction of a fast-acting DMT has been associated with disease rebound after 3 to 4 months.[92] Alemtuzumab is a humanized monoclonal antibody directed at CD52, a protein on the surface of lymphocytes, which results in B-cell and T-cell lysis, as well as T-cell activation by an unclear mechanism.[46,77] It is known to cause profound and long-lasting alterations in lymphocyte counts (up to 2 years or more). It also carries an almost 40% of secondary autoimmunity (mainly thyroid) with potential long-term risk of malignancy.[85] Ocrelizumab is a humanized monoclonal antibody that targets CD20 on B-cells through mechanisms that induce antibody-dependent cell-mediated cytotoxicity and/or the induction of apoptosis.[5] Ocrelizumab became the first therapy approved in the United States for PPMS based on its observed benefits on the timed 25-foot walk test, changes in the number of brain MRI lesions, Expanded Disability Status Scale (EDSS) score, and mean percent brain volume during preplanned hierarchical testing of secondary endpoints.[93]

TREATMENT GOALS

The primary goal of the treatment in MS is to delay disease progression and limit the accrual of disability over time by reducing the inflammatory component of the disease. Epidemiologic studies and clinical trials suggest that this window of opportunity closes relatively early in the disease course (an EDSS score of 3.0 or less).[94] This concept is primarily based on prior observations that disability progression in MS may be driven mainly by focal inflammation and incomplete recovery from clinical relapses before reaching an EDSS score of 3.0 and by diffuse inflammation and neurodegeneration thereafter.[95]

APPROACH TO TREATMENT

With the expanding therapeutic landscape in MS, there is ongoing debate concerning which therapeutic agent should be initiated first. Although this is a considerable oversimplification, the overall treatment strategies can be divided into an escalation and early use of a highly effective therapy approach.[96] The escalation approach favors the initiation of moderate-efficacy DMTs, which generally have favorable safety profiles, followed by a period of clinical and radiological surveillance after which treatment may be escalated to a high-efficacy drug in the face of continued disease activity.[97] A common argument for this approach is based on concerns of overexposure to potentially more complex safety profiles of some high-efficacy DMTs. Alternatively, the early use of a highly effective therapy approach postulates that there is a short therapeutic window early in the disease process during which DMTs can significantly alter long-term disease outcomes.[98] Although arguments can be made for each of these approaches, treatment should always be tailored to each patient individually.

The TRaditional versus Early Aggressive Therapy for MS (TREAT-MS, NCT03500328) trial is an ongoing randomized controlled trial that aims to evaluate, jointly and independently, among patients deemed at higher versus lower risk for disability accumulation, whether early use of highly effective therapy versus a traditional lower efficacy therapy influences the intermediate-term risk of disability, and to evaluate if, among patients deemed at lower risk for disability who start on lower efficacy therapies but experience breakthrough disease, those who switch to a higher-efficacy versus a new first-line therapy have a different intermediate-term risk of disability. An additional ongoing randomized clinical trial, Determining the Effectiveness of earLy Intensive versus Escalation approaches for the Treatment of Relapsing-remitting Multiple Sclerosis (DELIVER-MS, NCT03535298), aims to determine whether early treatment with highly effective DMT improves the prognosis for patients with RRMS. These trials promise to provide higher quality data to help guide treatment decision-making in MS.

PROGRESSIVE DISEASE

Currently available DMTs primarily target inflammatory disease activity, which is present to a lesser degree in progressive disease.[5] Patients with both primary and secondary progressive MS can have clinical and radiologic evidence of disease activity, such as superimposed relapses on a progressive clinical decline or MRI activity with evidence of new or enhancing lesions, respectively.[99] Following the approval of siponimod in 2019 for RRMS and active SPMS based on its observed efficacy in secondary progressive disease with clinical and radiologic activity,[100] the Food and Drug

Administration changed the approval of all DMTs to include both RRMS and active SPMS, reflecting a new understanding that inflammatory disease activity may also occur in progressive forms of MS in which current DMTs may be of use. In this regard, ocrelizumab is the only approved DMT for PPMS.[93] Although developments in progressive MS treatment have been relatively slow compared with the multitude of advances in the treatment of RRMS in recent years, remyelination and neuroprotective therapies with potential benefits for both relapsing and progressive forms of MS are currently under exploration.

EMERGING THERAPIES
Tyrosine Kinase Inhibitors

Tyrosine kinases are enzymes that mediate the phosphorylation of tyrosine residues of molecules that have crucial roles in cellular proliferation and differentiation, metabolism, survival, and apoptosis.[101] Bruton's tyrosine kinase (BTK) is expressed by B-cells and myeloid cells, suggesting that its modulation might provide therapeutic benefits for patients with MS.[102] Irreversible BTK inhibitors (evobrutinib, tolebrutinib, and orelabrutinib), reversible BTK inhibitors (fenebrutinib and BIIB091), and a selective tyrosine kinase inhibitor (masitinib) are currently under investigation in various phases of development.

Remyelination

Failed remyelination underpins neurodegeneration and CNS dysfunction with aging and disease progression in MS.[103] Various extrinsic and intrinsic factors, including mitochondrial dysfunction leading to neuronal hypoxia, and failure of oligodendrocyte differentiation, can lead to axonal degeneration and irreversible disability.[16] Remyelination is an essential target for emerging therapies due to its potential to halt disability accrual and reverse existing disability.

Biotin is a cofactor for oligodendrocyte-expressed carboxylases thought to support myelin repair by enhancing fatty acid synthesis and protecting against hypoxia-driven axonal degeneration.[104] It was shown to promote remyelination at high doses in early phase clinical trials but the definitive phase 3 trial showed no effect on disability improvement.[105]

Clemastine fumarate, a first-generation antihistamine, has been shown to promote remyelination through its effect on human oligodendrocyte precursor cells.[106] ReBUILD (NCT02040298), a small phase 2, randomized, placebo-controlled, crossover study showed a reduced latency delay in VEPs in MS patients with chronic optic neuropathy. However, whether this reduction translates to a clinically meaningful improvement in individuals remains unclear.

Opicinumab, a humanized monoclonal antibody against the leucine-rich repeat neuronal protein 1 (LINGO-1), a cell-surface glycoprotein that inhibits oligodendrocyte differentiation, myelination, neuronal survival, and axonal regeneration, is another potential remyelination target of recent interest.[106] However, 2 phase 2 trials, RENEW (NCT01721161) and SYNERGY (NCT01864148), failed to improve the primary outcome of VEPs in patients with optic neuritis and disability scores, respectively.

The role of immunoablation and autologous hematopoietic stem cell transplantation (AHSCT) in treatment-resistant relapsing MS is currently under investigation. A recent review of retrospective studies, clinical trials, and meta-analyses/systematic reviews reported an overall incidence of relapse-free survival at 5 years after transplant of 80% to 87%, with many studies showing high rates of relapse-free survival disability stability or improvement, and improved MRI measures.[107] Overall, AHSCT seems to be most effective in patients with active, relapsing disease despite DMT, and in younger patients with a relatively shorter disease duration who are still ambulatory and actively accruing disability. The BEst Available Therapy versus autologous hematopoietic stem cell transplant for Multiple Sclerosis (BEAT-MS, NCT04047628) study is an ongoing randomized trial evaluating the safety, efficacy, and cost-effectiveness of AHSCT compared with the best available therapy (natalizumab, CD20 monoclonal antibodies, and alemtuzumab) in treatment-refractory relapsing patients to determine the optimal use of this treatment (BEAT-MS, NCT04047628).

Mesenchymal stem cells (MSCs) have also been an area of interest in progressive disease due to their ability to differentiate into various types of cells and remyelination potential. They can be isolated from bone marrow, adipose tissue, umbilical cord, and other sources.[108] Although their presence within the CNS seems to be short-lived following intrathecal injection, their potential therapeutic benefits could stem from the secretion of neurotrophic factors, inducing axonal outgrowth and increasing cell survival.[108] There are several ongoing studies investigating the potential use of MSCs in progressive MS but their efficacy has not been shown in phase I clinical trials.[109] Important questions regarding appropriate dosing regimens, route of administration, cell culture protocols, and storage procedures remain unclear, and possible associated risks including infection, infusion-related toxicity, malignancy, and so forth should be considered in clinical practice. Current knowledge and limitations of different stem cell-based approaches to therapy are described in detail elsewhere.[110]

Other cell types play critical roles in establishing where a lesion is conducive for regeneration. In the last few years, several studies have described beneficial and detrimental roles played by astrocytes and microglia in remyelination.[111,112]

NEUROPROTECTION

The goal of neuroprotective therapies is to prevent irreversible disability and to slow disease progression. Studies to date have been limited and encompassing medications with a variety of mechanisms of action.

Alpha-lipoic acid (ALA), a mitochondrial oxidation–reduction cofactor with anti-inflammatory properties and potential neuroprotective effects, showed benefit in reducing the rate of brain atrophy with a trend toward improving the timed 25-foot walk compared with placebo in a small, randomized phase 2 study (Lipoic Acid for Progressive Multiple Sclerosis [LAMPMS]; NCT03161028).

Ibudilast, a cyclic nucleotide phosphodiesterase, toll-like receptor 4, and macrophage inhibitory factor, was found to promote a slower rate of brain atrophy in patients with progressive MS compared with placebo in a phase 2 randomized clinical trial (Secondary and Primary progressive I budilast NeuroNEXT Trial in Multiple Sclerosis [SPRINT-MS], NCT01982942). However, its impact on clinical measures of disability progression remains unclear.

Metformin, a metabolic inhibitor that alters whole-body and cellular energy metabolism, exhibited neuroprotective effects in animal studies, presumably by mitigating mitochondrial dysfunction and oxidative stress and inducing an anti-inflammatory lymphocytic profile.[113] It is currently under investigation in combination with clemastine in a phase 2a randomized, placebo-controlled, clinical trial to determine whether the combination of these 2 agents can promote remyelination in patients with MS (CCMR Two; NCT05131828).

Phenytoin, a voltage-gated sodium channel inhibitor with neuroprotective properties in preclinical trials, was shown to reduce retinal nerve fiber layer thinning by 30% in patients with acute optic neuritis when given within 2 weeks of onset in a randomized, placebo-controlled, phase 2 trial (NCT01451593). However, the clinical relevance of these findings remains to be determined.

Simvastatin, a 3-hydroxy-3-methyl-glutaryl-coenzyme A reductase inhibitor has also been studied as a potential neuroprotective agent based on evidence from a phase 2 randomized clinical trial showing that simvastatin-treated patients with SPMS experienced a decrease in whole-brain atrophy rate compared with placebo (MS-STAT2, NCT03387670).

Finally, the efficacy of amiloride, fluoxetine, and riluzole as potential neuroprotective agents in patients with progressive MS was evaluated in a phase 2, multiarm, randomized clinical trial. However, none of these medications was superior to placebo for the primary outcome of percentage brain volume change (Multiple sclerosis-Secondary progressive Multi-Arm Randomisation Trial [MS-SMART], NCT01910259).

Despite these developments, it is important to note that none of these medications (ALA, amiloride, fluoxetine, ibudilast, metformin, phenytoin, riluzole, and simvastatin) should be used as a putative treatment of MS outside of clinical trials.

DISCUSSION

Remarkable advances in basic immunology and neuroscience have contributed to a conceptual shift in the understanding of the fundamental principles of MS immunopathogenesis in recent years. With an increased awareness of the multidimensional construct of phenotypic differences in clinical expression and long-term outcomes across racial groups due to complex interactions between social, environmental, and genetic factors, the evolving nature of the therapeutic landscape has favorably changed the long-term outlook for many patients. Optimization of treatment approaches and delivery of tailored interventions and personalized treatment to maximize benefits and minimize risks represent 2 of the most significant challenges within the field and 2 of the greatest opportunities, particularly as new treatments focused on remyelination neuroprotection, and neuronal repair emerge.

CLINICS CARE POINTS

- A diagnosis of MS is made through a combination of clinical history, neurologic examination, MRI, and exclusion of other diagnostic possibilities.

- The primary goal of currently available treatments in multiple sclerosis is to delay disease progression and limit the accrual of disability over time by reducing the inflammatory component of the disease, which is present to a lesser degree in progressive forms of MS.

- Although developments in progressive MS treatment have been relatively slow compared with the multitude of advances in the treatment of RRMS in recent years, remyelination and neuroprotective therapies with potential benefits for both relapsing and progressive forms of MS are currently under exploratio

DISCLOSURE

C.A. Pérez received postgraduate fellowship support from Genentech and has participated in advisory boards for Sanofi. F.X. Cuascut received research funding from Genentech and Biogen and has participated in advisory boards for Genentech, Biogen, Horizon, and Pharma Novartis and Horizon. G.J. Hutton received research funding from Biogen, Hoffman-La Roche, Sanofi, MedImmune, and Novartis and has participated in advisory boards for Novartis and Horizon.

REFERENCES

1. Thompson AJ, Baranzini SE, Geurts J, et al. Multiple Sclerosis. Lancet Neurol 2018;391:1622–36.
2. Brownlee WJ, Hardy TA, Fazekas F, et al. Diagnosis of multiple sclerosis: progress and challenges. Lancet 2017;389:1336–46.
3. Gelfand JM. Multiple sclerosis: diagnosis, differential diagnosis, and clinical presentation. Handb Clin Neurol 2014. https://doi.org/10.1016/B978-0-444-52001-2.00011-X.
4. Eriksson M, Andersen O, Runmarker B. Long-term follow up of patients with clinically isolated syndromes, relapsing-remitting and secondary progressive multiple sclerosis. Mult Scler 2003;9:260–74.
5. Ciotti JR, Cross AH. Disease-modifying treatment in progressive multiple sclerosis. Curr Treat Options Neurol 2018;20:12.
6. Krieger SC. New approaches to the diagnosis, clinical course, and goals of therapy in multiple sclerosis and related disorders. Continuum (Minneap Minn) 2016;22:723–9.
7. Confavreux C, Vukusic S. Natural history of multiple sclerosis. Brain 2006;129: 606–16.
8. Lublin FD, Reingold SC, Cohen J a, et al. Defining the clinical course of multiple sclerosis: the 2013 revisions. Neurology 2014;83:278–86.
9. Wang CX, Greenberg BM. Pediatric multiple sclerosis. Neurol Clin 2018;36: 135–49.
10. Hintzen RQ. Pediatric acquired CNS demyelinating syndromes. Neurology 2016;87:s67–73.
11. Wallin MT, Culpepper WJ, Campbell JD, et al. The prevalence of MS in the United States. Neurology 2019;92:e1029. LP-e1040.
12. Carroll WM. 2017 McDonald MS diagnostic criteria: Evidence-based revisions. Mult Scler J 2018;24:92–5.
13. Hempel S, Graham GD, Fu N, et al. A systematic review of modifiable risk factors in the progression of multiple sclerosis. Mult Scler 2017;23:525–33.
14. Freedman MS, Rush CA. Severe, highly active, or aggressive multiple sclerosis. Continuum (Minneap Minn) 2016;22:761–84.
15. Scott TF, Schramke CJ. Poor recovery after the first two attacks of multiple sclerosis is associated with poor outcome five years later. J Neurol Sci 2010; 292:52–6.
16. Reich DS, Lucchinetti CF, Calabresi PA. Multiple Sclerosis. N Engl J Med 2018; 378:169–80.
17. Jacobs BM, Giovannoni G, Cuzick J, et al. Systematic review and meta-analysis of the association between Epstein–Barr virus, multiple sclerosis and other risk factors. Mult Scler J 2020;26:1281–97.
18. Bjornevik K, Cortese M, Healy BC, et al. Longitudinal analysis reveals high prevalence of Epstein-Barr virus associated with multiple sclerosis. Science 2022; 375:296–301.
19. Bordon Y. Linking Epstein-Barr virus infection to multiple sclerosis. Nat Rev Immunol 2022;7:41586.
20. Narula S, Banwell B. Pediatric demyelination. Continuum (Minneap Minn) 2016; 22:897–915.
21. Yamamoto E, Ginsberg M, Rensel M, et al. Pediatric-onset multiple sclerosis: a single center study. J Child Neurol 2018;33:98–105.

22. Rostásy K, Bajer-Kornek B. Paediatric multiple sclerosis and other acute demyelinating diseases. Curr Opin Neurol 2018;31:244–8.

23. Kozhieva M, Naumova N, Alikina T, et al. Primary progressive multiple sclerosis in a Russian cohort: relationship with gut bacterial diversity. BMC Microbiol 2019;19:309.

24. Katz Sand I, Zhu Y, Ntranos A, et al. Disease-modifying therapies alter gut microbial composition in MS. Neurol Neuroimmunol Neuroinflammation 2018;6:e517.

25. Amezcua L, Conti D, Liu L, et al. Place of birth, age of immigration, and disability in Hispanics with multiple sclerosis. Mult Scler Relat Disord 2015;4:25–30.

26. Pérez CA, Salehbeiki A, Zhu L, et al. Assessment of Racial/Ethnic Disparities in Volumetric MRI Correlates of Clinical Disability in Multiple Sclerosis: A Preliminary Study. J Neuroimaging 2021;31:115–23.

27. Mercado V, Dongarwar D, Fisher K, et al. Multiple sclerosis in a multi-ethnic population in houston, texas: A retrospective analysis. Biomedicines 2020;8:1–11.

28. Amezcua L, Oksenberg JR, McCauley JL. MS in self-identified Hispanic/Latino individuals living in the US. Mult Scler J 2017;3. 205521731772510.

29. Amezcua L, Lund BT, Weiner LP, et al. Multiple sclerosis in Hispanics: A study of clinical disease expression. Mult Scler J 2011;17:1010–6.

30. Hillert J. Socioeconomic status and multiple sclerosis outcome. Nat Rev Neurol 2020. https://doi.org/10.1038/s41582-020-0329-3.

31. Pérez CA, Lincoln JA. Racial and ethnic disparities in treatment response and tolerability in multiple sclerosis: A comparative study. Mult Scler Relat Disord 2021;56:103248.

32. Nakamura Y, Gaetano L, Matsushita T, et al. A comparison of brain magnetic resonance imaging lesions in multiple sclerosis by race with reference to disability progression. J Neuroinflammation 2018;15. https://doi.org/10.1186/s12974-018-1295-1.

33. Amezcua L, Smith JB, Gonzales EG, et al. Race, ethnicity, and cognition in persons newly diagnosed with multiple sclerosis. Neurology 2020;94:1–9.

34. Amezcua L, McCauley JL. Race and ethnicity on MS presentation and disease course. Mult Scler J 2020;1–7.

35. Song X, Li D, Qiu Z, et al. Correlation between EDSS scores and cervical spinal cord atrophy at 3T MRI in multiple sclerosis: A systematic review and meta-analysis. Mult Scler Relat Disord 2019. https://doi.org/10.1016/j.msard.2019.101426.

36. Avasarala J. Inadequacy of Clinical Trial Designs and Data to Control for the Confounding Impact of Race/Ethnicity in Response to Treatment in Multiple Sclerosis. JAMA Neurol 2014;71:943–4.

37. Schwid SR, Panitch HS. Full results of the Evidence of Interferon Dose-Response-European North American Comparative Efficacy (EVIDENCE) study: a multicenter, randomized, assessor-blinded comparison of low-dose weekly versus high-dose, high-frequency interferon beta-1a for rela. Clin Ther 2007;29:2031–48.

38. Kappos L, Edan G, Freedman MS, et al. The 11-year long-term follow-up study from the randomized BENEFIT CIS trial. Neurology 2016;87:978–87.

39. Barkhof F, de Jong R, Sfikas N, et al. The influence of patient demographics, disease characteristics and treatment on brain volume loss in Trial Assessing Injectable Interferon vs FTY720 Oral in Relapsing-Remitting Multiple Sclerosis (TRANSFORMS), a phase 3 study of fingolimod in multiple sc. Mult Scler 2014;20:1704–13.

40. O'Connor P, Comi G, Freedman MS, et al. Long-term safety and efficacy of teri-flunomide: Nine-year follow-up of the randomized TEMSO study. Neurology 2016;86:920–30.

41. Koch M, Kingwell E, Rieckmann P. The natural history of primary progressive multiple sclerosis. Neurology 2009;73:1996–2002.

42. Miller DH, Chard DT, Ciccarelli O. Clinically isolated syndromes. Lancet Neurol 2012;11:157–69.

43. van der Vuurst de Vries RM, Mescheriakova JY, Wong YYM, et al. Application of the 2017 Revised McDonald Criteria for Multiple Sclerosis to Patients With a Typical Clinically Isolated Syndrome. JAMA Neurol 2018;75:1392–8.

44. Hou Y, Jia Y, Hou J. Natural Course of Clinically Isolated Syndrome: A Longitu-dinal Analysis Using a Markov Model. Sci Rep 2018;8:10857.

45. McDonald WI, Compston A, Edan G, et al. Recommended diagnostic criteria for multiple sclerosis: guidelines from the International Panel on the diagnosis of multiple sclerosis. Ann Neurol 2001;50:121–7.

46. Tillery EE, Clements JN, Howard Z. What's new in multiple sclerosis? Ment Heal Clin 2017;7:213–20.

47. Thompson AJ, Banwell BL, Barkhof F, et al. Diagnosis of multiple sclerosis: 2017 revisions of the McDonald criteria. Lancet Neurol 2018;17:162–73.

48. Olek MJ. Differential diagnosis, clinical features, and prognosis of multiple scle-rosis. In: Current clinical neurology: multiple sclerosis. Totowa, NJ: Humana Press Inc; 2005. p. 15–53.

49. Miller DH, Leary SM. Primary-progressive multiple sclerosis. Lancet Neurol 2007;6:903–12.

50. Vollmer TL, Nair KV, Williams IM, et al. Multiple Sclerosis Phenotypes as a Con-tinuum. Neurol Clin Pract 2021;11:342–51.

51. De Stefano N, Giorgio A, Tintoré M, et al. Radiologically isolated syndrome or subclinical multiple sclerosis: MAGNIMS consensus recommendations. Mult Scler J 2018;23:214–21.

52. Lebrun C. Radiologically isolated syndrome should be treated with disease-modifying therapy – commentary. Mult Scler J 2017;23:1821–3.

53. Okuda DT, Siva A, Kantarci O, et al. Radiologically isolated syndrome: 5-year risk for an initial clinical event. PLoS One 2014;9. https://doi.org/10.1371/journal.pone.0090509.

54. Matute-Blanch C, Villar LM, Álvarez-Cermeño JC, et al. Neurofilament light chain and oligoclonal bands are prognostic biomarkers in radiologically isolated syn-drome. Brain 2018;141:1085–93.

55. Yamout B, Al Khawajah M. Radiologically isolated syndrome and multiple scle-rosis. Mult Scler Relat Disord 2017;17:234–7.

56. Filippi M, Preziosa P, Meani A, et al. Prediction of a multiple sclerosis diagnosis in patients with clinically isolated syndrome using the 2016 MAGNIMS and 2010 McDonald criteria: a retrospective study. Lancet Neurol 2018;17:133–42.

57. Palace J. Making the diagnosis of multiple sclerosis. J Neurol Neurosurg Psychi-atry 2001;71. ii3–ii8.

58. McMahon KL, Cowin G, Galloway G. Magnetic resonance imaging: The under-lying principles. J Orthop Sports Phys Ther 2011;41:806–19.

59. Ge Y. Multiple sclerosis: the role of MR imaging. AJNR Am J Neuroradiol 2006;27:1165–76.

60. Wingerchuk DM. Immune-mediated myelopathies. Continuum (Minneap Minn) 2018;24:497–522.

61. Wildner P, Stasiołek M, Matysiak M. Differential diagnosis of multiple sclerosis and other inflammatory CNS diseases. Mult Scler Relat Disord 2020;37:101452.
62. Schäffler N, Köpke S, Winkler L, et al. Accuracy of diagnostic tests in multiple sclerosis - a systematic review. Acta Neurol Scand 2011;124:151–64.
63. Weinshenker BG, Wingerchuk DM. Neuromyelitis Spectrum Disorders. Mayo Clin Proc 2017;92:663–79.
64. Shukla NM, Lotze TE, Muscal E. Inflammatory Diseases of the Central Nervous System. Neurol Clin 2021;39:811–28.
65. Dixon GA, Pérez CA. Multiple sclerosis and the choroid plexus: emerging concepts of disease immunopathophysiology. Pediatr Neurol 2019. https://doi.org/10.1016/j.pediatrneurol.2019.08.007.
66. Lucchinetti CF, Guo Y, Popescu BFG, et al. The pathology of an autoimmune astrocytopathy: lessons learned from neuromyelitis optica. Brain Pathol 2014;24:83–97.
67. Borisow N, Mori M, Kuwabara S, et al. Diagnosis and Treatment of NMO Spectrum Disorder and MOG-Encephalomyelitis. Front Neurol 2018;9. https://doi.org/10.3389/fneur.2018.00888.
68. Lana-Peixoto MA, Talim N. Neuromyelitis optica spectrum disorder and anti-MOG syndromes. Biomedicines 2019;7:1–24.
69. Wynford-Thomas R, Jacob A, Tomassini V. Neurological update: MOG antibody disease. J Neurol 2019;266:1280–6.
70. Zhou L, Huang Y, Li H, et al. MOG-antibody associated demyelinating disease of the CNS: A clinical and pathological study in Chinese Han patients. J Neuroimmunol 2017. https://doi.org/10.1016/j.jneuroim.2017.01.007.
71. Shor N, Deschamps R, Cobo Calvo A, et al. MRI characteristics of MOG-Ab associated disease in adults: An update. Rev Neurol (Paris) 2021;177:39–50.
72. Menge T, Hemmer B, Nessler S, et al. Acute Disseminated Encephalomyelitis: An Update. Arch Neurol 2005;62:1673–80.
73. Tenembaum S, Chamoles N, Fejerman N. Acute disseminated encephalomyelitis: A long-term follow-up study of 84 pediatric patients. Neurology 2002;59:1224–31.
74. Weinshenker BG, O'Brien PC, Petterson TM, et al. A randomized trial of plasma exchange in acute central nervous system inflammatory demyelinating disease. Ann Neurol 1999;46:878–86.
75. Harding K, Williams O, Willis M, et al. Clinical outcomes of escalation vs early intensive disease-modifying therapy in patients with multiple sclerosis. JAMA Neurol 2019;76:536–41.
76. Group TIMSS. Interferon beta-1b is effective in relapsing-remitting multiple sclerosis. Neurology 1993;43(655). LP – 655.
77. Cross AH, Naismith RT. Established and novel disease-modifying treatments in multiple sclerosis. J Intern Med 2014;275:350–63.
78. Zhang J, Hutton G, Zang Y. A comparison of the mechanisms of action of interferon beta and glatiramer acetate in the treatment of multiple sclerosis. Clin Ther 2002;24:1998–2021.
79. Kappos L, Freedman MS, Polman CH, et al. Long-term effect of early treatment with interferon beta-1b after a first clinical event suggestive of multiple sclerosis: 5-year active treatment extension of the phase 3 BENEFIT trial. Lancet Neurol 2009;8:987–97.
80. La Mantia L, Di Pietrantonj C, Rovaris M, et al. Interferons-beta versus glatiramer acetate for relapsing-remitting multiple sclerosis. Cochrane Database Syst Rev 2016. https://doi.org/10.1002/14651858.CD009333.pub3.

81. Schrempf W, Ziemssen T. Glatiramer acetate: mechanisms of action in multiple sclerosis. Autoimmun Rev 2007;6:469–75.
82. Rae-Grant A, Day GS, Marrie RA, et al. Practice guideline recommendations summary: Disease-modifying therapies for adults with multiple sclerosis. Neurology 2018;90:777–88.
83. Liu Z, Liao Q, Wen H, et al. Disease modifying therapies in relapsing-remitting multiple sclerosis: A systematic review and network meta-analysis. Autoimmun Rev 2021;20:102826.
84. Cotchett KR, Dittel BN, Obeidat AZ. Comparison of the Efficacy and Safety of Anti-CD20 B Cells Depleting Drugs in Multiple Sclerosis. Mult Scler Relat Disord 2021;49. https://doi.org/10.1016/j.msard.2021.102787.
85. Eriksson I, Komen J, Piehl F, et al. The changing multiple sclerosis treatment landscape: impact of new drugs and treatment recommendations. Eur J Clin Pharmacol 2018;74:663–70.
86. Wingerchuk DM, Carter JL. Multiple sclerosis: current and emerging disease-modifying therapies and treatment strategies. Mayo Clin Proc 2014;89:225–40.
87. Naismith RT, Wundes A, Ziemssen T, et al. Diroximel Fumarate Demonstrates an Improved Gastrointestinal Tolerability Profile Compared with Dimethyl Fumarate in Patients with Relapsing–Remitting Multiple Sclerosis: Results from the Randomized, Double-Blind, Phase III EVOLVE-MS-2 Study. CNS Drugs 2020;34:185–96.
88. Singer BA. Initiating oral fingolimod treatment in patients with multiple sclerosis. Ther Adv Neurol Disord 2013;6:269–75.
89. Leist TP, Weissert R. Cladribine: Mode of Action and Implications for Treatment of Multiple Sclerosis. Clin Neuropharmacol 2011;34:28–35. Available at: https://journals.lww.com/clinicalneuropharm/Fulltext/2011/01000/Cladribine__Mode_of_Action_and_Implications_for.7.aspx.
90. Neema M, Stankiewicz J, Arora A, et al. MRI in multiple sclerosis: what's inside the toolbox? Neurotherapeutics 2007;4:602–17.
91. Feinstein A, Freeman J, Lo AC. Treatment of progressive multiple sclerosis: what works, what does not, and what is needed. Lancet Neurol 2015;14:194–207.
92. Rocca MA, Messina R, Filippi M. Multiple sclerosis imaging: recent advances. J Neurol 2013;260:929–35.
93. Montalban X, Hauser SL, Kappos L, et al. Ocrelizumab versus Placebo in Primary Progressive Multiple Sclerosis. N Engl J Med 2016;376:209–20.
94. Coles AJ, Cox A, Le Page E, et al. The window of therapeutic opportunity in multiple sclerosis: evidence from monoclonal antibody therapy. J Neurol 2006;253:98–108.
95. Leray E, Yaouanq J, Le Page E, et al. Evidence for a two-stage disability progression in multiple sclerosis. Brain 2010;133:1900–13.
96. Ontaneda D, Tallantyre E, Kalincik T, et al. Early highly effective versus escalation treatment approaches in relapsing multiple sclerosis. Lancet Neurol 2019;18:973–80.
97. Grand'Maison F, Yeung M, Morrow SA, et al. Sequencing of disease-modifying therapies for relapsing–remitting multiple sclerosis: a theoretical approach to optimizing treatment. Curr Med Res Opin 2018;34:1419–30.
98. Filippi M, Rocca MA. Rethinking multiple sclerosis treatment strategies. Lancet Neurol 2020;19:281–2.
99. Willis MA, Fox RJ. Progressive multiple sclerosis. Continuum (Minneap Minn) 2016;22:785–98.

100. Kappos L, Bar-Or A, Cree BAC, et al. Siponimod versus placebo in secondary progressive multiple sclerosis (EXPAND): a double-blind, randomised, phase 3 study. Lancet 2018;391:1263–73.

101. Vermersch P, Brieva-Ruiz L, Fox RJ, et al. Efficacy and Safety of Masitinib in Progressive Forms of Multiple Sclerosis. Neurol Neuroimmunol Neuroinflammation 2022;9:e1148.

102. Correale J. BTK inhibitors as potential therapies for multiple sclerosis. Lancet Neurol 2021;20:689–91.

103. Podbielska M, Banik NL, Kurowska E, et al. Myelin recovery in multiple sclerosis: the challenge of remyelination. Brain Sci 2013;3:1282–324.

104. Cree BAC, Cutter G, Wolinsky JS, et al. Safety and efficacy of MD1003 (high-dose biotin) in patients with progressive multiple sclerosis (SPI2): a randomised, double-blind, placebo-controlled, phase 3 trial. Lancet Neurol 2020;19:988–97.

105. Sedel F, Papeix C, Bellanger A, et al. High doses of biotin in chronic progressive multiple sclerosis: A pilot study. Mult Scler Relat Disord 2015;4:159–69.

106. Green AJ, Gelfand JM, Cree BA, et al. Clemastine fumarate as a remyelinating therapy for multiple sclerosis (ReBUILD): a randomised, controlled, double-blind, crossover trial. Lancet 2017;390:2481–9.

107. Cohen JA, Baldassari LE, Atkins HL, et al. Autologous Hematopoietic Cell Transplantation for Treatment-Refractory Relapsing Multiple Sclerosis: Position Statement from the American Society for Blood and Marrow Transplantation. Biol Blood Marrow Transplant 2019;25:845–54.

108. Mansoor SR, Zabihi E, Ghasemi-Kasman M. The potential use of mesenchymal stem cells for the treatment of multiple sclerosis. Life Sci 2019;235:116830.

109. Cohen JA, Imrey PB, Planchon SM, et al. Pilot trial of intravenous autologous culture-expanded mesenchymal stem cell transplantation in multiple sclerosis. Mult Scler 2018;24:501–11.

110. Cuascut FX, Hutton GJ. Stem Cell-Based Therapies for Multiple Sclerosis: Current Perspectives. Biomedicines 2019;7:26.

111. Rawji KS, Gonzalez Martinez GA, Sharma A, et al. The Role of Astrocytes in Remyelination. Trends Neurosci 2020;43:596–607.

112. Traiffort E, Kassoussi A, Zahaf A, et al. Astrocytes and Microglia as Major Players of Myelin Production in Normal and Pathological Conditions. Front Cell Neurosci 2020;14. https://doi.org/10.3389/fncel.2020.00079.

113. Nath N, Khan M, Paintlia MK, et al. Metformin attenuated the autoimmune disease of the central nervous system in animal models of multiple sclerosis. J Immunol 2009;182:8005–14.

Trigeminal Neuralgia
Diagnosis and Treatment

Anthony K. Allam, Himanshu Sharma, MD, PhD,
M. Benjamin Larkin, MD, PharmD, Ashwin Viswanathan, MD*

KEYWORDS

- Facial pain • Neuropathic pain • Trigeminal neuralgia • Trigeminal nerve
- Surgical treatment • Pharmacologic management

KEY POINTS

- Trigeminal neuralgia is frequently mis-/underdiagnosed in the population.
- Pharmacologic management of trigeminal neuralgia remains the first-line treatment.
- The gold standard for the surgical treatment of classic trigeminal neuralgia secondary to neurovascular impingement is microvascular decompression.
- Percutaneous modalities offer additional treatment options for secondary causes of trigeminal neuralgia.
- Stereotactic radiosurgery offers a favorable pain relief for patients without vascular compression or who would like to avoid craniotomy.

INTRODUCTION

Trigeminal neuralgia (TN), the most common craniofacial neuralgia, results in intense, debilitating facial pain and can profoundly affect quality of life. In this article, the authors summarize the characteristics, pathophysiology, and management of TN in both primary and secondary care settings.

Definition and Classification

TN classically presents with "recurrent unilateral brief electric shocklike pains, abrupt in onset and termination, limited to the distribution of one or more divisions of the trigeminal nerve and triggered by innocuous stimuli."[1] More recently, it has been understood that up to 30% of patients may present with continuous pain of moderate

We have no granting organizations or grant numbers, contract numbers, or other sources of financial or material support to disclose.
Conflicts of interests: none.
Department of Neurosurgery, Baylor College of Medicine, 7200 Cambridge St, Suite 9A, Houston, TX 77030, USA
* Corresponding author. Neurosurgery Department, Baylor College of Medicine, 7200 Cambridge St Ste 9B, Houston, TX 77030.
E-mail address: ashwinv@bcm.edu

Neurol Clin 41 (2023) 107–121
https://doi.org/10.1016/j.ncl.2022.09.001
0733-8619/23/Published by Elsevier Inc.

neurologic.theclinics.com

intensity within the same distribution as the affected nerve division.[1] Various classification methods have been proposed for facial pain. The International Headache Society has divided TN into 3 main categories: classic, secondary/symptomatic, and idiopathic.[1] Classic TN is associated with neurovascular compression (NVC) of the trigeminal nerve root with associated morphologic changes on MRI.[1] Secondary/symptomatic trigeminal (STN) neuralgia is associated with an underlying disease. The most common causes include multiple sclerosis (MS), space-occupying lesions, skull-base bone deformity, connective tissue diseases, arteriovenous malformations, dural arteriovenous fistulae, or genetic causes of neuropathy.[1] Idiopathic TN (ITN) is a diagnosis of exclusion, when neither classic nor secondary TN is identified through appropriate testing (eg, MRI and electrophysiological tests).[1] Both classic TN and ITN can further be classified based on the presence of concomitant pain.

Symptomology

TN is usually unilateral with an increased prevalence of right-sided pain.[1–5] The few cases in which TN presents bilaterally are often secondary TN, and pain in one of the sides exhibits temporal separation from the other side.[5–8] The location of pain in TN is divided based on the 3 distributions of the trigeminal nerve: V1 (ophthalmic), V2 (maxillary), and V3 (mandibular). Approximately 36% to 42% of patients exhibit pain in one distribution alone, with V2/V3 representing the most common distributions. In 35% of patients, pain is found in both V2 and V3 distributions with 14% of patients experiencing pain in all 3 distributions.[2,4,5,9–13] Given these distributions, patients frequently initially present to dentists with tooth pain. Another characteristic of TN is the evocable nature of the pain. Common daily activities (eg, chewing, talking, shaving, brushing teeth, and light touch) in the affected distribution can trigger TN pain.[1,3,4] Although patients may report spontaneous pain, it is debated whether the pain is truly spontaneous or if subtle sensory stimulation outside of conscious awareness triggers the attack. Pain is often followed by refractory period in which a new attack cannot be elicited. The pathophysiology of the refractory period is poorly understood, but the intensity and duration of an attack seems to correlate with the duration of the refractory period.[14] TN does not frequently present with sensory deficits on gross examination; however, advanced sensory testing (ie, quantitative sensory testing) can elicit subtle findings.[15,16] Indeed, a recent large series identified sensory abnormalities in 30% of patients. Autonomic symptoms were traditionally not considered a part of TN; however, recent work has shown that autonomic symptoms, in particular lacrimation and rhinorrhea, can occur in a large proportion of patients with TN.[2,4,17–21] The presence of autonomic symptoms can make the diagnosis of TN challenging, given overlap between short-lasting unilateral neuralgiform headaches with autonomic signs (SUNHA).[5,20,21] In fact, elucidating between SUNHA and TN with lacrimation can be so difficult that the patient may be assigned both diagnoses initially.[1,5]

Pathophysiology

Despite variable TN causes, the prevailing pathophysiologic theory remains similar. ITN results in a focal demyelination whose cause is unknown, whereas primary demyelination or demyelination secondary as a result of external insults has been linked to the hyperexcitability of primary afferents, leading to several downstream effects at the neuronal level that is thought to be responsible for symptom onset.[22] Animal models and patient biopsies suggest a cause to be related to the dysregulation of voltage-gated sodium channels (Na_v).[22,23] Specifically, both the $Na_v1.3$ and $Na_v1.1$ channels are upregulated, whereas $Na_v1.7$ is downregulated.[22,24–26]

Advancements in the histopathologic and electrophysiologic understanding of TN led Devor and colleagues, in 2002, to propose the original theory for the cause of symptoms of TN, which was termed the "ignition hypothesis."[27] Electrophysiological recordings obtained from the root entry zone of the trigeminal nerve demonstrated an ectopic generation of action potentials.[22,28–31] Dysfunctional ephaptic transmissions of the various types of demyelinated neurons was thought to be the result of a collective summation of the up-and-down regulation among the aforementioned sodium channels. It was this dysfunctional sensory transmission that was thought to be the source for the propagation of numerous amplified ectopic action potentials and the overall functional hyperexcitability responsible for the characteristic shocklike symptoms patients experienced.[22,32–34]

Numerous studies have since pointed to the demyelination of primary trigeminal afferents near the entry of the trigeminal root into the pons (dorsal root entry zone) as the pathophysiological mechanism of TN.[19,35–37] In particular, the transition from oligodendrocyte to Schwann cell myelination within the proximal 25% of the trigeminal nerve is particularly susceptible to insult representing a *locus minoris resistentiae*.[38] Furthermore, the hyperexcitability of afferent trigeminal nerves causes the sensitization of multiple areas within the central nervous system, including the spinal trigeminal nucleus, thalamus, and somatosensory cortices, leading to the further perpetuation of pain.[22,39,40]

In classic TN, it has been most commonly attributed to NVC by the superior cerebellar artery, located within the cerebellopontine cistern, which is thought to result in focal demyelination and hyperexcitability of the involved nerve.[19,41,42] Although in some cases, simply the mere contact of the artery to the nerve, even in the absence of morphologic changes, can lead to symptoms.[43,44] Burchiel and colleagues found that the association of classic TN with NVC was insignificant, as 99.94% of compression in the general population was asymptomatic. In addition, patients aged 20 to 40 years who presented with classic TN were much less likely to have evidence of NVC than patients older than 50 years.[45] Thus neither the presence nor absence of NVC is sufficient to diagnose TN; the patient must be symptomatic. Patients with TN can go for years at a time without a recurrence of pain between episodes. It has been suggested that a partial remyelination of the affected neurons may be attributable to this phenomenon as well as the spontaneous remission of pain described in some patients.[32]

In secondary TN, demyelination occurs because of other causes such as MS or space-occupying lesions. More specifically, in patients with multiple sclerosis, intrapontine demyelination can be an additional cause for the TN symptom onset.[5,19] In some cases, patients may present with a demyelinating plaque in addition to NVC at the root entry zone, representing a "double-crush" mechanism. Most of the patients undergoing a microvascular decompression have been shown to have severe NVC intraoperatively. However, in these patients, microvascular decompression is generally reported to be less effective.[46]

Trigeminal Neuralgia in Multiple Sclerosis

Compared with the general population, patients with MS have a 20-fold increased risk of developing TN. Typically, the pain symptoms associated with TN become apparent 12 years after the initial onset of MS symptoms.[47–49] MS-associated secondary TN differs significantly in regard to classic TN. In general, it often presents at a younger age and more commonly, occurs in the trigeminal distribution bilaterally.[50] As a result, the treatment pathway for the associated secondary TN symptoms in MS differs from those with the classic form. Patients tend to undergo surgical interventions earlier, as pharmacologic options can further exacerbate MS symptoms.[51] In addition, patients also tend to have an increased number and more frequent surgeries than patients with classic TN.[51]

DIAGNOSIS OF TRIGEMINAL NEURALGIA

A proper and thorough patient history is of the utmost importance when diagnosing TN, as it is a partially exclusionary diagnosis that is based on specific clinical features, whereas subsequent testing may be used to further elucidate the specific cause.[1]

The third edition of the International Classification of Headache Disorders (ICHD-3) by the International Headache Society, published in 2018, defined the features necessary for the diagnosis of TN.

Diagnostic Criteria

A. Recurrent unilateral facial pain in one or more distributions of the trigeminal nerve with no radiation beyond and fulfilling criteria B and C
B. Pain has the following characteristics:
1. Lasts from a fraction of a second to 2 minutes
2. Severe intensity
3. Electric shocklike, shooting, stabbing, or sharp in quality
C. Precipitated by innocuous stimuli within the affected trigeminal distribution
D. Is not accounted for by another ICHD-3 diagnosis[1]

A diagnosis of classic TN fulfills the aforementioned criteria and demonstrates NVC of the trigeminal nerve root with associated morphologic changes seen either on preoperative MRI or by direct visualization intraoperatively.

Classic TN can further be broken down into classic TN with purely paroxysmal pain in which the interval between attacks is pain free and classic TN with concomitant continuous pain in which there is continuous or near-continuous pain between attacks in the affected distribution.

Secondary TN is diagnosed based on the fulfillment of the criteria for TN highlighted earlier along with the pain attributed to a separate causative comorbid condition. Within secondary TN, there are 3 subdiagnoses: TN attributed to MS, TN attributed to space-occupying lesions, and TN attributed to other causes.

Finally, ITN is diagnosed when the criterion for TN is met, but neither classic nor secondary TN can be diagnosed based on MRI and electrophysiological tests. Similarly, to classic TN, idiopathic TN can be subdivided into purely paroxysmal pain or TN with concomitant continuous pain.

TN is frequently both mis- and under-diagnosed in the primary and secondary care settings. Although clear diagnostic criteria exist, the variable presentation of symptoms as well as their distribution and sometimes subtle pain qualities can lead to misdiagnosis in various clinical environments. Patients with TN consult a variety of medical professionals for their pain including primary care physicians, dentists, otolaryngologists, neurosurgeons, neurologists and/or headache specialists.[5,52] It is important to consider as well as exclude alternative diagnoses before arriving at TN as the final diagnosis.

The differential diagnoses for TN pain are expansive. The following list, although not complete, lists those that should be considered most often: glossopharyngeal neuralgia, painful posttraumatic trigeminal neuropathy, persistent idiopathic facial pain, painful trigeminal neuropathy attributed to acute herpes zoster, burning mouth syndrome, short-lasting unilateral neuralgiform headache attacks with autonomic symptoms, short-lasting unilateral neuralgiform headache attacks with conjunctival injection and tearing, migraine variants, paroxysmal hemicrania, cluster headaches, giant cell arteritis, occipital neuralgia, nervus intermedius neuralgia, perineural head and neck malignancies, trigeminal nerve or tract lesions, cavernous or cerebellopontine angle lesion, dental pain, temporomandibular joint dysfunction, osteomyelitis, glaucoma, sinus disease, and otitis media.[5,19,52,53] A careful patient history should provide particular characteristics of the location, onset, character, and duration of pain. Further questioning should seek to identify any associated symptoms in order to rule out alternative diagnoses (**Table 1**) before the diagnosis of TN.

MANAGEMENT AND TREATMENT OF TRIGEMINAL NEURALGIA

Pharmacologic agents are considered first line for the treatment of TN regardless of cause. Surgical or interventional procedure modalities are considered only when either pharmacologic measures are contraindicated or when the pain becomes refractory to medication therapy. Postoperatively, patients will often continue medical therapy albeit at lower doses.[42]

Pharmacologic Management Options

Before treatment, electrocardiogram and laboratory testing are done to ensure proper heart, liver, and kidney function. Furthermore, most medications used to treat TN pain are teratogenic. Women who expect to become pregnant or are of child-bearing age should be appropriately counseled. There are currently 10 Food and Drug Administration–approved medications for the treatment of TN: carbamazepine, oxcarbazepine, baclofen, lamotrigine, pimozide, gabapentin ± ropivacaine, phenytoin, tizanidine, and botulinum toxin A. In addition, pregabalin, topiramate, levetiracetam, and vixotrigine, according to various case series and reports, suggest some treatment response but their use remains off-label.

Carbamazepine/Oxcarbazepine

Carbamazepine is a sodium channel blocker with level A evidence for its use and is the most commonly prescribed first-line medication for the management of symptoms associated with TN.[54–58] Initial dosage is generally 100 to 200 mg twice a day, and escalations are done gradually (100 mg every other day up to 1600 mg) to avoid adverse reactions until pain relieved or side effects occur.[59] The number needed to treat (NNT) for any pain relief is 1.9 and 2.6 for significant pain relief,[5,60,61] whereas the number needed to harm is 3.4 for minor reactions and 24 for serious events.[55,59]

Among severe adverse events, Stevens-Johnson syndrome (SJS) and toxic epidermal necrolysis (TEN) have been shown to be associated with individuals who harbor the HLA-B*1502 allele when taking carbamazepine and is more commonly found in certain Asian populations. Carbamazepine is contraindicated in patients with atrioventricular conduction abnormalities and before its use all patients should undergo an electrocardiogram. It can also result in several other conditions including hyponatremia, certain blood disorders, and multiple neurologic side effects (eg, tiredness, sleepiness, memory problems, disturbed sleep, difficulty concentrating, and unsteadiness).[59,62] Routine blood sampling is necessary to monitor cell count and organ function.

Oxcarbazepine is a derivative of carbamazepine and has also been shown to be effective in reducing pain from TN. Daily dose ranges are between 300 and 1200 mg.[59] Although oxcarbazepine has the benefit of having far fewer side effects, when compared with carbamazepine, the body of evidence is lacking (level B evidence) and as a result is generally considered a second-line treatment option.[54,55,62]

Table 1
List of alternative diagnoses for trigeminal neuralgia sorted by characteristic features

Characteristic of Pain	Distinguishing Features	Alternative Diagnoses
Onset	Recent rash related to herpes zoster infection	Painful trigeminal neuropathy attributed to acute herpes zoster
	Injury or accident	Painful posttraumatic trigeminal neuropathy
Location	Pain in the jaw or teeth	Cracked tooth or carries/pulpitis
	Pain in the scalp or occipital region	Occipital neuralgia, primary stabbing headaches, or paroxysmal hemicrania
	Pain in the back of the tongue or soft palate	Glossopharyngeal neuralgia
	Pain deep in the ear	Nervus intermedius neuralgia
	Bilateral pain	Tension-type headaches, temporomandibular joint disorder, or persistent idiopathic facial pain
Duration	Constant pain	Otitis, giant cell arteritis, osteomyelitis, burning mouth syndrome, or trigeminal neuropathy
Associated symptoms	Autonomic symptoms	SUNA, SUNCT, or paroxysmal hemicrania

Recent pharmacodynamic and pharmacokinetic studies for these medications have shown gender-specific differences that become important and should be considered when determining the rate and extent of dose escalations. Women demonstrate adverse effects at significantly lower doses. The potential toxic daily dose in women was 800 mg and 1200 mg of carbamazepine and oxcarbazepine, respectively. Conversely, the toxic daily dose for men was 1200 mg and 1800 mg of carbamazepine and oxcarbazepine, respectively.[5,63]

Other Medications

Baclofen, lamotrigine, gabapentin ± ropivacaine, pimozide, phenytoin, tizanidine, and botulinum toxin A are all supported by randomized controlled trials (level C evidence). However, they are used most commonly as therapeutic adjunct or after first- and second-line medications have failed.[54,55]

Baclofen is a γ-aminobutyric acid type B receptor agonist with a relatively safe side-effect profile. The NTT is 1.4, with most patients requiring 50 to 80 mg daily. Because of its mechanism of action, it important to wean off the drug slowly to avoid withdrawal-like symptoms. Baclofen demonstrates synergistic effects with carbamazepine and is regularly used in combination therapy.[64,65]

Lamotrigine is another second-line medication, with daily dosing between 200 and 400 mg and can be used in combination with carbamazepine.[59,66,67] Similar to carbamazepine and oxcarbazepine, lamotrigine requires gradual dose escalation to avoid SJS, TEN, and DRESS syndrome.

Gabapentin exerts its effects on voltage-activated calcium channels, limiting neurotransmitter release and has been shown to significantly reduce neuropathic pain in multiple randomized controlled trials. But there has been only one study that has specifically investigated the use of gabapentin, albeit in conjunction with ropivacaine, for TN.[68] Gabapentin has several advantages favoring its use: faster dose titration ability and a favorable side-effect profile with limited concern for severe drug or adverse skin reactions seen with the other medications. It is generally also used in combination therapy with other drugs.

Pimozide is a dopamine receptor antagonist that has been tested in a randomized double-blind crossover trial for refractory TN. Despite excellent pain control outcomes, it is rarely used due to its severe side-effect profile that includes risk of arrhythmias, extrapyramidal symptoms, and Parkinsonism.[69]

Phenytoin, another sodium channel blocker, is generally used adjunctively with carbamazepine with daily dose ranges between 200 and 300 mg. It has a large side-effect profile, and its routine use for chronic symptom management has fallen out of favor. However, it remains effective option in acute settings because intravenous boluses allow for rapid therapeutic serum levels.

Tizanidine is an alpha-adrenergic agonist with limited evidence to support its use. In a small trial all treated patients (n = 10) who initially had good pain relief developed recurrence of symptoms within 3 months.[70]

Botulinum toxin A (BTA) has been useful for the treatment of other pain conditions such as migraines, tension headaches, occipital headaches, and postherpetic neuralgias. To date, there has been one randomized controlled trial and 5 prospective open-label studies that have investigated the use of BTA for the treatment of TN.[71–76] In these studies, patients were injected between 5 and 75 units. Most of the patients received a dose of between 20 and 50 units.[5] Four weeks postprocedures, pain relief was reported in 70% to 100% of all patients, and there was a 60% to 100% reduction in the mean pain intensity and frequency. In another study following injection of BTA, 47% of patients did not require any further treatment, 33% of patients continued use of nonsteroidal antiinflammatory drugs, and the remaining 20% had good response with the use of traditional pharmacologic therapy.[73] Initial studies have yield significant pain relief outcomes; however, further investigation is necessary to better understand its indications as well as any long-term recurrence and complication rates.

Some medications have shown some evidence for use in small, lower evidence studies. In an open-label study, pregabalin, a medication structurally similar to gabapentin, showed a reduction in TN-associated pain in 50% to 74% of patients.[77] Similarly, a small study showed pain reduction in 75% taking topiramate for symptoms of classic TN.[78] But when carbamazepine alone was compared with the combination therapy of carbamazepine and topiramate, there was no additional benefit.[79] Levetiracetam is a newer antiepileptic medication that inhibits presynaptic calcium channels thereby decreasing neurotransmitter release. In 2 small studies investigating its use, patients reported 50% to 90% improvement in pain and a 62% reduction in daily attacks.[80,81] Lastly, vixotrigine is a $Na_v1.7$ selective sodium channel blocker that is currently undergoing a phase III randomized controlled trial.[82] Preliminary evidence from a phase 2a withdrawal randomized controlled trial indicated that vixotrigine had a moderate effect.[83]

Surgical and Radiosurgical Treatment Options

Although there are no specific guidelines for the selection and timing, it is recommended that patients be managed as part of a multidisciplinary team. In general, surgical options should be considered after the patient has either failure or had an adequate trial of medication management. In addition, the patient's age, general health, surgeon's level of expertise, and the available facilities may further influence the consideration and/or timing of any surgical intervention.

Percutaneous Treatment Options

Percutaneous procedures seek to create a focal injury to trigeminal nerve afferents within the gasserian ganglion. These procedures include the most commonly performed thermocoagulation via radiofrequency ablation, as well as chemical neurolysis via glycerol injection, mechanical neurolysis via balloon compression nerve blocks, and cryotherapy. Historically these procedures have been used most in patients older than 65 years, as well as patients with MS, pontine infarct, or local mass lesions affecting the dorsal root entry zone.

Radiofrequency (RF) ablation is performed typically under short-acting general anesthesia or deep sedation, whereas a cannula and RF probe are inserted into the trigeminal ganglion through foramen ovale. The entry point is 2.5 cm lateral to the corner of the mouth and 1 cm inferior with a trajectory aimed toward a point 3 cm anterior to the ipsilateral external auditory meatus and in the plane of the mid-pupillary line. Glycopyrrolate may be give before entering the foramen ovale with the cannula to avoid the vagal effects that can occur with dural puncture. The initial placement of the probe is determined based on the dermatomal distribution of pain as well as the relationship of the cannula to the clival line with the use of intra-operative fluoroscopy. The patient is then partially awoken to confirm proper placement with the use of sensory test stimulation (100 Hz, 1 msec pulse width, 0.1–0.15 V amplitude). Afterward the patient is placed back under general anesthesia for the ablation. The ablation typically consists of 2 lesions made at 70 to 80°C for 90 seconds each. The use of sensory test stimulation can help improve the selectivity of the procedure. Nearly 100% of patients with an adequate ablation will experience immediate pain relief. It is expected that patients have some numbness within the prior pain distribution area.

The technique for glycerol rhizotomy is similar to RF ablation in terms of obtaining access to the trigeminal cistern. Once access is obtained, the patient is repositioned to a sitting position with their head flexed. A cisternogram is then performed to estimate the volume of the trigeminal cistern. Afterward glycerol is slowly injected to the appropriate volume, and the patient remains upright, sitting with their head flexed for at least 1 to 2 hours. The effect is not immediate, and it can in some instances take up to 2 weeks for pain relief.[84]

Balloon compression does not require the patient to be awake and can be done under general anesthesia. The foramen ovale is similarly accessed as previously described, at which point a No. 4 Fogarty balloon catheter is placed through the cannula and inflated to an intraluminal pressure of 1200 to 1500 mm Hg and maintained for 1 to 2 minutes; this results in compression of the nerve with presumed sparing of the small unmyelinated fibers responsible for corneal reflex and is thought to provide additionally an aspect of dural stretching, resulting in some *decompression* of the trigeminal ganglion. Most patients experience pain relief immediately or within 1 to 2 days following the procedure.

A pooled analysis showed that 19% to 58% of patients were pain free at 4 to 11 years after glycerol injection, 26% to 82% after radiofrequency ablation, and 55% to 80% after balloon compression.[85] Although pain-free rates are promising, large variations between institutions prevent strong conclusions from being drawn. Multiple treatments can improve outcomes but at the risk of increased morbidity, most notably dysesthesias and anesthesia dolorosa.

Nerve blocks can be helpful in an acute setting. Their effect typically lasts only hours but can be helpful in managing severe exacerbations, allowing time for other administered medications to start working.[86,87]

Microvascular Decompression

Microvascular decompression remains the gold-standard primary surgical treatment of patients suffering from classic TN symptoms caused by neurovascular conflict. For secondary TN that remains refractory to pharmacologic management or treatment of the underlying cause and for idiopathic TN any of the percutaneous ablative procedure of the gasserian ganglion described earlier may be performed.

The goal of microvascular decompression (MVD) is to separate the trigeminal nerve root from the blood vessels that are in contact with the nerve root; this is done through a retrosigmoid craniotomy to gain access to the trigeminal nerve root within the posterior cranial fossa. Although this procedure is the most invasive technique for the treatment of TN, it has been shown to provide the lowest rate of pain recurrence and the highest patient satisfaction.[88] Greater than 73% of patients maintained pain relief 5 years after the procedure, with 62% to 89% of patients with classic TN pain free at 3 to 11 years.[54,55,85] In general, the average TN recurrence rate is approximately 4% per year.[89]

Complications from an MVD are rare, and morbidity ranges from 0.3% to 3% and mortality from 0.2% to 0.5%. The lowest complications are seen at high-volume hospital centers where the procedure is done routinely.[90] Complications can include cerebral spinal fluid leak, aseptic meningitis, cerebral infarcts, hematomas, unilateral hearing loss, facial weakness, and facial sensory loss.[54,55,91]

Stereotactic Radiosurgery

Stereotactic radiosurgery is another ablative procedure that can help treat TN. One common modality, Gamma Knife, uses radiation (75–85 Gy) from a cobalt-60 gamma emission source to target the root entry zone of the trigeminal nerve root and can be used in patients with or without vascular compression. Because of the destructive nature of radiosurgery, patients often endorse sensory loss following the procedure. Higher radiation doses resulted in better pain relief outcomes but come at the expense of an increase in the area of sensory loss.[54,55] Pooled analysis demonstrates that 30% to 66% of patients remained pain free 4 to 11 years after surgery.[85] Because of mechanistic action of radiation therapy, pain relief on average is delayed 1 month. Other studies have shown that the proportion of patients who have pain relief can continue to increase for up to 24 months after radiation.[5,92–94]

Although microvascular decompression has been shown to have longer period of pain relief and lower rates of recurrence (70%–74% relief at 10 years; 18% recurrence at 25 years) compared with Gamma Knife Radiosurgery (GKRS) (67% relief at 3 years), the less-invasive nature of radiosurgery allows it to be offered to patients who may be ineligible for the more invasive microvascular decompression while still offering favorable pain relief.[95,96]

SUMMARY

In recent years, the classic definitions for TN have been revised as a result of improved mechanistic understanding of the pathophysiology. Initially, the pain management and treatment of TN begins with an accurate diagnosis among myriad of differential diagnoses, followed by an adequate trial of one of the many effective pharmacologic options currently available. Percutaneous and open microvascular surgical decompression or radiosurgery of the trigeminal nerve are often reserved for those patients who continue to have symptoms despite a period of nonsurgical management. Surgical interventions must be individually tailored in terms of the type of TN present and taking into consideration the treatment goals of the patient. Despite the volume of research currently available of this topic, there is still a need for continued research into the pathophysiology and management of TN.

CLINICS CARE POINTS

- It is important to consider all alternative diagnoses and exclude them before diagnosing a patient with TN.
- Carbamazepine is a first-line treatment of TN with level A evidence supporting its use.
- Surgical treatments of TN are considered when pain is refractory to medications or medications are not indicated.

REFERENCES

1. Vincent M, Wang S jiun. Headache Classification Committee of the International Headache Society (IHS) The International Classification of Headache Disorders, 3rd edition. Cephalalgia 2018;38(1):1–211.
2. Haviv Y, Khan J, Zini A, et al. Trigeminal neuralgia (part I): Revisiting the clinical phenotype. Cephalalgia 2016;36(8):730–46.
3. Bowsher D. Trigeminal neuralgia: A symptomatic study of 126 successive patients with and without previous interventions. Pain Clinic 2000;12(2):93–101.
4. Maarbjerg S, Gozalov A, Olesen J, et al. Trigeminal neuralgia–a prospective systematic study of clinical characteristics in 158 patients. Headache 2014;54(10): 1574–82. https://doi.org/10.1111/head.12441.
5. Maarbjerg S, Benoliel R. The changing face of trigeminal neuralgia—A narrative review. Headache: The J Head Face Pain 2021;61(6):817–37.
6. Maarbjerg S, Gozalov A, Olesen J, et al. Concomitant persistent pain in classical trigeminal neuralgia–evidence for different subtypes. Headache 2014;54(7): 1173–83. https://doi.org/10.1111/head.12384.
7. Kuncz A, Vörös E, Barzó P, et al. Comparison of clinical symptoms and magnetic resonance angiographic (MRA) results in patients with trigeminal neuralgia and persistent idiopathic facial pain. Medium-term outcome after microvascular decompression of cases with positive MRA findings. Cephalalgia 2006;26(3): 266–76.
8. Tacconi L, Miles JB. Bilateral trigeminal neuralgia: a therapeutic dilemma. Br J Neurosurg 2000;14(1):33–9.
9. Katusic S, Beard CM, Bergstralh E, et al. Incidence and clinical features of trigeminal neuralgia, Rochester, Minnesota, 1945-1984. Ann Neurol 1990;27(1): 89–95.
10. Tan CY, Shahrizaila N, Goh KJ. Clinical Characteristics, Pain, and Quality of Life Experiences of Trigeminal Neuralgia in a Multi-Ethnic Asian Cohort. J Oral Facial Pain Headache 2017;31(4):e15–20. https://doi.org/10.11607/ofph.1793.
11. Benoliel R, Zadik Y, Eliav E, et al. Peripheral painful traumatic trigeminal neuropathy: clinical features in 91 cases and proposal of novel diagnostic criteria. J Orofac Pain 2012;26(1):49–58. http://www.ncbi.nlm.nih.gov/pubmed/22292140.

12. Siqueira SR, Teixeira MJ, Siqueira JT. Clinical characteristics of patients with trigeminal neuralgia referred to neurosurgery. Eur J Dent 2009;3(3):207–12. http://www.ncbi.nlm.nih.gov/pubmed/19756195.
13. Rasmussen P. Facial pain. II. A prospective survey of 1052 patients with a view of: character of the attacks, onset, course, and character of pain. Acta Neurochir (Wien) 1990;107(3–4):121–8.
14. KUGELBERG E, LINDBLOM U. The mechanism of the pain in trigeminal neuralgia. J Neurol Neurosurg Psychiatr 1959;22(1):36–43.
15. Younis S, Maarbjerg S, Reimer M, et al. Quantitative sensory testing in classical trigeminal neuralgia-a blinded study in patients with and without concomitant persistent pain. Pain 2016;157(7):1407–14.
16. Maier C, Baron R, Tölle TR, et al. Quantitative sensory testing in the German Research Network on Neuropathic Pain (DFNS): somatosensory abnormalities in 1236 patients with different neuropathic pain syndromes. Pain 2010;150(3): 439–50.
17. Rasmussen P. Facial pain. IV. A prospective study of 1052 patients with a view of: precipitating factors, associated symptoms, objective psychiatric and neurological symptoms. Acta Neurochir (Wien) 1991;108(3–4):100–9.
18. Simms HN, Honey CR. The importance of autonomic symptoms in trigeminal neuralgia. Clinical article. J Neurosurg 2011;115(2):210–6.
19. Maarbjerg S, di Stefano G, Bendtsen L, et al. Trigeminal neuralgia – diagnosis and treatment. Cephalalgia 2017;37(7):648–57.
20. Benoliel R, Sharav Y. Trigeminal neuralgia with lacrimation or SUNCT syndrome? Cephalalgia 1998;18(2):85–90.
21. Benoliel R, Sharav Y, Haviv Y, et al. Tic, Triggering, and Tearing: From CTN to SU-NHA. Headache 2017;57(6):997–1009.
22. Chen Q, Yi DI, Perez JNJ, et al. The Molecular Basis and Pathophysiology of Trigeminal Neuralgia. Int J Mol Sci 2022;23(7):3604.
23. Gambeta E, Chichorro JG, Zamponi GW. Trigeminal neuralgia: An overview from pathophysiology to pharmacological treatments. Mol Pain 2020;16. https://doi.org/10.1177/1744806920901890. 174480692090189.
24. Liu M, Zhong J, Xia L, et al. The expression of voltage-gated sodium channels in trigeminal nerve following chronic constriction injury in rats. Int J Neurosci 2019; 129(10):955–62.
25. Siqueira SRDT, Alves B, Malpartida HMG, et al. Abnormal expression of voltage-gated sodium channels Nav1.7, Nav1.3 and Nav1.8 in trigeminal neuralgia. Neuroscience 2009;164(2):573–7.
26. Xu W, Zhang J, Wang Y, et al. Changes in the expression of voltage-gated sodium channels Nav1.3, Nav1.7, Nav1.8, and Nav1.9 in rat trigeminal ganglia following chronic constriction injury. NeuroReport 2016;27(12):929–34.
27. Devor M, Amir R, Rappaport ZH. Pathophysiology of Trigeminal Neuralgia: The Ignition Hypothesis. Clin J Pain 2002;18(1):4–13.
28. Burchiel KJ. Abnormal impulse generation in focally demyelinated trigeminal roots. J Neurosurg 1980;53(5):674–83.
29. Calvin WH, Loeser JD, Howe JF. A neurophysiological theory for the pain mechanism of tic douloureux. Pain 1977;3(2):147–54.
30. Puil E, Spigelman I. Electrophysiological responses of trigeminal root ganglion neurons in vitro. Neuroscience 1988;24(2):635–46.
31. Rappaport HZ, Devor M. Trigeminal neuralgia: The role of self-sustaining discharge in the trigeminal ganglion. Pain 1994;56(2):127–38.

32. Love S, Coakham HB. Trigeminal neuralgia: pathology and pathogenesis. Brain 2001;124(Pt 12):2347–60.

33. Rasminsky M. Ectopic generation of impulses and cross-talk in spinal nerve roots of ?dystrophic? mice. Ann Neurol 1978;3(4):351–7.

34. Amir R, Devor M. Functional cross-excitation between afferent A- and C-neurons in dorsal root ganglia. Neuroscience 1999;95(1):189–95.

35. Rappaport ZH, Govrin-Lippmann R, Devor M. An electron-microscopic analysis of biopsy samples of the trigeminal root taken during microvascular decompressive surgery. Stereotact Funct Neurosurg 1997;68(1–4 Pt 1):182–6.

36. Lutz J, Thon N, Stahl R, et al. Microstructural alterations in trigeminal neuralgia determined by diffusion tensor imaging are independent of symptom duration, severity, and type of neurovascular conflict. J Neurosurg 2016;124(3):823–30.

37. Obermann M, Yoon MS, Ese D, et al. Impaired trigeminal nociceptive processing in patients with trigeminal neuralgia. Neurology 2007;69(9):835–41.

38. Peker S, Kurtkaya Ö, Üzün İ, et al. Microanatomy of the Central Myelin-Peripheral Myelin Transition Zone of the Trigeminal Nerve. Neurosurgery 2006;59(2):354–9.

39. Zhang C, Hu H, Das S, et al. Structural and Functional Brain Abnormalities in Trigeminal Neuralgia: A Systematic Review. J Oral Facial Pain Headache 2020; 34(3):222–35.

40. Tang Y, Wang M, Zheng T, et al. Grey matter volume alterations in trigeminal neuralgia: A systematic review and meta-analysis of voxel-based morphometry studies. Prog Neuro-Psychopharmacology Biol Psychiatry 2020;98:109821.

41. Love S. Trigeminal neuralgia: Pathology and pathogenesis. Brain 2001;124(12): 2347–60.

42. Nurmikko TJ, Eldridge PR. Trigeminal neuralgia–pathophysiology, diagnosis and current treatment. Br J Anaesth 2001;87(1):117–32.

43. Maarbjerg S, Wolfram F, Gozalov A, et al. Association between neurovascular contact and clinical characteristics in classical trigeminal neuralgia: A prospective clinical study using 3.0 Tesla MRI. Cephalalgia 2015;35(12):1077–84.

44. Antonini G, di Pasquale A, Cruccu G, et al. Magnetic resonance imaging contribution for diagnosing symptomatic neurovascular contact in classical trigeminal neuralgia: a blinded case-control study and meta-analysis. Pain 2014;155(8): 1464–71.

45. Burchiel KJ. Trigeminal Neuralgia: New Evidence for Origins and Surgical Treatment. Neurosurgery 2016;63:52–5.

46. Di Stefano G, Maarbjerg S, Truini A. Trigeminal neuralgia secondary to multiple sclerosis: from the clinical picture to the treatment options. J Headache Pain 2019;20(1):20.

47. Osterberg A, Boivie J, Thuomas KA. Central pain in multiple sclerosis–prevalence and clinical characteristics. Eur J Pain 2005;9(5):531–42.

48. Foley PL, Vesterinen HM, Laird BJ, et al. Prevalence and natural history of pain in adults with multiple sclerosis: systematic review and meta-analysis. Pain 2013; 154(5):632–42.

49. Danesh-Sani SA, Rahimdoost A, Soltani M, et al. Clinical assessment of orofacial manifestations in 500 patients with multiple sclerosis. J Oral Maxillofac Surg 2013;71(2):290–4.

50. de Simone R, Marano E, Brescia Morra V, et al. A clinical comparison of trigeminal neuralgic pain in patients with and without underlying multiple sclerosis. Neurol Sci 2005;26(Suppl 2):s150–1.

51. Ferraro D, Annovazzi P, Moccia M, et al. Characteristics and treatment of Multiple Sclerosis-related trigeminal neuralgia: An Italian multi-centre study. Mult Scler Relat Disord 2020;37:101461.
52. Antonaci F, Arceri S, Rakusa M, et al. Pitfals in recognition and management of trigeminal neuralgia. J Headache Pain 2020;21(1):82.
53. van Vliet JA, Eekers PJE, Haan J, et al, Dutch RUSSH Study Group. Features involved in the diagnostic delay of cluster headache. J Neurol Neurosurg Psychiatry 2003;74(8):1123–5.
54. Cruccu G, Gronseth G, Alksne J, et al. AAN-EFNS guidelines on trigeminal neuralgia management. Eur J Neurol 2008;15(10):1013–28.
55. Gronseth G, Cruccu G, Alksne J, et al. Practice parameter: the diagnostic evaluation and treatment of trigeminal neuralgia (an evidence-based review): report of the Quality Standards Subcommittee of the American Academy of Neurology and the European Federation of Neurological Societies. Neurology 2008;71(15): 1183–90.
56. Nicol CF. A four year double-blind study of tegretol(r)in facial pain. Headache: The J Head Face Pain 1969;9(1):54–7.
57. Killian JM. Carbamazepine in the Treatment of Neuralgia. Arch Neurol 1968; 19(2):129.
58. Campbell FG, Graham JG, Zilkha KJ. Clinical trial of carbazepine (tegretol) in trigeminal neuralgia. J Neurol Neurosurg Psychiatry 1966;29(3):265–7.
59. McMillan R. Trigeminal Neuralgia - A Debilitating Facial Pain. Rev Pain 2011;5(1): 26–34.
60. Wiffen P, Collins S, McQuay H, et al. Anticonvulsant drugs for acute and chronic pain. Cochrane Database Syst Rev 2005;3:CD001133.
61. Wiffen PJ, McQuay HJ, Moore RA. Carbamazepine for acute and chronic pain. Cochrane Database Syst Rev 2005;3:CD005451.
62. Besi E, Boniface DR, Cregg R, et al. Comparison of tolerability and adverse symptoms in oxcarbazepine and carbamazepine in the treatment of trigeminal neuralgia and neuralgiform headaches using the Liverpool Adverse Events Profile (AEP). J Headache Pain 2015;16:563.
63. Zakrzewska JM, Patsalos PN. Oxcarbazepine: a new drug in the management of intractable trigeminal neuralgia. J Neurol Neurosurg Psychiatry 1989;52(4): 472–6.
64. Fromm GH, Terrence CF, Chattha AS, et al. Baclofen in trigeminal neuralgia: its effect on the spinal trigeminal nucleus: a pilot study. Arch Neurol 1980;37(12): 768–71.
65. Fromm GH, Terrence CF, Chattha AS. Baclofen in the treatment of trigeminal neuralgia: double-blind study and long-term follow-up. Ann Neurol 1984;15(3):240–4.
66. Zakrzewska JM, Chaudhry Z, Nurmikko TJ, et al. Lamotrigine (lamictal) in refractory trigeminal neuralgia: results from a double-blind placebo controlled crossover trial. Pain 1997;73(2):223–30.
67. Lunardi G, Leandri M, Albano C, et al. Clinical effectiveness of lamotrigine and plasma levels in essential and symptomatic trigeminal neuralgia. Neurology 1997;48(6):1714–7.
68. Khan OA. Gabapentin relieves trigeminal neuralgia in multiple sclerosis patients. Neurology 1998;51(2):611–4.
69. Lechin F, van der Dijs B, Lechin ME, et al. Pimozide therapy for trigeminal neuralgia. Arch Neurol 1989;46(9):960–3.
70. Vilming ST, Lyberg T, Lataste X. Tizanidine in the Management of Trigeminal Neuralgia. Cephalalgia 1986;6(3):181–2.

71. Wu CJ, Lian YJ, Zheng YK, et al. Botulinum toxin type A for the treatment of trigeminal neuralgia: results from a randomized, double-blind, placebo-controlled trial. Cephalalgia 2012;32(6):443–50.
72. Piovesan EJ, Teive HG, Kowacs PA, et al. An open study of botulinum-A toxin treatment of trigeminal neuralgia. Neurology 2005;65(8):1306–8.
73. Bohluli B, Motamedi MHK, Bagheri SC, et al. Use of botulinum toxin A for drug-refractory trigeminal neuralgia: preliminary report. Oral Surg Oral Med Oral Pathol Oral Radiol Endod 2011;111(1):47–50.
74. Zúñiga C, Díaz S, Piedimonte F, et al. Beneficial effects of botulinum toxin type A in trigeminal neuralgia. Arq Neuropsiquiatr 2008;66(3A):500–3.
75. Türk U, Ilhan S, Alp R, et al. Botulinum toxin and intractable trigeminal neuralgia. Clin Neuropharmacol 2005;28(4):161–2. https://doi.org/10.1097/01.wnf.0000172497.24770.b0.
76. Borodic GE, Acquadro MA. The use of botulinum toxin for the treatment of chronic facial pain. J Pain 2002;3(1):21–7.
77. Obermann M, Yoon MS, Sensen K, et al. Efficacy of pregabalin in the treatment of trigeminal neuralgia. Cephalalgia 2008;28(2):174–81.
78. Domingues RB, Kuster GW, Aquino CCH. Treatment of trigeminal neuralgia with low doses of topiramate. Arq Neuropsiquiatr 2007;65(3B):792–4.
79. Wang QP, Bai M. Topiramate versus carbamazepine for the treatment of classical trigeminal neuralgia: a meta-analysis. CNS Drugs 2011;25(10):847–57.
80. Jorns TP, Johnston A, Zakrzewska JM. Pilot study to evaluate the efficacy and tolerability of levetiracetam (Keppra) in treatment of patients with trigeminal neuralgia. Eur J Neurol 2009;16(6):740–4.
81. Mitsikostas DD, Pantes G v, Avramidis TG, et al. An observational trial to investigate the efficacy and tolerability of levetiracetam in trigeminal neuralgia. Headache 2010;50(8):1371–7.
82. Kotecha M, Cheshire WP, Finnigan H, et al. Design of Phase 3 Studies Evaluating Vixotrigine for Treatment of Trigeminal Neuralgia. J Pain Res 2020;13:1601–9.
83. Zakrzewska JM, Palmer J, Morisset V, et al. Safety and efficacy of a Nav1.7 selective sodium channel blocker in patients with trigeminal neuralgia: a double-blind, placebo-controlled, randomised withdrawal phase 2a trial. Lancet Neurol 2017;16(4):291–300.
84. Jho HD, Lunsford LD. Percutaneous retrogasserian glycerol rhizotomy. Current technique and results. Neurosurg Clin N Am 1997;8:63–74.
85. Bendtsen L, Zakrzewska JM, Abbott J, et al. European Academy of Neurology guideline on trigeminal neuralgia. Eur J Neurol 2019;26(6):831–49.
86. Seo HJ, Park CK, Choi MK, et al. Clinical Outcome of Percutaneous Trigeminal Nerve Block in Elderly Patients in Outpatient Clinics. J Korean Neurosurg Soc 2020;63(6):814–20.
87. Peters G, Nurmikko TJ. Peripheral and gasserian ganglion-level procedures for the treatment of trigeminal neuralgia. Clin J Pain 2002;18(1):28–34.
88. Tatli M, Satici O, Kanpolat Y, et al. Various surgical modalities for trigeminal neuralgia: literature study of respective long-term outcomes. Acta Neurochir (Wien) 2008;150(3):243–55.
89. Burchiel KJ, Clarke H, Haglund M, et al. Long-term efficacy of microvascular decompression in trigeminal neuralgia. J Neurosurg 1988;69(1):35–8.
90. Kalkanis SN, Eskandar EN, Carter BS, et al. Microvascular decompression surgery in the United States, 1996 to 2000: mortality rates, morbidity rates, and the effects of hospital and surgeon volumes. Neurosurgery 2003;52(6):1251–61 [discussion: 1261-2].

91. Barker FG, Jannetta PJ, Bissonette DJ, et al. The Long-Term Outcome of Micro-vascular Decompression for Trigeminal Neuralgia. New Engl J Med 1996;334(17): 1077–84.
92. Jawahar A, Wadhwa R, Berk C, et al. Assessment of pain control, quality of life, and predictors of success after gamma knife surgery for the treatment of trigeminal neuralgia. Neurosurg Focus 2005;18(5):E8.
93. Loescher AR, Radatz M, Kemeny A, et al. Stereotactic radiosurgery for trigeminal neuralgia: outcomes and complications. Br J Neurosurg 2012;26(1):45–52.
94. Tuleasca C, Carron R, Resseguier N, et al. Patterns of pain-free response in 497 cases of classic trigeminal neuralgia treated with Gamma Knife surgery and followed up for least 1 year. J Neurosurg 2012;117(Suppl):181–8.
95. Pollock BE. Comparison of posterior fossa exploration and stereotactic radiosurgery in patients with previously nonsurgically treated idiopathic trigeminal neuralgia. Neurosurg Focus 2005;18(5):E6.
96. Sanchez-Mejia RO, Limbo M, Cheng JS, et al. Recurrent or refractory trigeminal neuralgia after microvascular decompression, radiofrequency ablation, or radiosurgery. Neurosurg Focus 2005;18(5):e12.

Management of Psychiatric Symptoms in Dementia

Yavuz Ayhan, MD[a,b,c,d,*], Selam A. Yoseph, MD[a,b,c,e], Bruce L. Miller, MD[a,b,c]

KEYWORDS

- Dementia • Neuropsychiatric
- Behavioral and psychological symptoms of dementia (BPSD) • Agitation • Apathy
- Psychosis • Depression

KEY POINTS

- BPSD are associated with excess morbidity and mortality, rapid disease progression, increased nursing home placement, increased caregiver burden, and increased health care costs.
- BPSD are frequent in dementia, and reflect the neuroanatomy and neurochemistry of the disease process.
- BPSD may be triggered by medical illnesses, medications, unmet patient needs, pain, caregiving approach, and the physical environment of the patient. Potential triggers and causes should be evaluated as a part of the management plan.
- Nonpharmacologic approaches to BPSD include cognitive therapies, cognitive behavioral therapies, massage, reminiscence, music or art therapy, and animal-assisted therapies. Caregiver interventions are beneficial for the caregiver, and by improving caregiver health one can improve the patients' outcome.
- Pharmacologic approach starts for Alzheimer disease (AD) with optimizing the use of cholinesterase inhibitors and memantine where indicated.
- The studies evaluating the effects of specific drugs for BPSD have shown limited efficacy, and are primarily focused to AD.
- Harm-benefit should be carefully considered before initiating drugs, especially antipsychotics. Drug treatment should start with low doses, with gradual increments and frequent monitoring of efficiency and side effects.

[a] Department of Neurology, Memory and Aging Center, Weill Institute for Neurosciences, University of California, 675 Nelson Rising Lane, Suite 190, San Francisco, CA 94158, USA; [b] Global Brain Health Institute, University of California, San Francisco (UCSF), 1651 4th St, 3rd Floor, San Francisco, CA 94143, USA; [c] Trinity College Dublin, Dublin, Ireland; [d] Department of Psychiatry, Hacettepe University Faculty of Medicine, 06230, Sihhiye/ Altindag/ Ankara, Turkey; [e] Department of Psychiatry, Addis Ababa University, Addis Ababa, Ethiopia
* Corresponding author. Department of Psychiatry, Hacettepe University Faculty of Medicine, 06230, Sihhiye/ Altindag/ Ankara, Turkey.
E-mail address: yavuz.ayhan@gbhi.org

Neurol Clin 41 (2023) 123–139
https://doi.org/10.1016/j.ncl.2022.05.001
0733-8619/23/© 2022 Elsevier Inc. All rights reserved.

INTRODUCTION

Behavioral and psychological symptoms of dementia (BPSD) are highly prevalent in neurodegenerative dementias. The most common symptoms are apathy, depression, anxiety, sleep disturbances, and agitation.[1,2] All these symptoms have their own unique disease profile in dementia and reflect specific anatomic and chemical changes in the brain. The course of BPSD changes with the disease state and tends to occur more frequently as the disease progresses.[3] Mood symptoms, apathy, irritability, sleep disorders, and even psychosis may occur before the emergence of cognitive symptoms, representing a prodrome.[4,5] Comorbid diseases, constipation, pain, unmet needs of the patient, diminished nutritional status, new traumatic events, and poor care environment may prompt the emergence of BPSD,[6] and these triggers need to be sought and treated when present. BPSD are associated with rapid progression of dementia,[7] increased nursing home placement,[8] hospitalization,[9] caregiver burden,[10] and societal cost.[11] These complications can be reduced with proper treatment.[12]

When possible, BPSD should be screened for and graded with a questionnaire.[13] The most commonly used instruments for clinical practice are the Neuropsychiatric Inventory (NPI) and Behavioral Pathology in Alzheimer's Disease Rating Scale (BEHAVE-AD).[14,15] Both are based on the caregiver-derived information, but a clinician rated version of the NPI is available for which the physicians use their own clinical impression for ratings.

Multiple BPSD symptoms often co-occur, further increasing their burden. When the symptoms co-occur, management can be prioritized based on the distress and potential harm of a specific symptom; however, a single approach may not suffice.[16]

It is important to remember that the types of psychiatric symptoms that emerge, particularly in the early stages of the illness, help with diagnosis. The early presence of anxiety, depression, and rapid eye movement (REM)-behavior disorder should suggest the diagnosis of Parkinson disease/dementia with Lewy bodies (PD/DLB).[17] Euphoria, disinhibition, lack of empathy, overeating, and repetitive motor behaviors characterize frontotemporal dementia (FTD).[18] Social withdrawal can occur early in Alzheimer disease (AD), but patients, at least in the early stages, may exhibit a normal psychiatric profile. As AD progresses, BPSD become more common and happen in most patients with advanced disease.[3]

This review focuses on the outpatient treatment of BPSD. Even though this article is based on published evidence, it offers a selective, not a comprehensive, review, which is influenced by the collective experiences of the authors. Sadly, for most BPSD domains, the evidence is not conclusive, and the treatment options are still limited. The authors summarize their recommendations in **Box 1** and **Table 1**.

GENERAL PRINCIPLES FOR THE TREATMENT OF BEHAVIORAL AND PSYCHOLOGICAL SYMPTOMS OF DEMENTIA

It is beneficial to follow a structured framework for the management of BPSD. Describe, investigate, create, evaluate (DICE) is an evidence-based systematized way of defining the symptom, investigating its causes, creating a plan, and evaluating the outcome.[19] Similarly, a structured approach for nursing homes is valuable.[20] These and other approaches help the physician to follow an organized management plan regardless of the symptoms.

The second principle is to use nonpharmacologic options whenever possible. Nonpharmacologic interventions are safe, many involve the caregivers, and may be effective even when the BPSD are severe.[21] The caveats are, many protocols require know-

---

Box 1
Do's and don'ts in the management of behavioral and psychological symptoms of dementia

Do
- Use a structured framework in the management: helps to keep track
- Search for and eliminate the triggers
- Inform the caregivers and involve them in the treatment process
- Optimize cholinesterase inhibitors and memantine
- Use nonpharmacologic approaches when available

Do not
- Ignore the needs of caregivers
- Directly start with the drugs
- Use psychotropics indefinitely
- Use antipsychotics liberally
- Use drugs that affect mental status, especially anticholinergics and benzodiazepines

---

how, and either due to efficiency or availability reasons, many patients end up using psychotropics.[22] Nonpharmacologic treatment options will be presented under their appropriate headings, and the readers are referred to the references for further information.

The third principle for care of BPSD is to ensure that the primary treatment of dementia is provided. For example, acetylcholinesterase inhibitors (AChEIs) and memantine, alone and in combination, may help BPSD[23-25] while simultaneously improving cognition. Note that both AChEIs and memantine have side effects and are associated with behavioral disturbances in a small number of patients. Memantine should be reserved for patients with moderate to severe AD and can be used in combination with cholinesterase inhibitors or in isolation.

The fourth principle relates to the demographics and vulnerability of the patient population. Elders with dementia can be extremely sensitive to psychotropic medications, leading frequently to unwanted and unexpected side effects. Psychotropics should be started at low doses, which may be effective, and increased gradually with frequent monitoring of efficacy and side effects, leading to halting the drugs when not necessary.

Finally, often, the nonpharmacologic or pharmacologic approaches deployed by the clinician for BPSD do not work. When beginning intervention, it is important to let the patient and their caregivers know that BPSD can be difficult to treat and that despite best intentions from the health care provider the patient's symptoms may persist. Sometimes the appearance of BPSD may require a change in the environment, such as placement in a nursing facility.

THE TREATMENT OF SPECIFIC BEHAVIORAL AND PSYCHOLOGICAL SYMPTOMS OF DEMENTIA
Depression

Depressive symptoms can be the first manifestation of a neurodegenerative disorder,[26] with late-life depression posing a significant risk.[27,28] In AD, depressive symptoms might be prodromal as a part of the disease process.[29,30] In particular, late-life depression is a risk factor or early prodromal feature of PD/DLB.[31]

Cognitive behavioral therapy (CBT), interpersonal therapy, and mindfulness-based interventions may be effective for depressive symptoms, particularly for those patients with mild cognitive impairment.[32-34] Also, structured sleep hygiene programs, massage and touch therapy, occupational therapy, reminiscence, exercise, art and music

| | Why Is This Question | |
Questions to Ask	Relevant?	Recommendations
Table 1		
Questions to Ask, Probes to Follow		
What are you dealing with?	Deconstructing the problematic behavior and identifying the target symptoms will help to get better treatment response	General and specific screening tools are available to better identify the symptoms.
Are there any triggering factors?	The problem behavior might be due to external or internal factors. By ignoring the potential triggers, your management will only suppress the expression of the symptom, if it works at all.	Concomitant illnesses, pain, emotional and social problems, unmet needs, too many or too few stimuli, and caregiving problems may contribute to the symptom formation. Address these as much as possible.
How can you better organize the caregiving environment?	Improvements of care quality and the caregiving environment positively affect BPSD. Caregiver well-being is directly related to your patients' status.	Inform the caregivers, help them to overcome their problems associated with the burden. Assess the daily life and the environment of the patient for necessary adjustments
Are AChEls and memantine optimally used in the treatment of your patient?	AChEls and memantine are associated not only with better cognition but also with improvements in BPSD.	The use of dementia drugs solely for BPSD is not rationalized, but when indicated as a primary treatment, use these drugs. Be aware that on occasion, these might be associated with BPSD too.
Is there a nonpharmacologic approach you can use?	Nonpharmacologic approaches are safe; they may be effective. Some studies suggest comparable effectiveness to psychotropics.	Choose the appropriate approach based on the target symptom. Effective use of nonpharmacologic approach may reduce the need for psychotropics.
Is pharmacologic treatment required?	Presence of symptoms may not always require pharmacologic treatment. In fact, less severe symptoms may be less responsive to the treatment. Psychotropics are not immune from side effects.	Assess the severity of the target symptom by its potential harm risk, the distress to the patient and the caregiver, and potential negative effects on daily living
What is the suitable pharmacologic approach?	Patients with dementia are generally elderly, and the neurodegenerative	• Monotherapy better than combination • Start low

(continued on next page)

Questions to Ask	Why Is This Question Relevant?	Recommendations
Table 1 (*continued*)		
	disease process makes them vulnerable to the medication effects.	• Increase the dose gradually • Monitor for the efficacy and the adverse events • Use minimum effective dose • Discontinue when not needed
What is important in choosing the drug for BPSD?	Drugs that affect sensorium and cognition will impair the clinical status of your patient. Many patients with dementia are more prone to falls and under more risk of vascular events, risks that may increase with certain psychotropics. Antipsychotics are associated with increased morbidity and mortality risk.	Avoid drugs with high anticholinergic properties. Avoid benzodiazepines and Z-drugs. Use antipsychotics only when highly necessary. Keep drug interactions in mind.

Abbreviation: AChEI, acetylcholinesterase inhibitor.

therapies, and bright light may show efficacy for carefully selected patients.[35,36] Bright light was useful in nursing homes.[37] More placebo-controlled studies are still needed to truly determine the efficacy of these nonpharmacologic interventions.

Selective Serotonin Reuptake Inhibitors (SSRIs) are the safest pharmacologic option for many of the BPSD. Positive studies exist with sertraline, citalopram, and escitalopram in AD and FTD; however, the efficacy seems to be somewhat limited.[38–40] The doses of citalopram and escitalopram are constrained due to their arrhythmogenic effects. Of note, some studies with positive outcome used higher doses, which resulted in QTc prolongation.

The evidence for other antidepressants is less robust. In one study, trazodone was effective for depressive symptoms (and other BPSD) in behavioral variant FTD (bvFTD).[41] In another cohort study, trazodone was associated with cognitive decline.[42] The efficacy of mirtazapine is also questionable and might be limited to a subgroup of patients.[43] Mianserin had similar efficacy to citalopram in an early small study.[44] Venlafaxine and duloxetine are used for geriatric depression, but the studies in dementia are scarce and the results suggest mild efficacy at best.[45,46] Vortioxetine was beneficial in an open label study of depressed patients with AD.[47] One argument for the limited efficacy in most studies is that antidepressants are more effective in clinically depressed patients[39] and that prescribing for subthreshold symptoms might be associated with reduced effectiveness.[48]

Anxiety

Studies specifically addressing anxiety symptoms in dementia are sparse. Anxiety may be a risk factor or a prodromal symptom in AD and DLB.[49] Anxiety symptoms generally correlate with depression, irritability, and agitation.[50] CBT, exercise, music therapy, and aromatherapy can be effective in dementia.[51–53] SSRIs are preferred for long-term treatment. For acute anxiety, reassurance, support, or distraction might help. Buspirone has limited supportive evidence.[54] Generally, benzodiazepines should be avoided in patients with dementia, although there are some with severe agitation or anxiety who benefit from cautious use of benzodiazepines. Antipsychotics may reduce anxiety, but their use in dementia and in the elderly carries significant risks (see following discussion).

Agitation/Aggression

Agitation and aggression are frequent in dementia and may be long lasting or display a relapsing course.[55,56] Nonpharmacologic options include massage and touch therapy, music therapy, pet-assisted interventions, multidisciplinary care, and personally tailored interventions.[57,58] For long-term treatment, SSRIs are beneficial with small to medium effect sizes.[40] The response may occur late and is more prominent in the presence of depression and dysphoria.[40,59] Citalopram displayed comparable efficacy to antipsychotics,[60] but the effects may be partly due to sedation.[61] In limited number of studies, trazodone displayed effectiveness.[40] Mirtazapine was not efficacious with increased death rates.[62]

Antipsychotics should be used as a last resort[63] (see Psychosis section), but they are used frequently for agitation in various clinics.[64] Risperidone 1 to 2 mg/d was reported to be beneficial over quetiapine and haloperidol, although the extrapyramidal effects of risperidone are always a concern.[65] Risperidone is approved for aggression in patients with AD (in differing stages) in Europe, Canada, and Australia but not in the United States.[66–68] Aripiprazole when used for psychosis was also useful for agitation in institutionalized patients.[69]

There are small but positive studies with lithium,[70] medical cannabinoids,[71] pimavanserin,[72] and dextromethorphan-quinidine,[73] but all these compounds have adverse side effects.[74] Carbamazepine was useful in early studies, but there are few studies of this compound in recent years.[75] Beta blockers were tried with variable success but use with AChEIs is problematic due to cardiac rate-limiting effects. Overall, the trials for agitation have been criticized for high dropout rates and lack of control populations.[76]

Psychosis

Delusions and hallucinations occur in one-fifth to half of patients with dementia.[77,78] Delusions display a stable but sometimes relapsing course in AD.[56] The pharmacologic treatment of psychosis includes antipsychotics. Antipsychotics are associated with increased risk of mortality due to vascular events in dementia[79,80] and carry a black box warning. Fortunately, mortality risk diminishes with withdrawal.[81] Antipsychotics should only be considered after the evaluation of alternative approaches.[82,83] When required, antipsychotics should be first tried on a short-term basis with frequent reassessment as to dose and necessity. Typical antipsychotics are not recommended unless there is delirium and severe agitation.[84]

For dementia-related psychosis (DRP), risperidone, olanzapine, quetiapine, and aripiprazole are associated with slight improvement in symptoms with somnolence, motor side effects including parkinsonism, falls, metabolic and cardiovascular side effects, and increased risk of mortality.[85–87] Data are accumulating for pimavanserin in DRP.[88,89] Additional clinical experience and data on safety in DRP is needed.[90]

Psychosis in DLB/Parkinson disease dementia (PDD) is common and may occur in up to one-third of patients. In many cases the psychosis is associated with visual hallucinations, and delusional misidentification of people, buildings, or animals.[91] The nature of psychosis in DLB/PDD, PD, and AD may differ; however, the treatment approach is comparable for all 3.[92,93] Dopaminergics and anticholinergics should be reassessed as a trigger for the psychosis. Similarly, determining whether delirium is a cause for the psychosis is important. For DLB/PDD, AChEls may help improve symptoms and do not have the problem of sedation or increasing extrapyramidal symptoms.[94] If not, quetiapine, clozapine, and pimavanserin may be tried,[93] but the evidence for them is weak, and clozapine might be problematic due to its anticholinergic effects. Hallucinations, misperceptions, and even delusions may not always require treatment, and with treatment hallucinations may respond to lesser doses compared with delusions.[93]

Disinhibition

Disinhibition is a complex construct and more common in frontotemporal lobar dementia (FTLD) than AD.[95,96] In AD, disinhibition generally occurs with agitation, aggression, hyperactivity, and impulsivity cluster.[97]

The research on interventions is limited. Nonpharmacologic interventions include diversion and distraction tactics or engagement to hobbies.[97,98] In some instances, a paid assistant may be needed to prevent the patients with FTD from getting into trouble with disinhibition, and 40% of such patients commit antisocial behavior that do or could lead to incarceration.[99] SSRIs may be effective and safe, and this observation is supported by experimental data.[100–102] In practice, atypical antipsychotics are also used for disinhibition.[103,104] Aripiprazole was useful for sexual disinhibition in cases with AD and bvFTD.[105,106] The risk of antipsychotics in dementia applies here as well.

Apathy

Apathy is frequent, starts early, and is generally persistent in AD and many other dementias.[107] Apathy is a component of bvFTD, and this symptom is associated with caregiver burden.[108] Owing to its high frequency and treatment difficulty, apathy poses a challenge to clinicians.[109] Nonpharmacologic treatments for apathy include multisensory stimulation, music therapy, cognitive stimulation, and pet therapy.[110,111] Regarding the pharmacologic options, psychostimulants, in particular methylphenidate 20 mg/d, were reported to be effective in several studies.[112,113] In another study modafinil at 200 mg/d was not effective.[114] Generally, there is a risk for delirium, agitation, and exacerbation of bad behaviors with stimulants, which limits the enthusiasm of these investigators for their use.

The data on antidepressants are contradictory. Sertraline and citalopram improved apathy in AD in some studies,[115,116] and also SSRIs have been reported to cause apathy.[117] In general, antidepressants are not effective in FTLD.[101] Noradrenergic agents may be beneficial in theory, but there is little empirical evidence to support their use in dementia. Bupropion is not effective in AD[118] or in Huntington disease (HD).[119]

Sleep

Sleep problems are highly prevalent in dementia because the neurodegenerative process attacks brainstem, and diencephalic systems involved with sleep. Recent work suggests that both amyloid and tau are cleared from the brain during deep sleep, and any medications that diminish deep sleep like the benzodiazepines or antipsychotics carry the theoretic risk of triggering or exacerbating AD.[120,121] Tau accumulates early in wake promoting neurons in AD increasing the likelihood of sleepiness in these subjects.[121–123] Sleep-wake problems are integral in DLB.[124] REM behavior disorder or the acting out of dreams is often a prodromal feature. Up to 80% of these patients eventually develop this sleep syndrome. Orexinergic neuron degeneration with tau accumulation occurs in the lateral hypothalamus in PSP[123] where severe and persistent insomnia is common.

CBT directed to insomnia helped sleep in Mild Cognitive Impairment (MCI) and mild AD.[125] Lifestyle interventions including exercise, sleep hygiene, diet, and bright light therapy may be useful.[126] BPSD may be notable at night (sundowning), and environmental organization, daytime planning, exercise, and reducing the stimulation at evening hours may help prevent this.[127]

The evidence for pharmacologic treatments is scarce.[128] Orexin antagonists may be beneficial.[129] The efficacy of melatonin is uncertain with a few positive studies.[130] Trazodone 50 mg may improve sleep.[131,132] Mirtazapine had negative results in AD.[133] The authors suggest avoiding benzodiazepines, other GABAergics, and antipsychotics in patients with dementia.

Eating Disorders

Eating difficulties eventually occur in the late stages of dementia, leading to weight loss and malnourishment. Postural changes, modification of diet, and behavioral management strategies may be effective.[134]

Hyperphagia, pica, and oral explorative behaviors are seen in dementias,[135] more prominently in bvFTD.[136] Overeating was associated with hyperactive behaviors, longer institutionalization, caregiver approach, and antipsychotic use.[137,138] Cognitive techniques and topiramate 25 to 50 mg/d may help.[139,140]

Compulsive eating and carbohydrate craving can respond to serotonergic antidepressants.[14,141] "Messy" eating, rigid eating habits, passivity, and food faddism are also reported in FTLD.[136,142,143] These problems may be addressed by behavioral and environmental management (see Ref.[127,144])

OTHER PROBLEMATIC BEHAVIORS

Repetitive behaviors are part of the clinical criteria of bvFTD and frequent in FTLD syndromes[18,145] but are also seen in AD and HD.[1] Serotonergic antidepressants can be used, but evidence for their efficacy is limited.[146] Wandering is frequent and may become problematic. Caregiver education, environmental organization, increased control, and supervision may help to prevent harm associated with them.[127]

SUMMARY

BPSD are frequent, present as a component of dementia, and are associated with significant burden. Proper management may help reduce morbidity, the caregiver burden, and the health care cost. Eliminating potential triggers, nonpharmacologic management, and caregiver involvement is essential. There are no conclusive data on the treatment of many BPSD dimensions, and future research is needed.

CLINICS CARE POINTS

- The presentation of behavioral complaints may be complicated. Standardized tools may help the physician to identify target symptoms and generate a management plan.
- Potential environmental triggers should be assessed and addressed.
- Optimizing the use of cholinesterase inhibitors for AD and DLB and memantine for AD may help for the BPSD.

- Nonpharmacologic treatments may be helpful and reduce the need for psychotropics.
- Consider the severity of the symptoms and their effects on daily activities of living when planning drug treatments.
- Drugs specific to BPSD should be carefully monitored for safety and efficacy. Avoid indefinite use of psychotropics.
- Drugs that affect sensorium should be avoided as much as possible.
- Antipsychotics are associated with increased mortality in dementia and their use should be limited.

DISCLOSURE

The authors declare no conflict of interest.

ACKNOWLEDGEMENT

YA and SAY are Atlantic Fellows for Equity in Brain Health at the Global Brain Health Institute (GBHI), BLM is codirector and a faculty member at the GBHI.

REFERENCES

1. Zhao Q-F, Tan L, Wang H-F, et al. The prevalence of neuropsychiatric symptoms in Alzheimer's disease: systematic review and meta-analysis. J Affect Disord 2016;190:264–71.
2. Leung DKY, Chan WC, Spector A, et al. Prevalence of depression, anxiety, and apathy symptoms across dementia stages: A systematic review and meta-analysis. Int J Geriatr Psychiatry 2021;36(9):1330–44.
3. Eikelboom WS, van den Berg E, Singleton EH, et al. Neuropsychiatric and cognitive symptoms across the Alzheimer disease clinical spectrum: cross-sectional and longitudinal associations. Neurology 2021;97(13):e1276–87.
4. Ismail Z, Gatchel J, Bateman DR, et al. Affective and emotional dysregulation as pre-dementia risk markers: exploring the mild behavioral impairment symptoms of depression, anxiety, irritability, and euphoria. Int Psychogeriatr 2018;30(2): 185–96.
5. Bateman DR, Gill S, Hu S, et al. Agitation and impulsivity in mid and late life as possible risk markers for incident dementia. Alzheimers Dement (N Y). 2020; 6(1):e12016.
6. Gerlach LB, Kales HC. Managing behavioral and psychological symptoms of dementia. Psychiatr Clin North Am 2018;41(1):127–39.
7. Peters ME, Schwartz S, Han D, et al. Neuropsychiatric symptoms as predictors of progression to severe Alzheimer's dementia and death: the Cache County Dementia Progression Study. Am J Psychiatry 2015;172(5):460–5.
8. Toot S, Swinson T, Devine M, et al. Causes of nursing home placement for older people with dementia: a systematic review and meta-analysis. Int Psychogeriatr 2017;29(2):195–208.
9. Matsuoka T, Manabe T, Akatsu H, et al. Factors influencing hospital admission among patients with autopsy-confirmed dementia. Psychogeriatrics 2019; 19(3):255–63.
10. Liu S, Liu J, Wang X-D, et al. Caregiver burden, sleep quality, depression, and anxiety in dementia caregivers: a comparison of frontotemporal lobar

degeneration, dementia with Lewy bodies, and Alzheimer's disease. Int Psychogeriatr 2018;30(8):1131–8.

11. Angeles RC, Berge LI, Gedde MH, et al. Which factors increase informal care hours and societal costs among caregivers of people with dementia? A systematic review of Resource Utilization in Dementia (RUD). Health Econ Rev 2021; 11(1):37.

12. Burley CV, Livingston G, Knapp MRJ, et al. Time to invest in prevention and better care of behaviors and psychological symptoms associated with dementia. Int Psychogeriatr 2020;31:1–6.

13. van der Linde RM, Stephan BCM, Dening T, et al. Instruments to measure behavioural and psychological symptoms of dementia. Int J Methods Psychiatr Res 2014;23(1):69–98.

14. Cummings J. The neuropsychiatric inventory: development and applications. J Geriatr Psychiatry Neurol 2020;33(2):73–84.

15. Reisberg B, Monteiro I, Torossian C, et al. The BEHAVE-AD assessment system: a perspective, a commentary on new findings, and a historical review. Dement Geriatr Cogn Disord 2014;38(1–2):89–146.

16. Kales HC. Common sense: addressed to geriatric psychiatrists on the subject of behavioral and psychological symptoms of dementia. Am J Geriatr Psychiatry 2015;23(12):1209–13.

17. Seritan AL, Rienas C, Duong T, et al. Ages at onset of anxiety and depressive disorders in parkinson's disease. J Neuropsychiatry Clin Neurosci 2019;31(4): 346–52.

18. Rascovsky K, Hodges JR, Knopman D, et al. Sensitivity of revised diagnostic criteria for the behavioural variant of frontotemporal dementia. Brain 2011; 134(Pt 9):2456–77.

19. Kales HC, Gitlin LN, Lyketsos CG. Detroit expert panel on assessment and management of neuropsychiatric symptoms of dementia. Management of neuropsychiatric symptoms of dementia in clinical settings: recommendations from a multidisciplinary expert panel. J Am Geriatr Soc 2014;62(4):762–9.

20. Lichtwarck B, Selbaek G, Kirkevold Ø, et al. Targeted interdisciplinary model for evaluation and treatment of neuropsychiatric symptoms: A cluster randomized controlled trial. Am J Geriatr Psychiatry 2018;26(1):25–38.

21. Hsu T-J, Tsai H-T, Hwang A-C, et al. Predictors of non-pharmacological intervention effect on cognitive function and behavioral and psychological symptoms of older people with dementia. Geriatr Gerontol Int 2017;17(Suppl 1):28–35.

22. Vasudev A, Shariff SZ, Liu K, et al. Trends in psychotropic dispensing among older adults with dementia living in long-term care facilities: 2004-2013. Am J Geriatr Psychiatry 2015;23(12):1259–69.

23. Campbell N, Ayub A, Boustani MA, et al. Impact of cholinesterase inhibitors on behavioral and psychological symptoms of Alzheimer's disease: a meta-analysis. Clin Interv Aging 2008;3(4):719–28.

24. Kishi T, Matsunaga S, Oya K, et al. Memantine for Alzheimer's disease: an updated systematic review and meta-analysis. J Alzheimers Dis 2017;60(2): 401–25.

25. Tsoi KKF, Chan JYC, Leung NWY, et al. Combination therapy showed limited superiority over monotherapy for Alzheimer disease: a meta-analysis of 14 randomized trials. J Am Med Dir Assoc 2016;17(9):863.e1–8.

26. Brenowitz WD, Zeki Al Hazzouri A, Vittinghoff E, et al. Depressive symptoms imputed across the life course are associated with cognitive impairment and cognitive decline. J Alzheimers Dis 2021;83(3):1379–89.

27. Ly M, Karim HT, Becker JT, et al. Late-life depression and increased risk of dementia: a longitudinal cohort study. Transl Psychiatry 2021;11(1):147.
28. Lee ATC, Fung AWT, Richards M, et al. Risk of incident dementia varies with different onset and courses of depression. J Affect Disord 2021;282:915–20.
29. Grinberg LT, Rüb U, Ferretti REL, et al. The dorsal raphe nucleus shows phospho-tau neurofibrillary changes before the transentorhinal region in Alzheimer's disease. A precocious onset? Neuropathol Appl Neurobiol 2009; 35(4):406–16.
30. Robinson AC, Roncaroli F, Davidson YS, et al. Mid to late-life scores of depression in the cognitively healthy are associated with cognitive status and Alzheimer's disease pathology at death. Int J Geriatr Psychiatry 2021;36(5):713–21.
31. Kazmi H, Walker Z, Booij J, et al. Late onset depression: dopaminergic deficit and clinical features of prodromal Parkinson's disease: a cross-sectional study. J Neurol Neurosurg Psychiatr 2021;92(2):158–64.
32. Tay K-W, Subramaniam P, Oei TP. Cognitive behavioural therapy can be effective in treating anxiety and depression in persons with dementia: a systematic review. Psychogeriatrics 2019;19(3):264–75.
33. Orgeta V, Qazi A, Spector AE, et al. Psychological treatments for depression and anxiety in dementia and mild cognitive impairment. Cochrane Database Syst Rev 2014;(1):CD009125.
34. Wang FL, Tang QY, Zhang LL, et al. Effects of Mindfulness-based Interventions on Dementia Patients: a meta-analysis. West J Nurs Res 2020;42(12):1163–73.
35. Baruch N, Burgess J, Pillai M, et al. Treatment for depression comorbid with dementia. Evid Based Ment Health 2019;22(4):167–71.
36. Watt JA, Goodarzi Z, Veroniki AA, et al. Comparative efficacy of interventions for reducing symptoms of depression in people with dementia: systematic review and network meta-analysis. BMJ 2021;372:n532.
37. Kolberg E, Hjetland GJ, Thun E, et al. The effects of bright light treatment on affective symptoms in people with dementia: a 24-week cluster randomized controlled trial. BMC Psychiatry 2021;21(1):377.
38. Orgeta V, Tabet N, Nilforooshan R, et al. Efficacy of antidepressants for depression in Alzheimer's disease: systematic review and meta-analysis. J Alzheimers Dis 2017;58(3):725–33.
39. Dudas R, Malouf R, McCleery J, et al. Antidepressants for treating depression in dementia. Cochrane Database Syst Rev 2018;8:CD003944.
40. Hsu T-W, Stubbs B, Liang C-S, et al. Efficacy of serotonergic antidepressant treatment for the neuropsychiatric symptoms and agitation in dementia: A systematic review and meta-analysis. Ageing Res Rev 2021;69:101362.
41. Lebert F, Stekke W, Hasenbroekx C, et al. Frontotemporal dementia: a randomised, controlled trial with trazodone. Dement Geriatr Cogn Disord 2004; 17(4):355–9.
42. Sommerlad A, Werbeloff N, Perera G, et al. Effect of trazodone on cognitive decline in people with dementia: Cohort study using UK routinely collected data. Int J Geriatr Psychiatry 2021;25. https://doi.org/10.1002/gps.5625.
43. Zuidersma M, Chua K-C, Hellier J, et al, HTA-SADD Investigator Group. Sertraline and Mirtazapine Versus Placebo in Subgroups of Depression in Dementia: Findings From the HTA-SADD Randomized Controlled Trial. Am J Geriatr Psychiatry 2019;27(9):920–31.
44. Karlsson I, Godderis J, Augusto De Mendonça Lima C, et al. A randomised, double-blind comparison of the efficacy and safety of citalopram compared to

mianserin in elderly, depressed patients with or without mild to moderate dementia. Int J Geriatr Psychiatry 2000;15(4):295–305.

45. de Vasconcelos Cunha UG, Lopes Rocha F, Avila de Melo R, et al. A placebo-controlled double-blind randomized study of venlafaxine in the treatment of depression in dementia. Dement Geriatr Cogn Disord 2007;24(1):36–41.

46. Oslin DW, Ten Have TR, Streim JE, et al. Probing the safety of medications in the frail elderly: evidence from a randomized clinical trial of sertraline and venlafaxine in depressed nursing home residents. J Clin Psychiatry 2003;64(8):875–82.

47. Cumbo E, Cumbo S, Torregrossa S, et al. Treatment effects of vortioxetine on cognitive functions in mild Alzheimer's disease patients with depressive symptoms: a 12 month, open-label, observational study. J Prev Alzheimers Dis 2019;6(3):192–7.

48. Bobo WV, Grossardt BR, Lapid MI, et al. Frequency and predictors of the potential overprescribing of antidepressants in elderly residents of a geographically defined U.S. population. Pharmacol Res Perspect 2019;7(1):e00461.

49. Mendez MF. The relationship between anxiety and alzheimer's disease. J Alzheimers Dis Rep 2021;5(1):171–7.

50. Porter VR, Buxton WG, Fairbanks LA, et al. Frequency and characteristics of anxiety among patients with Alzheimer's disease and related dementias. J Neuropsychiatry Clin Neurosci 2003;15(2):180–6.

51. Dimitriou T-D, Verykouki E, Papatriantafyllou J, et al. Non-Pharmacological interventions for the anxiety in patients with dementia. A cross-over randomised controlled trial. Behav Brain Res 2020;390:112617.

52. van der Steen JT, Smaling HJ, van der Wouden JC, et al. Music-based therapeutic interventions for people with dementia. Cochrane Database Syst Rev 2018;7:CD003477.

53. Jin JW, Nowakowski S, Taylor A, et al. Cognitive behavioral therapy for mood and insomnia in persons with dementia: A systematic review. Alzheimer Dis Assoc Disord 2021;35(4):366–73.

54. Santa Cruz MR, Hidalgo PC, Lee MS, et al. Buspirone for the treatment of dementia with behavioral disturbance. Int Psychogeriatr 2017;29(5):859–62.

55. Marston L, Livingston G, Laybourne A, et al. Becoming or remaining agitated: the course of agitation in people with dementia living in care homes. The english longitudinal managing agitation and raising quality of life (MARQUE) study. J Alzheimers Dis 2020;76(2):467–73.

56. Vik-Mo AO, Giil LM, Borda MG, et al. The individual course of neuropsychiatric symptoms in people with Alzheimer's and Lewy body dementia: 12-year longitudinal cohort study. Br J Psychiatry 2020;216(1):43–8.

57. Leng M, Zhao Y, Wang Z. Comparative efficacy of non-pharmacological interventions on agitation in people with dementia: a systematic review and Bayesian network meta-analysis. Int J Nurs Stud 2020;102:103489.

58. Watt JA, Goodarzi Z, Veroniki AA, et al. Comparative efficacy of interventions for aggressive and agitated behaviors in dementia: a systematic review and network meta-analysis. Ann Intern Med 2019;171(9):633–42.

59. Weintraub D, Drye LT, Porsteinsson AP, et al. Time to response to citalopram treatment for agitation in Alzheimer disease. Am J Geriatr Psychiatry 2015;23(11):1127–33.

60. Viscogliosi G, Chiriac IM, Ettorre E. Efficacy and safety of citalopram compared to atypical antipsychotics on agitation in nursing home residents with alzheimer dementia. J Am Med Dir Assoc 2017;18(9):799–802.

61. Newell J, Yesavage JA, Taylor JL, et al. Sedation mediates part of Citalopram's effect on agitation in Alzheimer's disease. J Psychiatr Res 2016;74:17–21.
62. Banerjee S, High J, Stirling S, et al. Study of mirtazapine for agitated behaviours in dementia (SYMBAD): a randomised, double-blind, placebo-controlled trial. Lancet 2021;398(10310):1487–97.
63. Frederiksen KS, Cooper C, Frisoni GB, et al. A European Academy of Neurology guideline on medical management issues in dementia. Eur J Neurol 2020; 27(10):1805–20.
64. Aigbogun MS, Cloutier M, Gauthier-Loiselle M, et al. Real-world treatment patterns and characteristics among patients with agitation and dementia in the United States: findings from a large, observational, retrospective chart review. J Alzheimers Dis 2020;77(3):1181–94.
65. Kongpakwattana K, Sawangjit R, Tawankanjanachot I, et al. Pharmacological treatments for alleviating agitation in dementia: a systematic review and network meta-analysis. Br J Clin Pharmacol 2018;84(7):1445–56.
66. Schedule of Pharmaceutical Benefits, General Pharmaceutical Schedule - Volume 1, published by: Australian Government, Department of Health. Canberra, Commonwealth of Australia.January 2022. Available at: https://www.pbs.gov.au/publication/schedule/2022/07/2022-07-01-general-%20schedule-volume-1.pdf.
67. Committee for Medicinal Products for Human Use (CHMP). Opinion following an article 30 referral for risperdal and associated names. London: European Medicines Agency; 2008.
68. Risperidone - Restriction of the Dementia Indication - Recalls and safety alerts. Available at: https://healthycanadians.gc.ca/recall-alert-rappel-avis/hc-sc/2015/43797a-eng.php?_ga=1.262734028.1767095615.1458263529.   Accessed January 18, 2022.
69. Mintzer JE, Tune LE, Breder CD, et al. Aripiprazole for the treatment of psychoses in institutionalized patients with Alzheimer dementia: a multicenter, randomized, double-blind, placebo-controlled assessment of three fixed doses. Am J Geriatr Psychiatry 2007;15(11):918–31.
70. Devanand DP, Crocco E, Forester BP, et al. Low dose lithium treatment of behavioral complications in Alzheimer's disease: lit-AD randomized clinical trial. Am J Geriatr Psychiatry 2021. https://doi.org/10.1016/j.jagp.2021.04.014.
71. Stella F, Valiengo LCL, de Paula VJR, et al. Medical cannabinoids for treatment of neuropsychiatric symptoms in dementia: systematic review. Trends Psychiatry Psychother 2021. https://doi.org/10.47626/2237-6089-2021-0288.
72. Ballard CG, Coate B, Abler V, et al. Evaluation of the efficacy of pimavanserin in the treatment of agitation and aggression in patients with Alzheimer's disease psychosis: a post hoc analysis. Int J Geriatr Psychiatry 2020;35(11):1402–8. https://doi.org/10.1002/gps.5381.
73. Cummings JL, Lyketsos CG, Peskind ER, et al. Effect of dextromethorphan-quinidine on agitation in patients with Alzheimer disease dementia: a randomized clinical trial. JAMA 2015;314(12):1242–54.
74. Watt JA, Goodarzi Z, Veroniki AA, et al. Safety of pharmacologic interventions for neuropsychiatric symptoms in dementia: a systematic review and network meta-analysis. BMC Geriatr 2020;20(1):212.
75. Tariot PN, Erb R, Podgorski CA, et al. Efficacy and tolerability of carbamazepine for agitation and aggression in dementia. Am J Psychiatry 1998;155(1):54–61.
76. Liu KY, Borissova A, Mahmood J, et al. Pharmacological treatment trials of agitation in Alzheimer's disease: a systematic review of ClinicalTrials.gov registered trials. Alzheimers Dement (N Y). 2021;7(1):e12157.

77. Chen J, Bell S, Brain C. The incidence of dementia-related psychosis in people with dementia: Results from a survey of 302 U.S. healthcare providers. Alzheimers Dement 2020;16(S6). https://doi.org/10.1002/alz.047138.

78. Vilalta-Franch J, López-Pousa S, Calvó-Perxas L, et al. Psychosis of Alzheimer disease: prevalence, incidence, persistence, risk factors, and mortality. Am J Geriatr Psychiatry 2013;21(11):1135–43.

79. Maust DT, Kim HM, Seyfried LS, et al. Antipsychotics, other psychotropics, and the risk of death in patients with dementia: number needed to harm. JAMA Psychiatry 2015;72(5):438–45.

80. Yeh T-C, Tzeng N-S, Li J-C, et al. Mortality risk of atypical antipsychotics for behavioral and psychological symptoms of dementia: a meta-analysis, meta-regression, and trial sequential analysis of randomized controlled trials. J Clin Psychopharmacol 2019;39(5):472–8.

81. Ballard C, Hanney ML, Theodoulou M, et al. The dementia antipsychotic withdrawal trial (DART-AD): long-term follow-up of a randomised placebo-controlled trial. Lancet Neurol 2009;8(2):151–7.

82. APA. Five things physicians and patients should question. Philadelphia, PA: American Psychiatric Association Choosing wisely; 2013.

83. American Geriatrics Society | Choosing Wisely. Available at: https://www.choosingwisely.org/societies/american-geriatrics-society/. Accessed January 3, 2022.

84. Ballard C. Evidence-based treatment and monitoring strategies for dementia-related psychosis. J Clin Psychiatry 2021;82(3). https://doi.org/10.4088/JCP.AD19038BR4C.

85. Yunusa I, Rashid N, Abler V, et al. Comparative efficacy, safety, tolerability, and effectiveness of antipsychotics in the treatment of dementia-related psychosis (DRP): a systematic literature review. J Prev Alzheimers Dis 2021;8(4):520–33.

86. Yunusa I, Alsumali A, Garba AE, et al. Assessment of reported comparative effectiveness and safety of atypical antipsychotics in the treatment of behavioral and psychological symptoms of dementia: a network meta-analysis. JAMA Netw Open 2019;2(3):e190828.

87. Mühlbauer V, Möhler R, Dichter MN, et al. Antipsychotics for agitation and psychosis in people with Alzheimer's disease and vascular dementia. Cochrane Database Syst Rev 2021;12:CD013304.

88. Ballard C, Banister C, Khan Z, et al. Evaluation of the safety, tolerability, and efficacy of pimavanserin versus placebo in patients with Alzheimer's disease psychosis: a phase 2, randomised, placebo-controlled, double-blind study. Lancet Neurol 2018;17(3):213–22.

89. Tariot PN, Cummings JL, Soto-Martin ME, et al. Trial of Pimavanserin in Dementia-Related Psychosis. N Engl J Med 2021;385(4):309–19.

90. The Lancet Neurology. Difficult choices in treating Parkinson's disease psychosis. Lancet Neurol 2018;17(7):569.

91. Naasan G, Shdo SM, Rodriguez EM, et al. Psychosis in neurodegenerative disease: differential patterns of hallucination and delusion symptoms. Brain 2021;144(3):999–1012.

92. Badwal K, Kiliaki SA, Dugani SB, et al. Psychosis management in lewy body dementia: A comprehensive clinical approach. J Geriatr Psychiatry Neurol 2021;19. https://doi.org/10.1177/0891988720988916.

93. Kyle K, Bronstein JM. Treatment of psychosis in Parkinson's disease and dementia with Lewy Bodies: a review. Parkinsonism Relat Disord 2020;75:55–62.

94. Taylor J-P, McKeith IG, Burn DJ, et al. New evidence on the management of Lewy body dementia. Lancet Neurol 2020;19(2):157–69.

95. Borges LG, Rademaker AW, Bigio EH, et al. Apathy and disinhibition related to neuropathology in amnestic versus behavioral dementias. Am J Alzheimers Dis Other Demen 2019;34(5):337–43.

96. Magrath Guimet N, Miller BL, Allegri RF, et al. What do we mean by behavioral disinhibition in frontotemporal dementia? Front Neurol 2021;12:707799.

97. Keszycki RM, Fisher DW, Dong H. The hyperactivity-impulsivity-irritability-disinhibition-aggression-agitation domain in Alzheimer's disease: current management and future directions. Front Pharmacol 2019;10:1109.

98. Sarangi A, Jones H, Bangash F, et al. Treatment and management of sexual disinhibition in elderly patients with neurocognitive disorders. Cureus 2021; 13(10):e18463.

99. Liljegren M, Naasan G, Temlett J, et al. Criminal behavior in frontotemporal dementia and Alzheimer disease. JAMA Neurol 2015;72(3):295–300.

100. Trieu C, Gossink F, Stek ML, et al. Effectiveness of pharmacological interventions for symptoms of behavioral variant frontotemporal dementia: a systematic review. Cogn Behav Neurol 2020;33(1):1–15.

101. Nisar M, Abubaker ZJ, Nizam MA, et al. Behavioral and cognitive response to selective serotonin reuptake inhibitors in frontotemporal lobar degeneration: a systematic review and meta-analysis. Clin Neuropharmacol 2021;44(5):175–83.

102. Hughes LE, Rittman T, Regenthal R, et al. Improving response inhibition systems in frontotemporal dementia with citalopram. Brain 2015;138(Pt 7):1961–75.

103. Nagata T, Shinagawa S, Nakajima S, et al. Classification of neuropsychiatric symptoms requiring antipsychotic treatment in patients with Alzheimer's disease: analysis of the CATIE-AD study. J Alzheimers Dis 2016;50(3):839–45.

104. Lee KS, Kim S-H, Hwang H-J. Behavioral and Psychological symptoms of dementia and antipsychotic drug use in the elderly with dementia in korean long-term care facilities. Drugs Real World Outcomes 2015;2(4):363–8.

105. Nomoto H, Matsubara Y, Ichimiya Y, et al. A case of frontotemporal dementia with sexual disinhibition controlled by aripiprazole. Psychogeriatrics 2017; 17(6):509–10.

106. Sarikaya S, Sarikaya B. Aripiprazole for the Treatment of inappropriate sexual behavior: case report of an Alzheimer's disease patient known as heterosexual with recently shifted sexual orientation to same gender. J Alzheimers Dis Rep 2018;2(1):117–21.

107. Sherman C, Liu CS, Herrmann N, et al. Prevalence, neurobiology, and treatments for apathy in prodromal dementia. Int Psychogeriatr 2018;30(2):177–84.

108. Merrilees J, Dowling GA, Hubbard E, et al. Characterization of apathy in persons with frontotemporal dementia and the impact on family caregivers. Alzheimer Dis Assoc Disord 2013;27(1):62–7.

109. Mortby ME, Adler L, Agüera-Ortiz L, et al. Apathy as a treatment target in alzheimer's disease: implications for clinical trials. Am J Geriatr Psychiatry 2021. https://doi.org/10.1016/j.jagp.2021.06.016.

110. Cai Y, Li L, Xu C, et al. The effectiveness of non-pharmacological interventions on apathy in patients with dementia: a systematic review of systematic reviews. Worldviews Evid Based Nurs 2020;17(4):311–8.

111. Theleritis C, Siarkos K, Politis AA, et al. A systematic review of non-pharmacological treatments for apathy in dementia. Int J Geriatr Psychiatry 2018;33(2):e177–92.

112. Ruthirakuhan MT, Herrmann N, Abraham EH, et al. Pharmacological interventions for apathy in Alzheimer's disease. Cochrane Database Syst Rev 2018;5: CD012197.

113. Mintzer J, Lanctôt KL, Scherer RW, et al. Effect of methylphenidate on apathy in patients with alzheimer disease: the ADMET 2 randomized clinical trial. JAMA Neurol 2021;78(11):1324–32.

114. Frakey LL, Salloway S, Buelow M, et al. A randomized, double-blind, placebo-controlled trial of modafinil for the treatment of apathy in individuals with mild-to-moderate Alzheimer's disease. J Clin Psychiatry 2012;73(6):796–801.

115. Takemoto M, Ohta Y, Hishikawa N, et al. The efficacy of sertraline, escitalopram, and nicergoline in the treatment of depression and apathy in alzheimer's disease: the okayama depression and apathy project (ODAP). J Alzheimers Dis 2020;76(2):769–72.

116. Zhou T, Wang J, Xin C, et al. Effect of memantine combined with citalopram on cognition of BPSD and moderate Alzheimer's disease: A clinical trial. Exp Ther Med 2019;17(3):1625–30.

117. Padala PR, Padala KP, Majagi AS, et al. Selective serotonin reuptake inhibitors-associated apathy syndrome: A cross sectional study. Medicine (Baltimore) 2020;99(33):e21497.

118. Maier F, Spottke A, Bach J-P, et al. Bupropion for the treatment of apathy in alzheimer disease: a randomized clinical trial. JAMA Netw Open 2020;3(5): e206027.

119. Gelderblom H, Wüstenberg T, McLean T, et al. Bupropion for the treatment of apathy in Huntington's disease: a multicenter, randomised, double-blind, placebo-controlled, prospective crossover trial. PLoS One 2017;12(3):e0173872.

120. Insel PS, Mohlenhoff BS, Neylan TC, et al. Association of Sleep and β-Amyloid Pathology Among Older Cognitively Unimpaired Adults. JAMA Netw Open 2021;4(7):e2117573. https://doi.org/10.1001/jamanetworkopen.2021.17573.

121. Ju Y-ES, Ooms SJ, Sutphen C, et al. Slow wave sleep disruption increases cerebrospinal fluid amyloid-β levels. Brain 2017;140(8):2104–11.

122. Holth JK, Fritschi SK, Wang C, et al. The sleep-wake cycle regulates brain interstitial fluid tau in mice and CSF tau in humans. Science 2019;363(6429):880–4.

123. Oh J, Eser RA, Ehrenberg AJ, et al. Profound degeneration of wake-promoting neurons in Alzheimer's disease. Alzheimers Dement 2019;15(10):1253–63.

124. McKeith IG, Boeve BF, Dickson DW, et al. Diagnosis and management of dementia with Lewy bodies: Fourth consensus report of the DLB Consortium. Neurology 2017;89(1):88–100.

125. Cassidy-Eagle E, Siebern A, Unti L, et al. Neuropsychological functioning in older adults with mild cognitive impairment and insomnia randomized to CBT-I or control group. Clin Gerontol 2018;41(2):136–44.

126. Falck RS, Davis JC, Best JR, et al. Effect of a Multimodal Lifestyle Intervention on Sleep and Cognitive Function in Older Adults with Probable Mild Cognitive Impairment and Poor Sleep: A Randomized Clinical Trial. J Alzheimers Dis 2020;76(1):179–93.

127. Stages & Behaviors | Alzheimer's Association. Available at: https://www.alz.org/help-support/caregiving/stages-behaviors. Accessed January 24, 2022.

128. McCleery J, Sharpley AL. Pharmacotherapies for sleep disturbances in dementia. Cochrane Database Syst Rev 2020;11:CD009178.

129. Herring WJ, Ceesay P, Snyder E, et al. Polysomnographic assessment of suvorexant in patients with probable Alzheimer's disease dementia and insomnia: a randomized trial. Alzheimers Dement 2020;16(3):541–51.

130. Wade AG, Farmer M, Harari G, et al. Add-on prolonged-release melatonin for cognitive function and sleep in mild to moderate Alzheimer's disease: a 6-month, randomized, placebo-controlled, multicenter trial. Clin Interv Aging 2014;9:947–61.
131. Camargos EF, Pandolfi MB, Freitas MPD, et al. Trazodone for the treatment of sleep disorders in dementia: an open-label, observational and review study. Arq Neuropsiquiatr 2011;69(1):44–9.
132. Camargos EF, Louzada LL, Quintas JL, et al. Trazodone improves sleep parameters in Alzheimer disease patients: a randomized, double-blind, and placebo-controlled study. Am J Geriatr Psychiatry 2014;22(12):1565–74.
133. Scoralick FM, Louzada LL, Quintas JL, et al. Mirtazapine does not improve sleep disorders in Alzheimer's disease: results from a double-blind, placebo-controlled pilot study. Psychogeriatrics 2017;17(2):89–96.
134. Abdelhamid A, Bunn D, Copley M, et al. Effectiveness of interventions to directly support food and drink intake in people with dementia: systematic review and meta-analysis. BMC Geriatr 2016;16:26.
135. Shinagawa S, Honda K, Kashibayashi T, et al. Classifying eating-related problems among institutionalized people with dementia. Psychiatry Clin Neurosci 2016;70(4):175–81.
136. Ikeda M, Brown J, Holland AJ, et al. Changes in appetite, food preference, and eating habits in frontotemporal dementia and Alzheimer's disease. J Neurol Neurosurg Psychiatr 2002;73(4):371–6.
137. Wu H-S. Predictors of hyperphagia in institutionalized patients with dementia. J Nurs Res 2014;22(4):250–8.
138. Chi L-W, Lin S-C, Chang S-H, et al. Factors associated with hyperphagic behavior in patients with dementia living at home. Biol Res Nurs 2015;17(5):567–73.
139. Kao C-C, Lin L-C, Wu S-C, et al. Effectiveness of different memory training programs on improving hyperphagic behaviors of residents with dementia: a longitudinal single-blind study. Clin Interv Aging 2016;11:707–20.
140. Shinagawa S, Tsuno N, Nakayama K. Managing abnormal eating behaviours in frontotemporal lobar degeneration patients with topiramate. Psychogeriatrics 2013;13(1):58–61.
141. Swartz JR, Miller BL, Lesser IM, et al. Frontotemporal dementia: treatment response to serotonin selective reuptake inhibitors. J Clin Psychiatry 1997;58(5):212–6.
142. Lewis C, Walterfang M, Velakoulis D, et al. A review: mealtime difficulties following frontotemporal lobar degeneration. Dement Geriatr Cogn Disord 2018;46(5–6):285–97.
143. Rosen HJ, Allison SC, Ogar JM, et al. Behavioral features in semantic dementia vs other forms of progressive aphasias. Neurology 2006;67(10):1752–6.
144. Managing Care for Frontotemporal Degeneration (FTD) | AFTD. Available at: https://www.theaftd.org/living-with-ftd/managing-ftd/. Accessed January 18, 2022.
145. Benussi A, Premi E, Gazzina S, et al. Progression of behavioral disturbances and neuropsychiatric symptoms in patients with genetic frontotemporal dementia. JAMA Netw Open 2021;4(1):e2030194.
146. Gambogi LB, Guimarães HC, de Souza LC, et al. Treatment of the behavioral variant of frontotemporal dementia: a narrative review. Dement Neuropsychol 2021;15(3):331–8.

Chronic Migraine
Diagnosis and Management

Doris Kung, DO[a],*, Gage Rodriguez, MD[a], Randolph Evans, MD[b]

KEYWORDS

- Chronic migraine • Migraine • Headache • Preventive treatment
- CGRP antagonists • OnabotulinumtoxinA

KEY POINTS

- Chronic migraines (CM) are underrecognized and undertreated. CM treatment has expanded in the last decade and knowledge of the available options is necessary.
- New calcitonin gene-related peptide (CGRP) antagonists are available in oral and parenteral formulations.
- Developing an individualized treatment approach for chronic migraines is important for patient adherence and effectiveness.

INTRODUCTION

Although chronic migraine (CM) is one of the most common and debilitating neurological disorders, it is often underdiagnosed and undertreated. In one study, only 25% of patients with CM received a correct diagnosis and just 4.5% of individuals consulted a health care professional for migraine, received an accurate diagnosis, and were prescribed minimal acute and preventive pharmacological treatments.[1] Hopefully, this is improving as the introduction of new effective and more tolerable acute and preventive medications in the last 5 years is generating enthusiasm for diagnosis and treatment among health care professionals and persons with migraine.

EPIDEMIOLOGY OF CHRONIC MIGRAINE

Migraine is a highly prevalent neurological disorder affecting about 40 million people in the United States and over one billion people worldwide per year. It is one of the most common disorders treated by neurologists in the outpatient setting. According to the Global Burden of Disease study in 2019, migraine remains the second most common cause of disability. It is important to recognize that it is rated the first most common cause of disability in women ages 15–49 years old and the second most common cause

[a] Neurology Department, Baylor College of Medicine, 7200 Cambridge Street, Houston, TX 77030, USA; [b] Department of Neurology, Baylor College of Medicine, 1200 Binz Street Suite 1370, Houston, TX 77004, USA
* Corresponding author.
E-mail address: kung@bcm.edu

Neurol Clin 41 (2023) 141–159
https://doi.org/10.1016/j.ncl.2022.05.005
0733-8619/23/© 2022 Elsevier Inc. All rights reserved.

of disability in men ages 15–49 years old.[2] The global prevalence rates of migraine are 19% and 10% among women and men, respectively, when standardized for age.[3]

CM is estimated to have a prevalence of 1.4–2.2% in the general population and affects around 8% of all migraine patients.[4,5] Additionally, each year 2.5% of patients with EM transform to CM.[6] Patients with CM have a larger burden of medical and psychiatric comorbidities and are more resistant to treatment than patients with EM.[7] However, spontaneous or therapy-induced remission is possible in about 26% of patients with CM over a 2-year period.[8] Thus, the recognition of CM and reduction of migraine disability is crucial.

DEFINITION OF CHRONIC MIGRAINE

The International Classification of Headache Disorders Third Edition (ICHD-3) provides criteria for the classification of migraines with aura and migraines without aura (episodic migraines), as well as CM which requires a patient to meet criteria for either of the former disorders[9] (**Table 1**). Proper classification of CM requires a careful history of the number of headache days a patient experiences per month and the presence of a diagnosis of either migraine without aura or migraine with aura. This number includes both migraine headaches and tension-type headaches, as these patients with frequent headaches often have the presence of multiple headache types. ICHD-3 criteria do allow for the inclusion of medication overuse headaches (MOH) in the definition of CM and include all headache days, even those which are not considered severe, debilitating, or requiring rescue medication. Patients must report 15 or more days per a 30-day period where headache was present–in the case of a single headache lasting multiple days, it is counted as the number of days it occurred, rather than as a single episode. Within these 15 days at least 8 should meet the criteria for migraine with or without aura, or at least believed to be a migraine at onset and relieved by an acute medication. This headache frequency must be present for 3 or more months prior to diagnosis.

PATHOPHYSIOLOGY

The development of CM is not well understood but several experimental and animal models have provided insight into possible mechanisms, including the breakdown of the normal descending pain pathways, abnormal central sensitization, and altered communication within the trigeminal, autonomic, and thalamic networks. These disruptions combined with genetic and environmental stressors ultimately lower the patient's sensory threshold leading to increased susceptibility to migraines. Arguably, patients with CM may have an even lower threshold than patients with EM causing them to become more prone to cycle into or be unable to escape a CM state.[10]

Risk factors for progression from episodic to CM with moderate to strong strength of evidence include the following: obesity, frequent headache days, persistent-frequent nausea with migraine, cutaneous allodynia, depression, asthma, noncephalic

Table 1	
ICHD-3 criteria for chronic migraines	
A.	Headaches on $\geq$ 15 days out of the month for > 3 months, and
B.	Patient has had at least 5 attacks, and
C.	At least $\geq$ 8 of the headaches fulfill the criteria for Migraines without aura or Migraines with aura, and
D.	Are not better accounted for by another diagnosis.

pain, snoring, acute medication use/overuse, and acute migraine treatment efficacy.[11] Risk factors with fair strength of evidence include the following: female gender, caffeine intake, major life events, head and neck injury, and insomnia.

MEDICATION OVERUSE HEADACHES

There is often a large overlap of patients with CM who also meet the criteria for MOH, defined by headaches occurring on 15 or more days per month and a 3-month period of regular overuse of one or more acute medications.[11] Overuse is defined as the use of all acute medications for 10 or more days per month, except in the case of simple analgesics such as acetaminophen or ibuprofen which requires 15 or more days of use. Use of opiates for 8 or more days per month and butalbital-containing medications 5 or more days per month can result in MOH. Opiate and butalbital-containing medications are avoided due to the risk of medication overuse and habituation.

Treatment of MOH involves withdrawal of the offending agent. The patient may experience worsening headaches upon withdrawal. Transitional therapy with common headache preventive medications, slower tapering of the offending agent, or replacement medications are some strategies that have shown benefits. Preventive treatment without tapering as discussed later in discussion may also be effective.

DEVELOPING A TREATMENT PLAN

Treatment plans for both acute and preventive therapy should be individualized based on a multitude of factors. Individual choice of medication should consider the amount of available evidence of efficacy, tolerability of side effects, childbearing potential, co-morbid disease, and patient preference. All patients with a diagnosis of migraine should be offered a trial of rescue medication, beginning with options with established efficacy. Patients with migraine who have frequent or severe attacks–including by definition all patients with CM –or those who cannot tolerate acute treatment should be considered for preventive therapy. Nonpharmacologic therapy for both acute and preventive treatment such as neuromodulation, biobehavioral treatment, and nutraceuticals may be used alone or in combination with pharmacologic therapy. Patients should be educated on the use of medications, asked to maintain a headache diary, and be given recommendations for good sleep, regular exercise, proper nutrition, adequate hydration, and stress management.[12]

ACUTE TREATMENT OF MIGRAINE

Acute treatment of migraines in patients with CM is the same as in patients with EM. A variety of pharmacologic and nonpharmacologic therapies are available for acute treatment including simple over-the-counter analgesics, prescription-strength NSAIDs, targeted migraine medications such as triptans, ergot derivatives, gepants, ditans, and various neuromodulation devices. Given the significant degree of disability and functional impairment that may accompany migraine attacks, it is important to devise a plan for abortive treatments in every patient who presents with migraine. When EM remains untreated or unsuccessfully treated, they may have increasing duration and disability and increase the risk for disease progression to CM.[13] The American Headache Society (AHS) regularly publishes acute migraine treatment guidelines which stress that clinicians should devise treatment plans that are evidence based, utilize rescue medications early in migraine attacks, and provide medications that can be self-administered –preferably a nonoral route when patients have either the rapid onset of attacks or significant nausea and/or vomiting. Stratified care has been shown to be a more effective treatment strategy in which patients choose targeted migraine medications at the onset of a moderate to severe migraine instead of using a stepwise approach with the initial use of nonspecific analgesics and then adding targeted migraine medications if headaches are unrelieved.[14] A brief review of the newer acute medication options is provided here.

NEWER ACUTE THERAPIES
Ditans

Lasmiditan is a newer form of acute migraine treatment which works via selective agonism for 5-HT_{1F} receptors within the trigeminal system.[15] Due to low affinity for 5-HT_{1B} receptors, lasmiditan does not cause vasoconstriction that may be seen with triptans and ergots. Because of the lack of vasoconstriction, lasmiditan could be considered in patients with vascular risk factors who might otherwise have contraindications to other abortive medications though notably, studies excluded patients with coronary artery disease, uncontrolled hypertension, and arrhythmias.[16] Dosing is 50 mg, 100 mg, or 200 mg tablets, dosed only once in a 24-h period. Side effects include sedation, fatigue, dizziness, and paresthesia. Because of significant sedation seen with use, patients should be cautioned to avoid driving for up to 8 hours following use of this medication, and it may be more reasonable to use for later migraine onset or prior to sleep rather than earlier in the day. Due to studies indicating a low potential for abuse, lasmiditan is classified as a schedule V controlled substance.[17] Similar to triptans, lasmiditan should be used cautiously with other serotonergic medications. Medication overuse is still a risk with frequent use as with any acute medication options.[18]

Oral Small-Molecule Calcitonin Gene-Related Peptide Receptor Antagonists (Gepants)

Two small-molecule calcitonin gene-related peptide (CGRP) receptor antagonists, referred to as gepants, have been FDA approved for acute treatment of migraine in adults. Rimegepant and ubrogepant have established efficacy as acute migraine therapy with a lower side effect profile than traditional acute therapies, with common side effects including nausea and somnolence.[19–21] They should be considered for patients with moderate to severe migraine who have contraindications or inefficacy with triptan usage. Similar to triptans, gepants may be most effective when taken when the pain is mild rather than when moderate to severe.[22]

Contrary to lasmiditan, gepants have not been shown to be associated with MOH.[19] The mechanism of CGRP antagonism is not associated with vasoconstriction, so they should be safe for use in patients with stable cardiovascular disease; however, studies have not included their use in patients with recent vascular events (eg, within 6 months).[23] Mice studies have suggested that use of gepants shortly following MCA occlusion worsened infarct risk and neurological deficits, so they should be used with caution in patients with recent stroke or other high risk or unstable vascular events.[24] Studies thus far have shown that use of gepants as acute medications have been safe in patients also concurrently receiving CGRP monoclonal antibodies (mAbs) as preventive treatment.[23]

ORAL PREVENTIVE TREATMENT OF CHRONIC MIGRAINE

Preventive therapy should be considered in all patients with CM. Preventive treatment options for CM have largely been derived from treatments for EM. There are a few randomized controlled trials specifically addressing oral preventive treatments for CM. Of the trials in oral therapies, the most evidence has been for topiramate. Other randomized controlled trials have looked at divalproex sodium, amitriptyline, propran-olol, candesartan, tizanidine, flunarizine, and gabapentin.[25–28] Smaller open-label tri-als have shown benefits with memantine, duloxetine, zonisamide, olanzapine, atenolol, and pregabalin.[10] Newer oral therapies are available and are approved by the United States Food and Drug Administration (FDA) for CMs, most recently ato-gepant. Other parenteral options include Onabotulinumtoxin A, which has been a longstanding safe and effective treatment of CMs. CGRP mAbs have also now been well-established as CM treatment options in the last few years. Given the variety of medication options, it is important to start with medications that are proven effective, with the fewest side effects, and are accessible to the patient. A complete preventive treatment plan should be individualized to patients and include patient ed-ucation on lifestyle modifications and avoidance of migraine triggers. Realistic expec-tations can be established by reviewing the possible outcomes which would define the prevention success of a migraine preventive. Goals may include a 50% reduction in headache days, decrease in attack duration or severity as defined by the patient, improved efficacy of acute treatments, or reduction in migraine-related disability and improvements in functioning and quality of life.[29] The selection of medications should be based on the patient's comorbid conditions, personal preference, and likeli-hood for adherence to a preventive treatment. In general, clinicians should avoid pre-ventive pharmacotherapy in pregnant or lactating women and those who are trying to conceive due to the potential for adverse effects on the developing fetus. Patients who have shown a partial response to treatment at first reassessment, it is possible that they may continue to receive cumulative benefits over 6–12 months of continued use.

Oral medications should be started at a low dose, titrating slowly until patients reach a predetermined initial target dose, and stopping once patients have optimal efficacy, intolerable adverse effects from medication, or when they have reached the maximum safe dose for that medication.[30] Preventive treatment plans should begin first with a trial for at least 8 weeks after reaching target therapeutic dose of an oral preventive from one of the following categories later in discussion. If no significant response is seen by that time, patients may be switched to a second oral preventive medication. **Table 2** provides a list of common preventive options, trial designs that were applied, typical medication dosages, and common side effects.

Antiepileptic Drugs

Topiramate
Topiramate has established efficacy as a preventive for both EM and CM.[31] Several randomized placebo-controlled trials of topiramate have demonstrated significant re-ductions in patients with CM, particularly reduction in migraine days. In one study, monthly migraine days were reduced by 5.8 days in topiramate groups compared to −0.2 days in placebo groups.[32] In a separate study, mean migraine days were significantly reduced by 6.4 days in the topiramate group compared to 4.7 days in the placebo group and migraine days compared to baseline were also reduced by 5.6 days compared to 4.1 days in the topiramate and placebo groups, respectively.[33] Topiramate may be effective in MOH without withdrawal of the overused medication.[34]

Initial target dosing is either 100 mg once daily or 50 mg twice daily. Some patients may benefit from titration up to 200 mg daily as tolerated.

Topiramate may cause weight loss and should be considered in patients with co-morbid obesity. It may be more effective in patients with frequent migraine aura. Despite its potency, side effects may be a limiting factor for use in many patients, most notably with word-finding difficulties or memory deficits. It is contraindicated

Table 2
Chronic migraine preventive treatments

Medication	Trial Designs	Typical Doses	Common Side Effects
Topiramate	RCT	50–200 mg daily (oral)	Paresthesias, weight loss, fatigue, word-finding difficulties
Amitriptyline	RCT	50–100 mg daily (oral)	Fatigue, constipation, dizziness, somnolence, weight gain, QT prolongation
Candesartan	RCT	16 mg daily (oral)	Dizziness, lightheadedness, fatigue, nausea, hypotension
Divalproex sodium	RCT	250–500 mg twice daily or 500–1000 mg delayed release form once daily (oral)	Nausea, weight gain, tremor, fatigue, alopecia
Gabapentin	RCT	Up to 2400 mg daily in divided doses three times a day (oral)	Dizziness, drowsiness, fatigue, edema
Propranolol	RCT	Up to 160 mg oral daily	Fatigue, orthostatic intolerance, dizziness
Tizanidine	RCT	Up to 24 mg daily in divided doses three times a day (oral)	Somnolence, dizziness, dry mouth, hallucinations, bradycardia
Atogepant	RCT	10, 30, or 60 mg daily (oral)	Constipation, nausea
Eptinezumab	RCT	100 mg or 300 mg administered via intravenous infusion every 3 months	Nausea, nasopharyngitis, upper respiratory infection
Erenumab	RCT	70 mg or 140 mg subcutaneous (SQ) monthly	Injection-site pain, upper respiratory tract infection, nausea
Fremanezumab	RCT	225 mg monthly or 625 mg quarterly SQ	Injection-site pain
Galcanezumab	RCT	240 mg SQ loading dose, then 120 mg SQ monthly	Injection-site pain
OnabotulinumtoxinA	RCT	155 Units in divided doses of 5 units each in 31 sites intramuscular administered every 12 weeks	Blepharoptosis, muscle weakness, neck pain, injection site pain
Flunarizine	Prospective, randomized, open-label, blinded	10 mg daily (oral)	Somnolence, dizziness, increased appetite, Parkinsonism

(continued on next page)

Table 2 (continued)			
Medication	**Trial Designs**	**Typical Doses**	**Common Side Effects**
Atenolol	OLS	50–200 mg daily (oral)	Dizziness, fatigue, hypotension
Duloxetine	OLS	Up to 60 mg daily (oral)	Nausea, decreased appetite
Memantine	OLS	10–20 mg daily in divided doses twice daily (oral)	Dizziness, insomnia
Pregabalin	OLS	75–450 mg daily (oral)	Dizziness, drowsiness, fatigue, edema, weight gain
Olanzapine	OLS	2.5–35 mg daily (oral), most patients use 5-10 mg daily	Weight gain, somnolence, dizziness, tremor, edema
Zonisamide	OLS	100–400 mg daily (oral)	Nausea, loss of appetite, dizziness, paresthesias, kidney stones

Abbreviations: OLS, open-label study; RCT, randomized controlled trial.

in patients with a history of nephrolithiasis due to its potential to cause this condition, patients who are pregnant or have a possibility of pregnancy due to teratogenicity, and patients with narrow-angle glaucoma as this may be further exacerbated.[35]

Divalproex sodium
Divalproex sodium has established efficacy and is highly effective for the prevention of CM, but is often limited by the side effect profile. It is dosed at 250–500 mg twice daily or 500–1000 mg delayed release form once daily. Open-label studies and one randomized controlled trial of sodium valproate have demonstrated a significant reduction in migraine pain levels and pain frequency. Specifically, patients with CM reported at baseline 22.05 days of headache pain in a month and by the end of the first and third months the headaches had significantly reduced to 7 days and 5.2 days, respectively, in the valproic acid groups.[36,37] Sodium valproate should be avoided in patients who wish to avoid weight gain, and may cause somnolence, hair loss, hepatotoxicity, and thrombocytopenia. Monitoring labs should be obtained to assess for the latter 2 side effects in patients using this medication. It is contraindicated in pregnancy due to high teratogenicity.[35]

Gabapentin
Gabapentin is well-known for its use in neuralgia and is FDA-approved for adjunctive use in partial-onset seizures. Still, its use in neuropathic pain and particularly in headache treatment has continued to be explored. Clinical trials have shown modest benefit in the effect of gabapentin for migraines and may suggest this treatment to be an alternative if other therapies are ineffective for patients with CM. One multicenter randomized cross-over trial with 133 patients showed a 9.1% decrease in headache days in gabapentin-treated patients compared to placebo. In patients complaining of daily headaches prior to randomization a greater than 50% decrease in headache

days was seen in 23% of patients while taking gabapentin compared to 7% of patients while on placebo.[38]

Pregabalin

Pregabalin use has been well-established in neuropathic pain similar to gabapentin. An open-label study of 30 patients given doses of 75 mg per day up to 450 mg per day demonstrated significant reductions in headache frequency and severity. Patients on pregabalin had significant decreases in the use of acute medications and significant improvements in quality of life scores. Ultimately, 40% of patients were considered to have a significant response on the pain scale and these responses were seen within 4 weeks and sustained up to 12 weeks at the end of the study.[39]

Zonisamide

Zonisamide has support from a few small open-label studies as a preventive agent for CM and can be considered in patients who may have improved with topiramate therapy but cannot tolerate cognitive side effects.[40,41] Target dosing is around 100–400 mg per day dosed once or twice daily.[42] It may cause weight loss so should be considered in patients who desire this outcome. Zonisamide has about a 2.5% risk of kidney stones.[43]

Antidepressants

Amitriptyline

Amitriptyline is a tricyclic antidepressant and is one of the earliest medications studied for migraine prevention. Early studies in chronic daily headache showed decrease in migraine frequency with doses of 50–100 mg per day. Patients taking amitriptyline noted a more significant decrease in headache days, particularly at the 8- and 12-week intervals compared to placebo groups. Notably, the number of patients reporting a greater than 50% reduction in headache days was 25–46% in the amitriptyline group compared to 5–20% in the placebo group.[44] Amitriptyline is usually started at lower doses and increased slowly to avoid adverse effects. It has anticholinergic properties and can cause dry mouth, blurred vision, constipation, and difficulty urinating. It should be considered in patients with comorbid insomnia and avoided in those who cannot tolerate fatigue. It may cause weight gain and is contraindicated in patients with glaucoma as it may worsen this condition. Amitriptyline is a second-line preventive during pregnancy and may be considered in patients who require an oral preventive but cannot tolerate propranolol. Due to a potential for QT prolongation consider obtaining a baseline EKG in patients with a personal or family history of arrhythmia or structural heart defects.[45]

Duloxetine

Duloxetine has been studied in patients with concomitant depression and CMs and shows a significant decrease in headache days. An open-label study showed a decrease from 5.8 at baseline to 1.9 on the 10-point pain scale at the end of the 8-week study. Findings from this study also showed decreases in headache days per week from a baseline of 5.2 to 2.9 days.[46] Duloxetine has a low risk of withdrawal syndrome. Its target dosing is 60 mg once daily and should be considered in patients with comorbid pain conditions such as neuropathic pain as it may work better to treat a variety of conditions.[47]

Beta-Blockers and Antihypertensive Drugs

Propranolol

Propranolol is a nonselective beta-blocker with established efficacy and is the most commonly prescribed antihypertensive medication for migraine prevention.

A head-to-head trial, TOP-PRO, has shown that propranolol may be as effective and not inferior to topiramate for CM. Mean migraine days were reduced by 5.29 days and 7.28 days ($P = 0.226$) in the topiramate and propranolol groups, respectively.[25] It is the first-line oral preventive for pregnant patients or those with a possibility of pregnancy and can be considered for patients with comorbid anxiety as well as those with mild hypertension (and contraindicated in those with hypotension). It is contraindicated in patients with asthma. Due to potential exercise intolerance, propranolol should be avoided in active patients such as athletes and runners.[35]

Candesartan
Candesartan is an angiotensin receptor blocker with recently established efficacy for migraine prevention.[48,49] Due to its favorable side effect profile as compared to propranolol, it has been studied for use in patients with EM and CM.[50] In some retrospective studies, candesartan has shown positive responses in almost half of the patients with CM with reduction in monthly headache days.[28,51] Target dosing is 8–16 mg once daily. It is generally well-tolerated and is contraindicated in patients with preexisting hypotension. It is contraindicated for use in pregnancy due to teratogenic effects.

Atenolol
Atenolol is a selective beta-blocker and has been shown to be effective in doses of 50–200 mg per day for EM prevention. A small open-label study of 17 patients with CM did show a decrease in mean headache days per month from around 20 days to less than 9 days a month after 1.5 and 3 months of taking atenolol. Headache severity also decreased significantly and 29% of patients in the study had complete remission of their CMs by the third month.[52] Side effects of atenolol include dizziness, fatigue, depression, and hypotension.

Other Oral Therapies

Flunarizine
Flunarizine is a calcium entry blocker with pharmacological effects on serotonin modulation. It is commonly used in Asian countries and has had established efficacy in EM. A prospective, randomized open-label blinded endpoint trial of flunarizine compared to topiramate in patients with CM showed a reduction in total headache days and secondary outcomes showed a reduction in the use of acute migraine medications. Patients taking flunarizine had a significant reduction in their migraine days with a mean change of −4.1 days compared to patients taking topiramate of −1.7 days. In this same study, patients on flunarizine had a significant reduction in the use of acute medications with a mean change of −2.3 days compared to patients on topiramate of −0.2 days. Patients with CM with or without medication overuse in both groups (flunarizine and topiramate groups) had similar reductions in migraine headache days.[27]

Olanzapine
Olanzapine is an atypical antipsychotic with serotonin and dopamine antagonism effects. These effects are thought to be why olanzapine may be a good choice for migraine prevention. A retrospective study of olanzapine use in patients with chronic daily headaches showed a significant decrease in headache days from 27.5 to 21.1 days and a significant decrease in headache severity on a 10 scale from 8.7 to 2.2 after 3 months of use. Thirty-six percent of patients converted to episodic headaches and 74% of patients reported improvement in their headaches overall.[53] Side effects of olanzapine may include weight gain, somnolence, dizziness, and edema.

Tizanidine

Tizanidine is a central muscle relaxant that has been studied for use in patients with chronic daily headaches. Open-label studies have shown a significant reduction in headaches reported. A randomized controlled trial has also demonstrated a significant reduction in headache frequency in 55% versus 21%, headache duration in 35% versus 19%, and headache intensity in 35% versus 20% in the tizanidine versus placebo groups, respectively.[54]

Memantine

Memantine is an N-methyl-D-aspartate (NMDA) receptor antagonist approved for the treatment of Alzheimer's disease which is rated probably effective for migraine preventive.[49] Studies of memantine have examined its usefulness in refractory migraines and have shown a significant a decrease in migraine days. However, no randomized controlled trials to date have specifically addressed CMs.[55] Target dose of memantine is 10 mg twice daily. It is generally well-tolerated but should be avoided in patients with comorbid insomnia as it may exacerbate this condition.

Atogepant

Atogepant is the first gepant designed for use as a preventive agent, which is FDA approved for episodic migraine.[56] In a 12-week study for CM prevention, the 50% or greater reduction in mean monthly migraines days for 60 mg daily, 30 mg twice daily, and placebo were as follows, respectively: 41.0%, 42.7%, and 26%.[57] The most common side effects were constipation and nausea. The 10 mg dose is recommended in patients using concomitant strong CYP3A4 inhibitors or and those with severe renal impairment. Use is not recommended in those with severe hepatic impairment. As adequate safety information is not available, use during pregnancy and lactation is not recommended. As the half-life is 11 hours, the medication can be stopped 3 days before trying to get pregnant.

PARENTERAL PREVENTION FOR CHRONIC MIGRAINE

Parenteral treatments with established efficacy for the prevention of CM include onabotulinumtoxinA and 4 mAbs targeting CGRP: eptinezumab, erenumab, fremanezumab, and galcanezumab.[58,59] Patients should be considered for parenteral prevention once they have shown an inability to tolerate or an ineffective response after an 8-week trial of at least *two* separate categories of oral preventive medications. This should also consider patients who have coexisting medical conditions where oral preventives are contraindicated and documented. There is no contraindication to concurrent use of other migraine preventives while using CGRP mAbs or onabotulinumtoxinA, so prior oral preventive medications may be continued with their initiation.

OnabotulinumtoxinA was the first drug approved specifically for CM. CGRP mAbs may be used in patients with frequency as low as 4 monthly migraine days when episodes cause at least moderate disability, and otherwise as low as 8 monthly migraine days, as well as in patients with CM. The decision on which treatment class to begin should be made based on patient preference and insurance coverage. American Headache Society guidelines suggest efficacy trial periods of 3–6 months for mAbs and 6 months for onabotulinumtoxinA.[30]

Calcitonin Gene-Related Peptide Monoclonal Antibodies

Calcitonin gene-related peptide mAbs target CGRP, a neuropeptide present in the central and peripheral nervous system which is linked to migraine pathogenesis.[60] Erenumab, fremanezumab, and galcanezumab are given as self-administered subcutaneous injections on a monthly basis (or quarterly basis for fremanezumab only), while eptinezumab is given quarterly as an intravenous (IV) infusion. Studies have shown efficacy in both episodic and CM, as well as in patients who have a lack of response to two to four previous preventive medications, and efficacy may be sustained for several years.[61–63]

Compared to oral preventive medications CGRP mAbs have a potentially lower side effect burden and have a more convenient dosing schedule of monthly or quarterly. Usual side effects include injection site reactions, constipation, and upper respiratory symptoms such as nasopharyngitis. The mAbs should be used cautiously in those with Raynaud's phenomenon, which is comorbid with migraine, as exacerbation or new-onset Raynaud's with potential ulceration has been reported.[64,65] Due to their half-life of 27–31 days, side effects may take several months to resolve even though treatment is stopped. There are no significant interactions with other medications so they can be considered in patients with polypharmacy. They have a faster onset of efficacy compared to oral options, with patients seeing the benefit in trials as early as the first week of use.[63,66] A limiting factor with these medications is that they are expensive and insurance coverage may be difficult. They are FDA approved for ages 18 and older. As adequate safety data are not available, CGRP mAbs are avoided in pregnancy and lactation.[67] Given their long half-life, CGRP mAbs should be stopped approximately 6 months before conception is attempted.[68]

Eptinezumab
Eptinezumab is a humanized CGRP mAb that targets the CGRP ligand and can be given via IV infusion either at dosages of 100 mg or 300 mg every 3 months.[62,69] In CM, eptinezumab has shown reductions in headache frequency with a 50% reduction in mean migraine days in 63.4% versus 44.5% of patients in the treatment versus placebo groups, respectively. A 75% reduction in mean migraine days was reported in 42.3% versus 22.7% of patients in the treatment versus placebo groups, respectively.[70] Side effects noted in > 2% of patients included nausea, nasopharyngitis, and upper respiratory infections. As with all CGRP mAbs benefits can be seen rapidly, as soon as the first day following initial treatment.[71]

Erenumab
Erenumab is a human CGRP mAb that targets the CGRP receptor and is dosed as either 70 or 140 mg monthly subcutaneous injections.[72–75] Erenumab studies in patients with CM have also shown 50% responder rates of 40% versus 23% in treatment versus placebo groups, respectively.[76] Further studies in CM with medication overuse and CM with prior treatment failures have also shown consistently favorable results for erenumab. The most frequently reported side effects were injection-site pain, upper respiratory tract infection, and nausea. The risk of severe constipation is higher in this medication than in others in the class. Given reports of hypersensitivity reactions it should be avoided in patients with latex allergies. Erenumab may cause the development or worsening of underlying hypertension.[62]

Fremanezumab
Fremanezumab is a humanized CGRP mAb that targets the CGRP ligand and is dosed subcutaneously as either 225 mg monthly injections or 625 mg quarterly injections.[77,78] Randomized controlled trials of the two doses have shown a 50% reduction in mean migraine days in about 40% of treated patients compared to 18% of placebo groups.[79] The risk of injection site reaction is higher than seen with erenumab.[72]

Galcanezumab

Galcanezumab is a humanized CGRP mAb which targets the CGRP ligand and is given first as a 240 mg subcutaneous loading dose, then 120 mg subcutaneous monthly.[80–82] Monthly headache days have been shown to decrease significantly and 50% responder rates are also significant with about 28 percent of treated patients responding versus 15% in placebo groups using doses of either 120 mg or 240 mg monthly.[81] Responder rates of 75% and 100% have also shown significant reductions in treatment groups with galcanezumab. The risk of injection site reaction was the only side effect reported reaching significance when compared to placebo.

OnabotulinumtoxinA

OnabotulinumtoxinA has established efficacy for the prevention of CM when administered at 12-week intervals of 155 units consisting of 31 individual injections based on the PREEMPT trial protocol.[59,82] Results from the pivotal trial noted significant decreases in headache frequency with 47.1% compared to 35.1% in the placebo group reporting at least a 50% reduction in headache days at all-time points.[83] A $\geq$50% reduction in headache-day frequency first occurred during treatment cycle 1, 2, and 3, respectively, as follows: 49.3%, 11.3%, and 10.3%.[84] OnabotulinumtoxinA may be effective even in medication overuse without withdrawal of the overused agent.

OnabotulinumtoxinA binds to cholinergic neurons via a synaptic vesicle protein 2 in conjunction with gangliosides to be taken up into cells. It is primarily taken up by cholinergic neurons including motor and autonomic neurons, and animal studies have suggested that botulinum toxin may modulate the function of nociceptive neurons involved in migraine. Another possible mechanism of action suggests onabotulinumtoxinA may prevent the activation of C fibers reducing neuronal hyperexcitability, peripheral, and central hypersensitivity by inhibiting the release of CGRP, substance P, and glutamate from peripheral trigeminal nociceptive neurons as well as disrupting TRP channels.[85]

There have been few serious adverse effects reported in trials of botulinum toxin for headache. Headache or exacerbation of headache may sometimes be a consequence of injection.[86] Brief flu-like symptoms have also been reported as a possible adverse effect.[87] As there is minimal to no systemic absorption of the toxin, the safety period (the time between stopping treatment and conception), has not been established.[71] Because insurance coverage may limit usage, a detailed CM history and clear documentation of lack of efficacy or intolerance of at least 2 classes of oral preventatives can be helpful in ensuring approval of this treatment. A treatment algorithm to consider is provided in **Fig. 1**.

Combined therapy

Although a randomized placebo-controlled trial found no benefit of adding propranolol to topiramate in CM, anecdotally many headache specialists continue to combine oral preventive medications with suspected albeit unproven benefit.[88] Many headache specialists also combine oral and parenteral medications based on anecdotal evidence in refractory patients. Five studies find benefits from combining onabotulinumtoxinA with mAbs to CGRP for refractory CM.[89–93]

Neuromodulation therapies

Neuromodulatory devices can be used alone or concurrently with medication for acute and/or preventive treatment. Several open-label studies and randomized controlled trials using neuromodulatory stimulation show mixed results when specifically

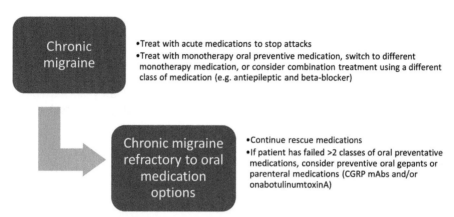

Fig. 1. Treatment algorithm for chronic migraines.

addressing CM. The only randomized controlled trial in CM was with noninvasive vagus nerve stimulation but did not show a significant reduction in migraine days.[94] Several single-center randomized controlled trials using repetitive transcranial magnetic devices in patients with CM have demonstrated a significant decrease in headache days. A few single-center randomized controlled trials have evaluated transcutaneous direct current stimulation in CM showing a significant decrease in migraine frequency, duration, and pain levels but due to variations in study design results have not been consistently replicated. Multiple devices have been studied in open-label trials with mixed results.[95] Clinicians should consider the use of neuromodulatory devices in patients who prefer nondrug therapies and those who have failed to respond to, have contraindications to or have poor tolerability with pharmacotherapy or concomitant medication. Use of these devices may be limited by insurance coverage and may be expensive out of pocket.

When to discontinue preventive medication?
There is little data to guide the discontinuation of successful preventive treatment in CM especially for those with baseline daily or almost daily headaches. Diener and colleagues[96] found that some patients with episodic migraine who improved on topiramate had sustained benefit when topiramate was discontinued after 6 months. A study of people with CM receiving onabotulinumtoxinA found that super-responders for 2 consecutive 12 weeks cycles may sustain benefit for at least 6 months following the discontinuation of onabotulinumtoxinA.[97] Patients with pretreatment daily headaches for more than 6 months were more likely to regress within 6 months of stopping treatment as compared to those with daily headaches of less than 6 months. An interesting large prospective longitudinal cohort study of patients on CGRP mAbs revealed the discontinuation of these medications could lead to temporary increases in headache frequency. Most patients (62.7%) in this study had CMs and headaches returned to baseline frequency four months after cessation.[98]

SUMMARY

Chronic migraines are often underdiagnosed and undertreated; moreover, they can be difficult to treat even for seasoned neurologist. It is important to recognize the clinical criteria for CMs, obtain a detailed history of symptoms and past medication treatment failures, identify possible lifestyle modifications, and establish clear expectations for improvement with the patient. In the last few years, novel treatment options for acute and preventive therapies have exploded providing a wide array of more tolerable options for a once largely underrecognized disease. Hopefully, future treatments will benefit the many incomplete and nonresponders. Although there is certainly room for further research in this area, the growing recognition of CMs by the physician community and the availability of newer treatment options in the last few years have given the physician and patient more options for targeted and holistic treatment of this condition.

CLINICS CARE POINTS

- Patients with chronic migraines have a larger burden of medical and psychiatric comorbidities and are more resistant to treatment than patients with episodic migraines.
- If a chronic migraine patient fails to respond to at least 2 different classes of preventative medications, parenteral medications may be effective.
- Newer oral gepants have also shown effectiveness in treating chronic migraines.

DISCLOSURE

The authors have nothing to disclose.

REFERENCES

1. Dodick DW, Loder EW, Manack Adams A, et al. Assessing barriers to chronic migraine consultation, diagnosis, and treatment: results from the chronic migraine epidemiology and outcomes (CaMEO) study. Headache 2016;56(5): 821–34.
2. Steiner TJ, Stovner LJ, Jensen R, et al. Migraine remains second among the world's causes of disability, and first among young women: findings from GBD2019. J Headache Pain 2020;21:137.
3. Reuter U. GBD 2016: still no improvement in the burden of Migraine. Lancet Neurol 2018;17(11):929–30.
4. Natoli JL, Manack A, Dean B, et al. Global prevalence of chronic migraine: a systematic review. Cephalalgia 2009;30(5):599–609.
5. Buse DC, Manack AN, Fanning KM, et al. Chronic migraine prevalence, disability, and sociodemographic factors: Results from the American migraine prevalence and Prevention Study. Headache 2012;52(10):1456–70.
6. Bigal ME, Serrano D, Buse D, et al. Acute migraine medications and evolution from episodic to chronic migraine: a longitudinal population-based study. Headache 2008;48(8):1157–68.
7. Burch RC, Buse DC, Lipton RB. Migraine. Neurol Clin 2019;37(4):631–49.
8. Manack A, Buse DC, Serrano D, et al. Rates, Predictors, and consequences of remission from chronic migraine to episodic migraine. Neurology 2011;76(8): 711–8.
9. Headache classification committee of the International Headache Society (IHS) the International Classification of Headache Disorders, 3rd Edition. Cephalalgia 2018;38(1):1–211.
10. May A, Schulte LH. Chronic migraine: risk factors, mechanisms and treatment. Nat Rev Neurol 2016;12(8):455–64.

11. Buse DC, Greisman JD, Baigi K, et al. Migraine progression: a systematic review. Headache 2019;59(3):306–38.
12. Robblee J, Starling AJ. Seeds for success: lifestyle Management in Migraine. Cleve Clin J Med 2019;86(11):741–9.
13. Lipton RB, Fanning KM, Serrano D, et al. Ineffective acute treatment of episodic migraine is associated with new-onset chronic migraine. Neurology 2015;84(7): 688–95.
14. Lipton RB, Stewart WF, Stone AM, et al. Stratified care vs step care strategies for migraine: the disability in strategies of care (DISC) study: a randomized trial. JAMA 2000;284(20):2599–605.
15. Goadsby PJ, Wietecha LA, Dennehy EB, et al. Phase 3 randomized, placebo-controlled, double-blind study of lasmiditan for acute treatment of Migraine. Brain 2019;142(7):1894–904.
16. Kuca B, Silberstein SD, Wietecha L, et al. Lasmiditan is an effective acute treatment for migraine. Neurology 2018;91(24):e2222–32.
17. Wilbraham D, Berg PH, Tsai M, et al. Abuse potential of lasmiditan: a phase 1 randomized, placebo- and alprazolam-controlled crossover study. J Clin Pharmacol 2019;60(4):495–504.
18. Rau JC, Navratilova E, Oyarzo J, et al. Evaluation of ly573144 (lasmiditan) in a preclinical model of medication overuse headache. Cephalalgia 2020;40(9): 903–12.
19. Lipton RB, Dodick DW, Ailani J, et al. Effect of ubrogepant vs placebo on pain and the most bothersome associated symptom in the acute treatment of Migraine. JAMA 2019;322(19):1887.
20. Croop R, Goadsby PJ, Stock DA, et al. Efficacy, safety, and tolerability of rimegepant orally disintegrating tablet for the acute treatment of Migraine: a randomised, phase 3, double-blind, placebo-controlled trial. The Lancet 2019; 394(10200):737–45.
21. Dodick DW, Lipton RB, Ailani J, et al. Ubrogepant for the treatment of Migraine. N Engl J Med 2019;381(23):2230–41.
22. Lipton RB, Dodick DW, Goadsby PJ, et al. Within-person analysis of ubrogepant treatment of mild versus moderate-severe headache pain during a phase 3 long-term safety extension trial (S31.006). Neurology 2022;98(18 Supplement):167.
23. Berman G, Croop R, Kudrow D, et al. Safety of Rimegepant, an oral CGRP receptor antagonist, plus CGRP monoclonal antibodies for Migraine. Headache. J Head Face Pain 2020;60(8):1734–42.
24. Mulder IA, Li M, Vries T, et al. Anti-migraine calcitonin gene–related peptide receptor antagonists worsen cerebral ischemic outcome in mice. Ann Neurol 2020;88(4):771–84.
25. Chowdhury D, Bansal L, Duggal A, et al. TOP-PRO Study: a randomized double-blind controlled trial of topiramate versus propranolol for prevention of chronic migraine. Cephalalgia 2022;42(4–5):396–408.
26. Jackson JL, Kuriyama A, Kuwatsuka Y, et al. Beta-blockers for the prevention of headache in adults, a systematic review and meta-analysis. PLoS One 2019; 14(3):e0212785.
27. Lai KL, Niddam DM, Fuh JL, et al. Flunarizine versus topiramate for chronic migraine prophylaxis: a randomized trial. Acta Neurol Scand 2017;135(4): 476–83.
28. Sánchez-Rodríguez C, Sierra A, Planchuelo-Gómez A, et al. Real world effectiveness and tolerability of candesartan in the treatment of migraine: a retrospective cohort study. Scientific Rep 2021;11(1):3846.

29. Silberstein SD. Preventive migraine treatment. Continuum 2015;21:973–89.
30. Ailani J, Burch RC, Robbins MS. The american headache society consensus statement: update on integrating new migraine treatments into clinical practice. Headache 2021;61(7):1021–39.
31. Schwedt TJ. Chronic migraine. BMJ 2014;348(mar24 5). https://doi.org/10.1136/bmj.g1416.
32. Diener H-C, Dodick D, Goadsby P, et al. Chronic migraine–classification, characteristics and Treatment. Nat Rev Neurol 2012;8(3):162–71.
33. Silberstein SD, Lipton R, Dodick D, et al. Efficacy and safety of topiramate for the treatment of chronic migraine: a randomized, double-blind, placebo-controlled trial. Headache 2007;47(2):170–80.
34. Diener HC, Bussone G, Oene JV, et al. Topiramate reduces headache days in chronic migraine: a randomized, double-blind, placebo-controlled study. Cephalalgia 2007;27:814–23.
35. Burch R. Preventive migraine treatment. Continuum 2021;27(3):613–32.
36. D'Amico D. Pharmacological prophylaxis of chronic migraine: a review of double-blind placebo-controlled trials. Neurol Sci 2010;31(Suppl 1):23–8.
37. Yurekli VA, Akhan G, Kutluhan S, et al. The effect of sodium valproate on chronic daily headache and its subgroups. J Headache Pain 2008;9:37–41.
38. Spira PJ, Beran RG. Gabapentin in the prophylaxis of chronic daily headache. Neurology 2003;61(12):1753–9.
39. Calandre EP, Garcia-Leiva JM, Rico-Villademoros F, et al. Pregabalin in the treatment of chronic migraine: an open-label study. Clin Neuropharmacol 2010;33(1):35–9.
40. Belvis R, Aceituno A, Martinez-Corral M. Zonisamide is effective in the preventive therapy of chronic migraine: doc 551. J Headache Pain 2013;14:1.
41. Villani V, Ciuffoli A, Prosperini L, et al. Zonisamide for migraine prophylaxis in topiramate-intolerant patients: An observational study. Headache 2011;51(2):287–91.
42. Bermejo PE, Dorado R. Zonisamide for migraine prophylaxis in patients refractory to topiramate. Clin Neuropharmacol 2009;32(2):103–6.
43. Jion YI, Raff A, Grosberg BM, et al. The risk and management of kidney stones from the use of topiramate and zonisamide in migraine and idiopathic intracranial hypertension. Headache 2015;55(1):161–6.
44. Couch JR. Amitriptyline in the prophylactic treatment of migraine and chronic daily headache. Headache 2011;51(1):33–51.
45. Doyle Strauss L, Weizenbaum E, Loder EW, et al. Amitriptyline dose and treatment outcomes in specialty headache practice: a retrospective cohort study. Headache 2016;56(10):1626–34.
46. Volpe FM. An 8-week, open-label trial of duloxetine for comorbid major depressive disorder and chronic headache. J Clin Psychiatry 2008;69(9):1449–54.
47. Young WB, Bradley KC, Anjum MW, et al. Duloxetine prophylaxis for episodic migraine in persons without depression: a prospective study. Headache 2013;53(9):1430–7.
48. Dorosch T, Ganzer CA, Lin M, et al. Efficacy of angiotensin-converting enzyme inhibitors and angiotensin receptor blockers in the preventative treatment of episodic migraine in adults. Curr Pain Headache Rep 2019;23(11):85–8.
49. Rau JC, Dodick DW. Other preventive anti-migraine treatments: ACE inhibitors, ARBS, calcium channel blockers, serotonin antagonists, and NMDA receptor antagonists. Curr Treat Options Neurol 2019;21(4):17.

50. Stovner LJ, Linde M, Gravdahl GB, et al. A comparative study of Candesartan versus propranolol for migraine prophylaxis: a randomised, triple-blind, placebo-controlled, double cross-over study. Cephalalgia 2013;34(7):523–32.

51. Messina R, Lastarria Perez CP, Filippi M, et al. Candesartan in migraine prevention: results from a retrospective real-world study. J Neurol 2020;267(11):3243–7.

52. Edvardsson B. Atenolol in the Prophylaxis of Chronic Migraine: a 3-Month Open-Label Study. SpringerPlus 2013;2(1):479.

53. Silberstein SD, Peres MFP, Hopkins MM, et al. Olanzapine in the treatment of refractory migraine and chronic daily headache. Headache 2002;42(6):515–8.

54. Saper JR, Lake AE III, Cantrell DT, et al. Chronic daily headache prophylaxis with tizanidine: a double-blind, placebo-controlled, multicenter outcome study. Headache 2002;42(6):470–82.

55. Huang L, Bocek M, Jordan JK, et al. Memantine for the prevention of primary headache disorders. Ann Pharmacother 2014;48(11):1507–11.

56. Goadsby PJ, Dodick DW, Ailani J, et al. Safety, tolerability, and efficacy of orally administered atogepant for the prevention of episodic migraine in adults: a double-blind, randomised phase 2B/3 trial. Lancet Neurol 2020;19(9):727–37.

57. Abbvie. Press release. AbbVie Announces Positive Phase 3 Atogepant (QULIPTA™) Data for the Preventive Treatment of Chronic Migraine. 2022. Available at: https://news.abbvie.com/news/press-releases/abbvie-announces-positive-phase-3-atogepant-qulipta-data-for-preventive-treatment-chronic-migraine.htm. Accessed March 10, 2022.

58. Silberstein SD, Holland S, Freitag F, et al. Evidence-based guideline update: Pharmacologic treatment for episodic migraine prevention in adults. Neurology 2012;78(17):1337–45.

59. Simpson DM, Hallett M, Ashman EJ, et al. Practice guideline update summary: botulinum neurotoxin for the treatment of blepharospasm, cervical dystonia, adult spasticity, and headache. Neurology 2016;86(19):1818–26.

60. Do TP, Guo S, Ashina M. Therapeutic novelties in Migraine: new drugs, new hope? J Headache Pain 2019;20(1):37.

61. Brandes JL, Diener H-C, Dolezil D, et al. The spectrum of response to erenumab in patients with chronic migraine and subgroup analysis of patients achieving ≥50%, ≥75%, and 100% response. Cephalalgia 2019;40(1):28–38.

62. Ashina M, Goadsby PJ, Reuter U, et al. Long-term safety and tolerability of erenumab: Three-plus year results from a five-year open-label extension study in episodic migraine. Cephalalgia 2019;39(11):1455–64.

63. Tepper SJ. History and review of anti-calcitonin gene-related peptide (CGRP) therapies: from Translational Research to treatment. Headache 2018;58:238–75.

64. Evans RW. Raynaud's phenomenon associated with calcitonin gene-related peptide monoclonal antibody antagonists. Headache 2019;59(8):1360–4.

65. Breen ID, Brumfield CM, Patel MH, et al. Evaluation of the safety of calcitonin gene-related peptide antagonists for migraine treatment among adults with raynaud phenomenon. JAMA Netw Open 2021;4(4):e217934.

66. Schwedt T, Reuter U, Tepper S, et al. Early onset of efficacy with erenumab in patients with episodic and chronic migraine. J Headache Pain 2018;19(1):92.

67. Rayhill M. Headache in pregnancy and lactation. Continuum (Minneap Minn) 2022;28(1):72–92.

68. Tinsley A, Rothrock JF. Safety and tolerability of preventive treatment options for chronic migraine. Expert Opin Drug Saf 2021;20(12):1523–33.

69. Lipton RB, Goadsby PJ, Smith J, et al. Efficacy and safety of eptinezumab in patients with chronic migraine. Neurology 2020;94(13):e1365–77.

70. Ray JC, Walter S, Rapoport AM, et al. Calcitonin gene related peptide in migraine: current therapeutics, future implications and potential off-target effects. J Neurol Neurosurg Psychiatr 2021;92(12):1325–34.

71. Dodick DW, Lipton RB, Silberstein S, et al. Eptinezumab for prevention of chronic migraine: a randomized phase 2B clinical trial. Cephalalgia 2019;39(9):1075–85.

72. Dodick DW, Ashina M, Brandes JL, et al. Arise: a phase 3 randomized trial of erenumab for episodic migraine. Cephalalgia 2018;38(6):1026–37.

73. Goadsby PJ, Reuter U, Hallström Y, et al. A controlled trial of erenumab for episodic migraine. N Engl J Med 2017;377(22):2123–32.

74. Tepper S, Ashina M, Reuter U, et al. Safety and efficacy of erenumab for preventive treatment of chronic migraine: a randomised, double-blind, placebo-controlled phase 2 trial. Lancet Neurol 2017;16(6):425–34.

75. Kudrow D, Pascual J, Winner PK, et al. Vascular safety of erenumab for migraine prevention. Neurology 2019;94(5):1052.

76. Lipton RB, Tepper SJ, Reuter U, et al. Erenumab in chronic migraine: patient-reported outcomes in a randomized double-blind study. Neurology 2019;92(19): e2250–60.

77. Dodick DW, Silberstein SD, Bigal ME, et al. Effect of fremanezumab compared with placebo for prevention of episodic migraine. JAMA 2018;319(19):1999.

78. Silberstein SD, Dodick DW, Bigal ME, et al. Fremanezumab for the preventive treatment of chronic migraine. N Engl J Med 2017;377(22):2113–22.

79. Detke HC, Goadsby PJ, Wang S, et al. Galcanezumab in chronic migraine. Neurology 2018;91(24):e2211–21.

80. Skljarevski V, Oakes TM, Zhang Q, et al. Effect of different doses of galcanezumab vs placebo for episodic migraine prevention. JAMA Neurol 2018;75(2):187.

81. Stauffer VL, Dodick DW, Zhang Q, et al. Evaluation of galcanezumab for the prevention of episodic migraine. JAMA Neurol 2018;75(9):1080.

82. Frampton JE, OnabotulinumtoxinA SS. A review in the prevention of chronic migraine. Drugs 2018;78(5):589–600.

83. Diener HC, Dodick DW, Turkel CC, et al. OnabotulinumtoxinA for treatment of chronic migraine: pooled results from the double-blind, randomized, placebo-controlled phases of the PREEMPT clinical program. Headache 2010;50(6): 921–36.

84. Silberstein SD, Dodick DW, Aurora SK, et al. Percent of patients with chronic migraine who responded per onabotulinumtoxinA treatment cycle: PREEMPT. J Neurol Neurosurg Psychiatr 2015;86(9):996–1001.

85. Burstein R, Zhang XC, Levy D, et al. Selective inhibition of meningeal nociceptors by botulinum neurotoxin type A: Therapeutic implications for migraine and other pains. Cephalalgia 2014;34(11):853–69.

86. Alam M. Pain associated with injection of botulinum a exotoxin reconstituted using isotonic sodium chloride with and without preservative. Arch Dermatol 2002; 138(4):510.

87. Baizabal-Carvallo JF, Jankovic J, Pappert E. Flu-like symptoms following botulinum toxin therapy. Toxicon 2011;58(1):1–7.

88. Silberstein SD, Dodick DW, Lindblad AS, et al. Chronic Migraine Treatment Trial Research Group. Randomized, placebo-controlled trial of propranolol added to topiramate in chronic migraine. Neurology 2012;78(13):976–84.

89. Boudreau GP. Treatment of chronic migraine with erenumab alone or as an add on therapy: a real-world observational study. Anesth Pain Res 2020;4(1):1–4.

90. Armanious M, Khalil N, Lu Y, et al. Erenumab and OnabotulinumtoxinA combination therapy for the prevention of intractable chronic migraine without aura: a retrospective analysis. J Pain Palliat Care Pharmacother 2021;35(1):1–6.
91. Cohen F, Armand C, Lipton RB, et al. Efficacy and tolerability of calcitonin gene-related peptide targeted monoclonal antibody medications as add-on therapy to OnabotulinumtoxinA in patients with chronic migraine. Pain Med 2021;22(8):1857–63.
92. Blumenfeld AM, Frishberg BM, Schim JD, et al. Real-World evidence for control of chronic migraine patients receiving CGRP monoclonal antibody therapy added to OnabotulinumtoxinA: a retrospective chart review. Pain Ther 2021;10(2):809–26.
93. Blazek A, Dafer R, Rhyne C, et al. Combined Prophylactic treatment of chronic migraine with OnabotulinumtoxinA and Anti-CGRP monoclonal antibodies (P14-2.001). Neurology 2022;98(18 supplement):14.
94. Silberstein SD, Calhoun AH, Lipton RB, et al. Chronic migraine headache prevention with noninvasive vagus nerve stimulation: the EVENT study. Neurology 2016;87(5):529–38.
95. Yuan H, Chuang T-Y. Update of neuromodulation in chronic migraine. Curr Pain Headache Rep 2021;25(11):71.
96. Diener H-C, Agosti R, Allais G, et al. Cessation versus continuation of 6-month migraine preventive therapy with topiramate (PROMPT): a randomised, double-blind, placebo-controlled trial. Lancet Neurol 2007;6(12):1054–62.
97. Ching J, Tinsley A, Rothrock J. Prognosis following discontinuation of OnabotulinumA Therapy in "Super-responding" Chronic Migraine Patients. Headache 2019;59(8):1279–85.
98. Raffaelli B, Terhart M, Overeem LH, et al. Migraine evolution after the cessation of CGRP(-receptor) antibody prophylaxis: a prospective, longitudinal cohort study. Cephalalgia 2022;42(4–5):326–34.

Postconcussional Syndrome
Clinical Diagnosis and Treatment

Ashley A. Taylor, MEd[a],[1], Stephen R. McCauley, PhD[b],[c],[d],[1],
Adriana M. Strutt, PhD, ABPP-CN[b],[e],*

KEYWORDS

- Postconcussion/postconcussional syndrome (PCS)
- Postconcussional disorder (PCD) • Mild traumatic brain injury (mTBI) • Concussion
- Neuropsychology

KEY POINTS

- Challenges and controversy exist related to the identification, confirmation, and treatment of PCS symptoms, because many symptoms mimic/overlap other diagnosable disorders and may be attributable to other factors (ie, medical conditions, psychiatric conditions, and psychosocial stressors).
- At present, uniform diagnostic criteria and specific treatments for PCS do not exist. Treatment approaches vary significantly and are largely aimed at symptom reduction and management.
- Despite limitations in diagnostic criteria, neuropsychological assessment of cognitive/psychiatric complaints is invaluable for individuals with PCS symptoms and is the only mechanism allowing medical professionals to obtain objective outcome data to be used for diagnostic purposes and tailored treatment recommendations.
- New evidence has emerged related to the similarities of many PCS symptoms and post-acute COVID-19 syndrome (PACS) or "long COVID," including but not limited to headaches, fatigue, and/or cognitive declines (ie, difficulties with concentration and memory), and mood changes.

DEFINITIONS

- *Traumatic brain injury (TBI)*: An alteration in brain function, or other evidence of brain pathology, caused by an external force and an injury that results from a

[a] Department of Psychological, Health, and Learning Sciences, Houston, TX, USA; [b] Department of Neurology, Baylor College of Medicine, Houston, TX 77030, USA; [c] H. Ben Taub Department of Physical Medicine & Rehabilitation, Baylor College of Medicine, Houston, TX 77030, USA; [d] Department of Pediatrics, Baylor College of Medicine, Houston, TX 77030, USA; [e] Department of Psychiatry & Behavioral Sciences, Baylor College of Medicine, Houston, TX, USA
[1] Present address: 7200 Cambridge, 9th Floor Houston, TX 77030.
* Corresponding author. UH College of Education, Stephen Power Farish Hall, 3657 Cullen Blvd, Room 491, Houston, TX 77204-5023.
E-mail address: adrianam@bcm.edu

Neurol Clin 41 (2023) 161–176
https://doi.org/10.1016/j.ncl.2022.08.003
0733-8619/23/© 2022 Elsevier Inc. All rights reserved.
neurologic.theclinics.com

bump, blow, or jolt to the head, or a penetrating head injury that disrupts normal brain function.[1,2]

- *Concussion:* A type of nonpenetrating TBI caused by a bump, blow, or jolt to the head, or by impact to the body causing the head and brain to move rapidly back and forth.[2] Concussion has also been referred to as a minimal TBI.[3]
- *Mild traumatic brain injury (mTBI):* mTBI and concussion are often used interchangeably in the literature; some research aims to classify a concussion as a less severe form of mTBI.[4]
  - To receive a diagnosis of mTBI, a patient must have had a traumatically induced physiological disruption of brain function, along with at least one of the following criteria:[5]
    1. Any period of loss of consciousness (LOC)
    2. Any loss of memory (ie, anterograde and/or retrograde)
    3. Focal neurologic deficits that can be transient or persistent in nature
    4. Impaired mental state at the time of accident (confusion, disorientation, and so on)
  - Furthermore, the severity of the injury must not exceed the following:
    1. LOC of less than or equal to 30 minutes
    2. Glasgow Coma Scale (GCS) of 13 to 15 at 30 minutes postinjury
    3. Posttraumatic amnesia less than 24 hours
  - Efforts to update the 1993 American Congress of Rehabilitation Medicine (ACRM) definition of mTBI by the Brain Injury Special Interest Group Mild Traumatic Brain Injury Task Force of the ACRM have been made. Survey findings from a study conducted by Silverberg and colleagues[6] suggest that an updated definition should:
    1. Consider a probabilistic framework that weighs observable signs more than subjective symptoms
    2. Incorporate research supporting objective cognitive, balance, and vestibular-oculomotor test findings
- Postconcussional syndrome (PCS)/postconcussional disorder (PCD): Clinically defined as the persistence (ie, greater than 3 months) of symptoms, which can encompass physical, cognitive, emotional, or sleep domains following a head injury (ie, mTBI or concussion).[7]
- Concussion grading: Multiple grading systems for mTBI have been proposed, but controversy exists regarding their value because they do not significantly assist the clinician in predicting outcome or necessarily modifying the treatment plan.[8]
- Secondary gain: Refers to external advantages (eg, social, financial, interpersonal) gained indirectly from illness or injury.[8]

POSTCONCUSSIONAL SYNDROME CRITERIA DEFINITIONS
Diagnostic and Statistical Manual of Mental Disorders (Fourth Edition, Text Revision) for Diagnosis of Postconcussional Disorder

- History of head trauma causing significant cerebral concussion
  - Manifestations include LOC, posttraumatic amnesia, and less commonly, posttraumatic seizure onset
- Cognitive deficit (identified via neuropsychological testing) in attention (concentration, shifting focus, multi-tasking) and/or memory (learning or recalling)
- Presence of at least 3 of 8 symptoms occurring shortly after injury and lasting at least 3 months: fatigue, sleep disturbance, headache, dizziness/vertigo, irritability/aggression, affective disturbance, personality change, and apathy

- Symptoms must appear after injury and persist for greater than or equal to 3 months.
- Symptoms must begin or worsen following injury
- Symptoms must interfere with social and/or occupational functioning
- Exclusion of dementia due to head trauma (code 294.1) and other disorders that better account for reported symptoms

Diagnostic and Statistical Manual of Mental Disorders (Fifth Edition) and Diagnostic and Statistical Manual of Mental Disorders (Fifth Edition, Text Revision) Criteria

- The criteria presented in *Diagnostic and Statistical Manual of Mental Disorders* (Fourth Edition) DSM-IV and DSM (Fourth Edition, Text Revision) for PCD (appendix of disorders for future research) was not included. DSM-V and DSM-V-TR present diagnostic criteria for mild or major neurocognitive disorder (NCD) due to TBI:
- Evidence of TBI
- LOC
- Posttraumatic amnesia
- Disorientation and confusion
- Neurological signs (eg, neuroimaging demonstrating injury, new onset of seizures, worsening of a preexisting seizure disorder, visual field cuts, anosmia, hemiparesis)
- NCD presents immediately following the occurrence of TBI or immediately following recovery of consciousness and persists past the acute postinjury period

International Classification of Diseases, Tenth Revision, Clinical Criteria

- History of head trauma with LOC precedes symptom onset by maximum of 4 weeks
- Presence of symptoms in 3 or more of the following categories:
  - Headache, dizziness, malaise, fatigue, noise tolerance
  - Irritability, depression, anxiety, emotional lability
  - Subjective concentration, memory, or intellectual difficulties without neuropsychological evidence of marked impairment
  - Insomnia
  - Reduced tolerance for alcohol
  - Preoccupation with aforementioned symptoms and fear of brain damage with hypochondriacal concern and adoption of sick role

International Classification of Diseases, Tenth Revision, Research Criteria

- History of head trauma resulting in LOC preceding symptom onset by less than or equal to 4 weeks
- Presence of at least 3 or more of the following 12 symptoms: headache, dizziness, fatigue, noise intolerance, irritability, emotional lability, depression and/or anxiety, subjective complaints of difficulty in concentration and/or memory problems (sans clear objective evidence from psychological tests), insomnia, reduced alcohol tolerance, preoccupation with the previous symptoms, and fear of permanent brain damage (even hypochondriacal) with the adoption of a sick role.

INTRODUCTION AND HISTORY

Postconcussional syndrome (PCS), a term coined by Strauss and Savitsky in 1934,[9] was used to describe the persistence of cognitive, physical, behavioral, emotional, and sleep symptoms lasting greater than 3 months following a head injury.[7] According to the American Congress of Rehabilitation Medicine,[10] the constellation of symptoms has previously been referred to by many names, such as minor head injury, postconcussive syndrome, traumatic head syndrome, traumatic cephalgia, post-brain injury syndrome, and posttraumatic syndrome. Much controversy has centered around the diagnosis and treatment of PCS, because the diagnosis largely depends on the criteria used, including those that are listed in the International Classification of Diseases, Tenth Revision (ICD-10), ICD-10 research criteria, and the DSM-IV. Moreover, newer versions of the DSM (ie, DSM-V and DSM-V-TR) exclude PCS as a diagnosis, thus creating additional challenges for treatment providers.

Treatment of PCS focuses on symptom-specific reduction and management, because there is currently no cure for this complex constellation of symptoms. Symptoms of PCS are not always predictable, and it is often unclear whether symptoms of this syndrome are physiogenic, psychogenic/functional neurological condition, or a combination of both.[11] The vast range of symptoms includes headache, sleep disturbance, fatigue, general malaise, short-term memory loss, posttraumatic amnesia, difficulty with concentration/disorientation, dizziness or vertigo, impaired reasoning/comprehension/confusion, tinnitus, personality change, apathy, irritability, affective disturbance, nervousness, difficulty shifting focus, and intolerance of alcohol, stress, noise, and/or emotion.[11–13] Furthermore, many symptoms associated with PCS mimic and overlap with other diagnosable conditions, which creates challenges for accurate diagnosis and treatment.[13] Diagnosis of PCS largely depends on many factors, including symptom duration, timing of assessment and evaluation, history of singular or multiple head injuries, premorbid functioning, and specific diagnostic criteria used.

PREVALENCE AND DIAGNOSIS OF POSTCONCUSSIONAL SYNDROME

The types of head injuries that contribute to PCS range in severity and include moderate (GCS 9–12) TBI, mild (GCS 13–15) TBI, and concussion.[3,14] Approximately 1.5 million Americans of all ages sustain a TBI annually, typically secondary to falls, motor vehicle accidents, assaults, or firearm injury with mTBIs accounting for 80% to 90% of these injuries.[15] Prevalence rates for PCS following TBI, specifically mTBI vary widely within the literature (11%–82%) and largely depend on the diagnostic criteria used (**Table 1**).[16–21]

At present, providers tend to rely on PCS diagnostic criteria from either the ICD-10 or the DSM-IV. Thus, diagnostic differences among providers remain.[22] Methodological frameworks implemented in research can further complicate a clinician's understanding of PCS because research studies have historically operationalized PCS/PCD in a study-dependent fashion, focusing on certain symptoms or symptom clusters, using different assessment tools, and forming unique definitions of the criteria. This study-specific methodology drastically limits comparisons and clouds the impact of moderating factors across samples.

Diagnosis of PCS requires a thoughtful and thorough approach via a multidisciplinary team, depending on the reported symptoms. When gathering patient history, head injury mechanism and mechanical force creating the head injury must be considered. Obtaining information pertaining to past head injuries is imperative, because those who have sustained multiple head injuries over the course of a lifetime may be at greater risk of developing PCS.[23] Providers should take special care to ask

Table 1
Prevalence and diagnosis of postconcussional syndrome/postconcussional disorder by reference criteria

Criteria for Diagnosis of PCS	Prevalence Rates and Prevalence-Related Factors

ICD-10 Clinical	• Among a *pediatric population* comparing children with mTBI with those with ECI:
	  ○ 11% (13.7% > 6 years of age) endorsed symptoms of PCS at 3 months postinjury compared with just under 1% diagnosed with ECI
	  ○ 2.3% of children with mTBI endorsed symptoms of PCS at 1 year postinjury[17]
	• Among *adults* diagnosed with mTBI prevalence rates at 1, 3, and 6 months postinjury were estimated to be 10.3%, 6%, and 0.9%, respectively.[18]
	  ○ 75% of the sample endorsed posttraumatic headache
	  ○ Slightly over half endorsed amnesia
	  ○ 42.5% endorsed LOC
	  ○ Before injury, 11% of their sample endorsed at least 1 PCS-related symptom
	  ○ At 1, 3, and 6 months postinjury, the rate of symptoms decreased to 27.3%, 18. 3%, and 6.3%, respectively
	• Another study found prevalence rates of PCS at 2 weeks postinjury to be 9.6%, and unchanged at 8.1% at 3 and 6 months postinjury[21]

ICD-10 Research	• Appears to be less sensitive when compared with ICD-10 clinical and DSM-IV criteria at 1 week postinjury[19]
ICD-10 & DSM-IV	• Among adults with mild to moderate TBI and a general trauma comparison group, prevalence rates for PCS were: ○ Six times higher when using ICD-10 criteria when compared with DSM-IV (64% vs 11%)[16]
ICD-10 Clinical, ICD-10 Research, & DSM-IV	• Prevalence rates of PCS among the sample varied significantly based on the criteria used at 1 week postinjury: 60.4% (ICD-10 clinical), 33.7% (ICD-10 research), and 27.7% (DSM-IV)[19] • Prevalence rates using all 3 criterion sets decreased at 3 months postinjury: 30.4%, 20.7%, and 13.0%, respectively.[19]

Abbreviation: ECI, extracranial injury.

questions related to the number, severity, and persistence of symptoms, including whether the patient experienced anterograde and/or retrograde amnesia.

In addition, it is important for providers to have the ability to decipher between concussion pathophysiology and a secondary process,[24,25] because many PCS symptoms mimic psychiatric disorders, namely, depression, apathy, and anxiety.[19]

Taking the time to assess and gain a thorough understanding of the patient's premorbid functioning (ie, before the first head injury) is crucial to making an accurate and well-informed diagnosis.[26]

Premorbid conditions such as elevated stress, depression, and anxiety tend to predict increased persistence of PCS symptoms and ultimately the diagnosis of PCS.[27–30] Furthermore, patients with premorbid traumatic stress, physical trauma, chronic pain, and fatigue are more likely to endorse symptoms and be diagnosed with PCS when compared with typically developing controls.[31] Differential diagnoses include depression, acute stress disorder or posttraumatic stress disorder (PTSD), fibromyalgia, migraines, tension-type headache, cluster-type headache, vertebral artery disease, and insomnia.

Providers must also remain keenly aware of the "good-old-days" bias (ie, the tendency to underestimate past problems and to view oneself as healthier before injury) when assessing for PCS symptoms. Research suggests that adult patients with mTBI tend to misperceive preinjury functioning as being better and endorse fewer preinjury symptoms when compared with the average person.[32,33] Findings among a pediatric sample yielded similar results.[34]

CAUSE, POPULATIONS AT RISK, AND MODERATING RISK FACTORS

For as long as PCS has been recognized, its cause has been widely debated.[35] When trying to understand overall health outcomes and prognosis, recognizing that symptom presentation is as unique and diverse as the patient population is imperative. Certain groups of individuals may be more vulnerable to the effects of head injury including long-term complications. These groups include racial/ethnic minorities, veterans, individuals who experience homelessness, those housed in correctional/detention facilities, survivors of intimate partner violence, and those residing in rural areas where timely and appropriate care may not be readily available.[15]

Several sociodemographic factors have been shown to impact prevalence rates of PCS, including biological sex, age, racial/ethnic status, education, and lifestyle.

- Studies suggest that women when compared with men were more likely to be diagnosed with PCS due to endorsements of headache, irritability, fatigue, and concentration problems.[12,16,36,37] Children seem to be less impacted by gender effects, and reasons for this remain inconclusive within the literature.[38,39]
- Older adults are more likely to endorse PCS symptoms in addition to adults with modest education levels.[38,39]
- One study documented that a higher percentage of Hispanic patients received diagnosis of PCS when compared with other racial/ethnically diverse groups.[40] Research examining PCS symptoms among a culturally diverse, nonconcussed sample found that the occurrence of PCS symptoms did not differ among groups stratified by cultural identity and language. However, findings from the same study revealed that higher rates of PCS symptoms were reported among non-White participants when compared with their White counterparts, including headaches, forgetfulness, dizziness, sensitivity to light and sound, difficulty with concentration, and depressed mood.[41]
- Research has elucidated the impact of lived experiences on symptom reporting.[42] Examined medical/scientific constructs may consist of multiple dimensions that result in varied interpretations and conceptualizations when working with non-English speakers or individuals from non-Western cultures.[40,41,43] Moreover, cultural values/traditions, including the amount of social support,

lifestyle/habits, and familial dynamics/roles/expectations may contribute either positively or negatively to PCS symptom duration and overall prognosis.

- Research suggests that many adults presenting with persistent PCS symptoms following mTBI are involved in litigation and may be prone to PCS symptom endorsement for secondary gain. Noteworthy to mention, as research suggests, more than 30% of individuals from this subgroup put forth suboptimal test taking effort, exhibit biases in their response patterns, and demonstrate other behaviors suggestive of symptom magnification or fabrication during formal neuropsychological testing.[8]

NEUROPSYCHOLOGICAL ASSESSMENT OF POSTCONCUSSIONAL SYNDROME

Thorough patient evaluation should consist of an open-ended or structured clinical interview, and/or checklists to obtain information associated with PCS symptoms. A structured interview approach seems to be more fruitful in symptom endorsement when compared with open-ended interview methods.[44] That said a combined approach may be of benefit. Using open-ended questions initially may help patients to freely express their concerns, thus providing an opportunity to build patient-provider rapport. Once rapport is established, moving to a more structured approach could prove more efficient, and this technique tends to limit patient-provider biases.

Several scales have been developed to measure the presence and severity of PCS symptoms. According to Sullivan and Garden,[45] the following 4 measures seem to have moderate to good reliability: Rivermead Post-Concussion Symptoms Questionnaire,[46] Post-Concussion Symptom Scale, Post-Concussion Syndrome Checklist,[47] and British Columbia Symptom Inventory.[48] As previously stated, many symptoms assessed by these instruments could be attributable to medical and psychiatric concerns, including but not limited to insomnia, depression, and anxiety, and few differences have been found between these conditions and PCS.[49] Moreover, self-report measures lack validity indicators (ie, scales used to examine underreporting and overreporting), which engenders challenges for providers in determining normal symptom variation when compared with both other clinical samples and the general population. Perhaps the utility of these measures is most beneficial toward tailoring clinical recommendations and intervention programs to improve overall patient functioning.

Neuropsychological testing conducted by a qualified neuropsychologist is necessary to determine the presence of neurocognitive deficits resulting from head injury and to obtain a better understanding of possible PCS symptoms. It is imperative that neuropsychologists remain mindful of the impact of culture and language on the neuropsychological process from the beginning until the end of the evaluation. Factors including bi/multilingualism, literacy, acculturation, and socioeconomic status are known to impact assessment performance.[8] In addition, variables such as communication style, use and understanding of neuropsychological/psychological constructs, values, beliefs, and social norms, test administration practices, test-taking strategies/testing naiveté, and chosen normative comparisons may significantly impact performance and subsequent diagnostic impressions.[8]

Thus, neuropsychological evaluations should be comprehensive and aim to measure motivation/testing engagement in addition to attention/concentration, working memory, learning and short-term memory, executive functions (eg, planning/organizing, abstraction, reasoning, problem solving), language, visual-spatial skills, and motor functions.[11] In addition, a neuropsychological assessment will screen for or sometimes examine in detail psychological symptoms, personality traits, and behavioral tendencies. Assessment tools may have linguistic and cultural limitations (instruments and normative data sets), and providers are advised to select the "most appropriate" tools that best generalize to the examinee.[8] This fact presents as a significant limitation in assessing for PCS symptoms among patients who are non-English speakers and/or who are of non-Western cultures.

Importantly, neuropsychological findings should be interpreted in conjunction with base rates and medical records. Specifically, neuroimaging studies should be used to bolster interpretation of the neurocognitive profile and results should be interpreted in context with sociodemographic factors (ie, education, acculturation, cultural and linguistic diversity).

PHARMACOLOGIC TREATMENT APPROACHES FOR POSTCONCUSSIONAL SYNDROME

At present, there is no universally agreed-upon treatment for PCS. Current treatment approaches center on symptom reduction and management and can be divided into 2 main categories: pharmacologic and nonpharmacologic. Furthermore, evidence to support the use of pharmacologic interventions for PCS symptoms is limited but promising; this is particularly true for headaches, sleep disturbance, depression, and anxiety.[50-55] Samples have been generally small (**Table 2**), and future research aimed at exploring the effects of new antidepressants on PCS symptoms could prove fruitful.

NONPHARMACOLOGIC TREATMENT APPROACHES FOR POSTCONCUSSIONAL SYNDROME

For patients not requiring the use of pharmacologic treatments, several nonpharmacologic intervention approaches are available, albeit with limited support related to their benefits. Studies have examined the use of vestibular physical therapy, cognitive rehabilitation, cognitive behavioral therapy, mindfulness-based/relaxation approaches, physical activity, health education, and rest.[56-67] Other, less studied, more costly, and time-intensive nonpharmacologic treatment approaches have also been examined (ie, hyperbaric oxygen therapy and repetitive transcranial magnetic stimulation) (**Table 3**).[68-71]

Addressing PCS symptoms via a multidisciplinary (neurologic, neuropsychological, and psychiatric/psychological) team approach may aid in understanding of symptoms, possible overlay between conditions, and expected prognosis. In addition, a multidisciplinary treatment approach would allow providers to address symptoms associated with their specialty fields and working in tandem would help to ensure expected patient recovery.

PROGNOSIS

Patients who present with PCS tend to have a good prognosis for recovery, because many symptoms are greatest during the initial week after head injury and tend to improve and sometimes completely resolve around the 1-month mark.[72]

For some patients, initial PCS symptoms tend to be more disabling several months postinjury when compared with immediately following. Symptoms associated with emotional well-being, including symptoms of depression and anxiety, tend to fall into this category, with depression accounting for a significant elevation in PCS symptom reporting. Longstanding PCS-type symptoms should, however, be interpreted with caution because the cause is unlikely to be a mild head injury/concussion, because there is evidence to suggest that there is a 90% likelihood for an individual

Table 2 Pharmacologic treatment approaches for postconcussional syndrome	
Pharmacologic Approach for the Treatment of PCS	**Treatment Results**
NSAIDs	• Reduction in PCS-related headaches (estimated to affect between 30% and 90% of patients following mTBI)[50]
Intravenous DHE & metoclopramide	• Good to excellent relief found among a small sample experiencing headache and at least 3 additional PCS-related symptoms[51]
Benzodiazepines[a] • Flurazepam • Lorazepam • Estazolam	• Increased total sleep time • Improved overall sleep quality
"Z-drugs"[a] • Zaleplon • Zolpidem • Zopiclone	• Increased total sleep time • Improved overall sleep quality
Melatonin & melatonin agonists[b] • Ramelteon • Tasimelteon	• Increase total sleep time • Decrease sleep latency
SSRIs • Sertraline • Citalopram	• Reduction in negative symptoms and cognitive impairments • Among patients diagnosed with major depression 3 to 24 months post-mTBI, statistically significant improvements with sertraline were found in the following areas: ○ psychological distress ○ anger and aggression ○ functioning ○ other PCS-related symptoms[53] • Prevention of depression following TBI when sertraline was administered shortly after injury[54] • Exploration of the effect of SSRIs on PCS-related cognitive impairments showed promise in the following: ○ Psychomotor speed ○ Cognitive efficiency ○ Recent memory ○ Flexible thinking[55]
Trazodone	• Effective in treating PCS-related insomnia comorbid with depression ○ Effects are comparable to SSRIs as well as TCAs[52]

Abbreviations: DHE, dihydroergotamine; NSAIDs nonsteroidal anti-inflammatory drugs; SSRIs, selective serotonin reuptake inhibitors; TCAs, tricyclic antidepressants.

[a] Concerns related to dependency and abuse exist, and patients should be closely monitored.

[b] Viable option for many patients presenting with PCS-related sleep problems (no risk of dependency or tolerance) and can be purchased affordably over the counter.[52].

with depression, as well as fibromyalgia, but no history of head injury to meet criteria for PCS as outlined in ICD-10.[35] Findings such as these highlight concerns related to the nonspecificity of available diagnostic criteria.

Nearly half of all individuals diagnosed with PCS following mTBI report symptoms lasting up to 3 months postinjury, and several studies have suggested that between

Table 3
Nonpharmacologic treatment approaches for postconcussional syndrome

Nonpharmacologic Approach for the Treatment of PCS	Treatment Description & Results
VPT	• Uses specialized exercises to stabilize gaze and gait[56] • PCS-related dizziness and vertigo were reported to improve following VPT initiation several days postinjury[57]

Cognitive rehabilitation	• Aims to address neurocognitive processes related to:
	  ○ attention
	  ○ memory
	  ○ executive functioning
	• Slight improvements in prospective memory and other PCS-related symptoms[58]
	• Conversely research conducted among patients with PCS found no significant impact on the long-term effects of PCS and no improvements were found between 1 and 10 years postinjury[59,60]

CBT	• When applied early, CBT may have some efficacy in reducing somatic symptoms, anxiety, and depression[61] • Early CBT intervention has shown to facilitate recovery and prevent longer-term PCS symptoms[62]
Mindfulness-based therapy/relaxation	• Improvements in overall quality of life have been reported[63] • Has been found to increase stress levels, which subsequently increased the severity of PCS-related symptoms[63–65] ○ Factors influencing findings include the notion that some individuals may feel more stressed when close attention is placed on their thoughts, as is the case with this approach
Health-related education	• Patients with head injury/those at risk of developing PCS benefitted from the receipt of health education regarding the effects of head injury accompanied with reassurance during the recovery process[66] • PCS-related education received before hospital discharge yielded shorter symptom duration, fewer symptoms/symptomatic days, and lower average severity levels[67]

HBOT	• Improvements in cognitive functions for patients with PCS, when compared with controls
	• Controls showed significant comparable improvements:
	  ○ memory
	  ○ executive functioning
	  ○ information processing speed
	  ○ attention
	• Cognitive functioning and quality of life improved for both groups[68]

(continued on next page)

Table 3 (continued)	
Nonpharmacologic Approach for the Treatment of PCS	**Treatment Description & Results**
rTMS	• Used to quantify excitation and inhibition of the primary motor cortex, spinal nerve roots, and the peripheral motor pathway (corticospinal)[69,70] • Four-week treatments with rTMS showed mild improvement in PCS symptoms but no change in cognitive function[71] • More research is necessary to identify the exact mechanisms behind rTMS-induced plasticity

Abbreviations: CBT, cognitive behavioral therapy; HBOT, hyperbaric oxygen therapy; rTMS, repetitive transcranial magnetic stimulation; VPT, Vestibular physical therapy.

10% and 15% report symptoms lasting greater than 1 year.[73] Alexander[74] found that at 1 year postinjury, approximately 15% of patients who sustained mTBI continued to report "disabling" symptoms. Similarly, findings from Rutherford and colleagues[75] revealed that 14.5% of patients with mild concussion endorsed symptoms 1 year postinjury. However, a more thorough review of available data from the two aforementioned investigators revealed issues related to symptom estimation and methodology, such that truer estimates of persistent PCS appear to be between 3% and 5%. In addition, nearly a quarter of patients with mTBI or concussion do not seek medical treatment, thus they remain unaccounted for in incidence estimates. Last, most of these individuals do not experience LOC or extended posttraumatic amnesia.[35]

Moderating factors such as biological sex, age, race/ethnicity, and other factors including sociodemographics (ie, employment, socioeconomic status), comorbid medical and/or psychiatric comorbidities (post–acute coronavirus disease 2019 (COVID-19) syndrome or "long COVID," personality disorders, poor coping mechanisms, and so on), and other factors (ie, litigation, secondary gains) may impact prognosis and recovery thus creating additional challenges for assessment, diagnosis, and estimating recovery.

DISCUSSION

Differences in PCS/PCD diagnostic criteria have resulted in heterogeneous results regarding prevalence, duration, and prognosis. As PCS symptoms tend to encompass many domains of functioning and often overlap with other diagnosable conditions, the need for standardization in diagnostic criteria, assessment methods, and research methodology is imperative for accurate diagnosis and treatment. Moreover, providers are responsible for the provision of patient care that is impartial and free of bias. Bias (ie, implicit bias) is well understood to perpetuate health care disparities and has the potential to influence patient-provider interaction, diagnosis, and treatment decisions.

Future PCS research should center on identifying and implementing a standard set of diagnostic criteria for PCS, using larger sample sizes, comparing patients with a history of head injury to healthy controls, and taking a patient-centered approach regarding the assessment and treatment of PCS. Last, there remains a dearth of literature related to the impact of culture, language, and lived experiences of non-English speakers and/or those from non-Western cultures on PCS symptom prevalence and prognosis.

CLINICS CARE POINTS

- PCS symptoms may mimic/overlap with those of other diagnosable medical conditions (ie, fibromyalgia and chronic fatigue), as well as psychiatric conditions (ie, major depressive disorder, generalized anxiety disorder, acute stress disorder, and PTSD).

- To differentiate between brain dysfunction resulting from head injury or another attributable cause, providers must consider the patient's psychiatric, behavioral, physical, and demographic factors. Patients with premorbid traumatic stress, physical trauma, chronic pain, and fatigue are more likely to endorse symptoms and be diagnosed with PCS when compared with normal controls.

- Treatment approaches should focus on mitigating PCS symptom severity through health education and pharmacologic and/or nonpharmacologic interventions.

- Clinicians have an obligation and responsibility to provide impartial care. Thus, addressing possible implicit bias and implementing neuropsychological assessment may reduce the likelihood of health care discrimination and enhance the ability to objectively measure PCS symptoms and severity.

- Clinical providers should be mindful of the possibility of litigation or other secondary gain because this may influence symptom presentation and duration. Neuropsychological assessment is warranted in these cases.

- Culture and language play an important role in all factors pertaining to PCS diagnosis and treatment, including prevalence rates, symptom reporting, test taking behavior, and accuracy of outcome data.

DISCLOSURE

The authors have nothing to disclose.

REFERENCES

1. Menon DK, Schwab K, Wright DW, et al. Position statement: definition of traumatic brain injury. Arch Phys Med Rehabil 2010;91(11):1637–40.
2. Traumatic brain injury/concussion. Centers for Disease Control and Prevention. 2022. Available at: https://www.cdc.gov/traumaticbraininjury/index.html. Accessed May 9, 2022.
3. McCrory P, Meeuwisse WH, Echemendia RJ, et al. What is the lowest threshold to make a diagnosis of concussion? Br J Sports Med 2013;47(5):268–71.
4. Mayer AR, Quinn DK, Master CL. The spectrum of mild traumatic brain injury. Neurology 2017;89(6):623–32.
5. Lefevre-Dognin C, Cogné M, Perdrieau V, et al. Definition and epidemiology of mild traumatic brain injury. Neurochirurgie 2021;67(3):218–21.
6. Silverberg ND, Iverson GL, Arciniegas DB, et al. Expert panel survey to update the American Congress of rehabilitation medicine definition of mild traumatic brain injury. Arch Phys Med Rehabil 2021;102(1):76–86.
7. Aminoff MJ, Josephson SA, Aminoff MJ. Aminoff's Neurology and General Medicine. Fifth Edition. Elsevier Science & Technology; 2014.
8. Stucky KJ, Kirkwood MW, Donders J. Clinical neuropsychology study guide and board review. New York, NY: Oxford University Press; 2020.
9. Strauss I, Savitsky N. THe sequelae of head injury. Am J Psychiatry 1934;91: 189–202.

10. https://www.acrm.org/wp-content/uploads/pdf/TBIDef_English_10-10.pdf (Accessed June 1, 2022).

11. Boyd WD. Post-concussion syndrome: an evidence based approach. United States: Xlibris; 2014.

12. Bazarian JJ, Atabaki S. Predicting postconcussion syndrome after minor traumatic brain injury. Acad Emerg Med 2001;8(8):788–95.

13. Ryan LM, Warden DL. Post concussion syndrome. Int Rev Psychiatry 2003;15(4): 310–6.

14. McCauley SR, Boake C, Pedroza C, et al. Postconcussional disorder: Are the DSM-IV criteria an improvement over the ICD-10? J Nerv Ment Dis 2005; 193(8):540–50.

15. Centers for Disease Control and Prevention. Report to congress: traumatic brain injury in the United States. Centers for Disease Control and Prevention. 2016. Available at: https://www.cdc.gov/traumaticbraininjury/pubs/tbi_report_to_congress.html#:~:text=Traumatic%20brain%20injury%20(TBI)%20is,people%20are%20hospitalized%20and%20survive. Accessed April 17, 2022.

16. Boake C, McCauley SR, Levin HS, et al. Diagnostic criteria for postconcussional syndrome after mild to moderate traumatic brain injury. J Neuropsychiatry Clin Neurosci 2005;17:350–6.

17. Barlow KM, Crawford S, Stevenson A, et al. Epidemiology of postconcussion syndrome in pediatric mild traumatic brain injury. Pediatrics 2010;126(2). https://doi.org/10.1542/peds.2009-0925.

18. Spinos P, Sakellaropoulos G, Georgiopoulos M, et al. Postconcussion syndrome after mild traumatic brain injury in Western Greece. J Trauma Inj Infect Crit Care 2010;69(4):789–94.

19. McCauley SR, Wilde EA, Miller ER, et al. Comparison of ICD-10 and DSM-IV Criteria for Postconcussion Syndrome/Disorder. La Revista Iberoamericana de Neuropsicología 2018;1:63–81.

20. Polinder S, Cnossen MC, Real RG, et al. A multidimensional approach to postconcussion symptoms in mild traumatic brain injury. Front Neurol 2018;9. https://doi.org/10.3389/fneur.2018.01113.

21. Balakrishnan B, Rus RM, Chan KH, et al. Prevalence of postconcussion syndrome after mild traumatic brain injury in young adults from a single neurosurgical center in east coast of malaysia. Asian J Neurosurg 2019;14(1):201–5.

22. Boake C, McCauley SR, Levin HS, et al. Limited agreement between criteria-based diagnoses of postconcussional syndrome. J Neuropsychiatry Clin Neurosciences 2004;16(4):493–9.

23. Permenter CM, Fernández-de Thomas RJ, Sherman Al. Postconcussive Syndrome. In: StatPearls [Internet]. Treasure Island (FL): StatPearls Publishing; 2022. Available at: https://www.ncbi.nlm.nih.gov/books/NBK534786/.

24. Dimberg EL, Burns TM. Management of common neurologic conditions in sports. Clin Sports Med 2005;24(3):637–62.

25. Kutcher JS, Eckner JT. At-risk populations in sports-related concussion. Curr Sports Med Rep 2010;9(1):16–20.

26. McCrory P, Meeuwisse W, Johnston K. Consensus statement on concussion in sport: 3rd International Conference on Concussion in Sport held in Zurich, November 2008. Clin J Sport Med 2009;19(3):185–200.

27. Paniak C. Patient complaints within 1 month of mild traumatic brain injury: a controlled study. Arch Clin Neuropsychol 2002;17(4):319–34.

28. Ettenhofer ML, Reinhardt LE, Barry DM. Predictors of neurobehavioral symptoms in a university population: a multivariate approach using a postconcussive symptom questionnaire. J Int Neuropsychological Soc 2013;19(9):977–85.

29. Meares S, Shores EA, Taylor AJ, et al. Mild traumatic brain injury does not predict acute postconcussion syndrome. J Neurol Neurosurg Psychiatry 2008;79(3): 300–6.

30. van der Horn HJ, Liemburg EJ, Scheenen ME, et al. Brain network dysregulation, emotion, and complaints after mild traumatic brain injury. Hum Brain Mapp 2016; 37(4):1645–54.

31. Ponsford J, Cameron P, Fitzgerald M, et al. Predictors of postconcussive symptoms 3 months after mild traumatic brain injury. Neuropsychology 2012;26(3): 304–13.

32. Lange RT, Iverson GL, Rose A. Post-concussion symptom reporting and the "good-old-days" bias following mild traumatic brain injury. Arch Clin Neuropsychol 2010;25(5):442–50.

33. Voormolen DC, Cnossen MC, Spikman J, et al. Rating of pre-injury symptoms over time in patients with mild traumatic brain injury: the good-old-days bias revisited. Brain Inj 2020;34(8):1001–9.

34. Brooks BL, Kadoura B, Turley B, et al. Perception of recovery after pediatric mild traumatic brain injury is influenced by the "Good Old Days" bias: tangible implications for clinical practice and outcomes research. Arch Clin Neuropsychol 2013;29(2):186–93.

35. McCrea MA. Mild traumatic brain injury and postconcussion syndrome: the new evidence base for diagnosis and treatment. New York: Oxford University Press; 2008.

36. Fenton G, McClelland R, Montgomery A, et al. The postconcussional syndrome: social antecedents and psychological sequelae. Br J Psychiatry 1993;162(4): 493–7.

37. Evans RW. The postconcussion syndrome and the sequelae of mild head injury. Neurol Clin 1992;10(4):815–47.

38. Zemek RL, Farion KJ, Sampson M, et al. Prognosticators of persistent symptoms following pediatric concussion. JAMA Pediatr 2013;167(3):259.

39. Ewing-Cobbs L, Cox CS Jr, Clark AE, et al. Persistent postconcussion symptoms after injury. Pediatrics 2018;142(5):e20180939.

40. Mollayeva T, Shapiro CM, Cassidy JD, et al. Assessment of concussion/mild traumatic brain injury-related fatigue, alertness, and daytime sleepiness: a diagnostic modelling study. Neuropsychiatry 2017;07(02). https://doi.org/10.4172/neuropsychiatry.1000184.

41. Zakzanis KK, Yeung E. Base rates of post-concussive symptoms in a nonconcussed multicultural sample. Arch Clin Neuropsychol 2011;26(5):461–5.

42. Valovich McLeod TC, Wagner AJ, Bacon CE. Lived experiences of adolescent athletes following sport-related concussion. Orthopaedic J Sports Med 2017; 5(12). https://doi.org/10.1177/2325967117745033. 232596711774503.

43. Kim SH, Olabarrieta-Landa L, Gilboa-Fried S, et al. Factor structure models for the post-concussion syndrome scale with monolingual Spanish-speaking adults from Colombia. Brain Inj 2019;33(11):1436–41.

44. Iverson GL, Brooks BL, Ashton VL, et al. Interview versus questionnaire symptom reporting in people with the postconcussion syndrome. J Head Trauma Rehabil 2010;25(1):23–30.

45. Sullivan K, Garden N. A comparison of the psychometric properties of 4 postconcussion syndrome measures in a nonclinical sample. J Head Trauma Rehabil 2011;26(2):170–6.
46. King NS, Crawford S, Wenden FJ, et al. The rivermead post concussion symptoms questionnaire: a measure of symptoms commonly experienced after head injury and its reliability. J Neurol 1995;242(9):587–92.
47. Gouvier W. Postconcussion symptoms and daily stress in normal and head-injured college populations. Arch Clin Neuropsychol 1992;7(3):193–211.
48. Iverson GL, Page JL, Koehler BE, et al. Test of memory malingering (TOMM) scores are not affected by chronic pain or depression in patients with fibromyalgia. Clin Neuropsychologist 2007;21(3):532–46.
49. Gunstad J, Suhr J. Perception of illness: Nonspecificity of postconcussion syndrome symptom expectation. J Int Neuropsychological Soc 2002;8(1):37–47.
50. Evans RW. Post-traumatic headaches. Neurol Clin 2004;22(1):237–49.
51. McBeath JG, Nanda A. Use of dihydroergotamine in patients with postconcussion syndrome. Headache: J Head Face Pain 1994;34(3):148–51.
52. Zhou Y, Greenwald BD. Update on Insomnia after Mild Traumatic Brain Injury. Brain Sci 2018;8(12):223.
53. Fann JR, Uomoto JM, Katon WJ. Sertraline in the treatment of major depression following mild traumatic brain injury. J Neuropsychiatry Clin Neurosciences 2000; 12(2):226–32.
54. Jorge RE, Acion L, Burin DI, et al. Sertraline for preventing mood disorders following traumatic brain injury: a randomized clinical trial. JAMA Psychiatry 2016;73(10):1041–7.
55. Fann JR, Uomoto JM, Katon WJ. Cognitive improvement with treatment of depression following mild traumatic brain injury. Psychosomatics 2001;42(1): 48–54.
56. Han BI, Song HS, Kim JS. Vestibular rehabilitation therapy: Review of indications, mechanisms, and key exercises. J Clin Neurol 2011;7(4):184.
57. Alsalaheen BA, Mucha A, Morris LO, et al. Vestibular rehabilitation for dizziness and balance disorders after concussion. J Neurol Phys Ther 2010;34(2):87–93.
58. Twamley EW, Jak AJ, Delis DC, et al. Cognitive Symptom Management and rehabilitation therapy (cogsmart) for veterans with traumatic brain injury: Pilot randomized controlled trial. J Rehabil Res Development 2014;51(1):59–70.
59. Elgmark Andersson E, Emanuelson I, Björklund R, et al. Mild traumatic brain injuries: the impact of early intervention on late sequelae. A randomized controlled trial. Acta Neurochirurgica 2007;149(2):151–60.
60. Elgmark Andersson E, Kärrdahl Bedics B, Falkmer T. Mild traumatic brain injuries: a 10-year follow-up. J Rehabil Med 2011;43(4):323–9.
61. Al Sayegh A, Sandford D, Carson AJ. Psychological approaches to treatment of Postconcussion Syndrome: a systematic review. J Neurol Neurosurg Psychiatry 2010;81(10):1128–34.
62. Silverberg ND, Hallam BJ, Rose A, et al. Cognitive-behavioral prevention of postconcussion syndrome in at-risk patients. J Head Trauma Rehabil 2013;28(4): 313–22.
63. Bedard M, Felteau M, Mazmanian D, et al. Pilot evaluation of a mindfulness-based intervention to improve quality of life among individuals who sustained traumatic brain injuries. Disabil Rehabil 2003;25(13):722–31.
64. Hanna-Pladdy B, Berry ZM, Bennett T, et al. Stress as a diagnostic challenge for postconcussive symptoms: Sequelae of mild traumatic brain injury or physiological stress response. Clin Neuropsychologist 2001;15(3):289–304.

65. McMillan T, Robertson IH, Brock D, et al. Brief mindfulness training for attentional problems after traumatic brain injury: a randomised control treatment trial. Neuropsychological Rehabil 2002;12(2):117–25.

66. Mittenberg W, Burton DB. A survey of treatments for post-concussion syndrome. Brain Inj 1994;8(5):429–37.

67. Mittenberg W, Tremont G, Zielinski RE, et al. Cognitive-behavioral prevention of postconcussion syndrome. Arch Clin Neuropsychol 1996;11(2):139–45. PMID 14588914.

68. Boussi-Gross R, Golan H, Fishlev G, et al. Hyperbaric oxygen therapy can improve post concussion syndrome years after mild traumatic brain injury - randomized prospective trial. PLoS One 2013;8(11). https://doi.org/10.1371/journal.pone.0079995.

69. Hallett M. Transcranial magnetic stimulation and the human brain. Nature 2000; 406(6792):147–50.

70. Kobayashi M, Pascual-Leone A. Transcranial magnetic stimulation in neurology. Lancet Neurol 2003;2(3):145–56.

71. Koski L, Kolivakis T, Yu C, et al. Noninvasive brain stimulation for persistent postconcussion symptoms in mild traumatic brain injury. J Neurotrauma 2015;32(1): 38–44.

72. Triebel KL, Martin RC, Novack TA, et al. Treatment consent capacity in patients with traumatic brain injury across a range of injury severity. Neurology 2012; 78(19):1472–8.

73. Iverson GL. Outcome from mild traumatic brain injury. Curr Opin Psychiatry 2005; 18(3):301–17.

74. Alexander MP. Mild traumatic brain injury: pathophysiology, natural history, and Clinical Management. Neurology 1995;45(7):1253–60.

75. Rutherford WH, Merrett JD, McDonald JR. Symptoms at one year following concussion from minor head injuries. Injury 1979;10(3):225–30.

Headache in Adolescents

Irene Patniyot, MD[a],*, William Qubty, MD[b,1]

KEYWORDS

- Adolescent headache • Adolescent migraine • Onabotulinumtoxin A • CGRP

KEY POINTS

- Migraine is a common neurologic disorder in adolescents, causing significant disability.
- Although NSAIDs and triptans are considered first-line therapies for short-term treatment of migraine attacks, clinical trials are evaluating the safety and efficacy of gepant use in the adolescent population.
- Several migraine preventive therapies are available, including calcitonin gene-related peptide (CGRP)-targeted therapies.
- Accompanying treatments include behavioral therapies, neuromodulation devices, and procedures for when symptoms are not improving.

INTRODUCTION

Migraine is a common neurologic disease that affects about 18% of women and 6% of men.[1] Prevalence increases with age, and by adolescence it affects 8% to 22% of individuals.[2] Although the degree to which migraine interferes with an individual's life varies, it is the second leading cause of years lived with disability (YLD) worldwide[3] and the leading cause of YLD in those aged 15 to 49 years.[4] It is therefore paramount to identify and address migraine symptoms in adolescence, in an effort to prevent escalation of symptoms in adulthood. In recent years there have been several advances in the areas of short-term and preventive medication treatments, behavioral therapies, and neuromodulation devices, which have provided more hope for treating migraine and reducing migraine-related disability. This article discusses headache classification, in addition to outpatient headache management strategies for meeting the needs of adolescent patients. Although the World Health Organization (WHO) considers years 10 to 19 as the period of adolescence,[5] in clinical practice the adolescent age group typically encompasses ages 12 to 17 years.

---

[a] Section of Neurology and Developmental Neuroscience, Department of Pediatrics, Texas Children's Hospital Pediatric Headache Clinic, Baylor College of Medicine, Houston, TX, USA;
[b] Division of Child Neurology, Minneapolis Clinic of Neurology, Minneapolis, MN, USA
[1] Present address: 9645 Grove Circle North Suite 100, Maple Grove, MN 55369.
* Corresponding author. Texas Children's Hospital, West Campus, 18200 Katy Freeway, Suite 360, Houston, TX 77094.
E-mail address: irene.patniyot@bcm.edu

Neurol Clin 41 (2023) 177–192
https://doi.org/10.1016/j.ncl.2022.08.001
0733-8619/23/© 2022 Elsevier Inc. All rights reserved.

HEADACHE CLASSIFICATION

The most common headache disorders in adolescence include tension-type headache (TTH), migraine, primary stabbing headache, new daily persistent headache (NDPH), and posttraumatic headache (PTH). The trigeminal autonomic cephalalgias (TACs) are quite uncommon in this population as a primary headache disorder. The frequency and features of these headache disorders in adolescents compared with the adult population may vary, and these differences are highlighted.

History taking is of particular importance in this age group. The adolescent developmental stage produces a wide range of behaviors, some of which results in vague, equivocal, or indifferent responses to the clinician's queries. Building rapport and asking questions in a variety of ways is crucial for obtaining the necessary history. The history should be directed toward the patient, although on rare occasion it may be necessary to rely more heavily on the parent/guardian.

Tension-Type Headache

TTH in adolescents is not significantly different from the adult presentation except that in the authors' experience, the bandlike sensation around the head is less common than a mid- to bifrontal pressure headache. The diagnostic criteria are found in **Box 1**. There are 4 variations of TTH based on headache frequency: infrequent episodic (<1 d/mo), frequent episodic (1–14 d/mo), chronic (>14 d/mo), and probable based on not meeting all the diagnostic criteria for TTH.

Migraine

Diagnosing migraine in adolescents is generally similar to that in adults with a few notable exceptions. Migraine in adolescents may be of shorter duration, lasting as little as 2 hours untreated versus 4 hours in adults. Also, the location of the headache is more likely to be bilateral instead of unilateral. It is the authors' opinion that the complete migraine diagnostic features early in the development of migraine may not all be present and that over time they may fully develop. Headache disability can be assessed using the validated pediatric migraine disability assessment (PedMIDAS)

Box 1
Tension-type headache diagnostic criteria

A. At least 10 episodes of headache occurring on [a]day(s)/month on average and fulfilling criteria B to D

B. Lasting from 30 minutes to 7 days

C. At least 2 of the following 4 characteristics:
   1. Bilateral location
   2. Pressing or tightening (nonpulsating) quality
   3. Mild or moderate intensity
   4. Not aggravated by routine physical activity such as walking or climbing stairs

D. Both of the following:
   1. No nausea or vomiting
   2. No more than 1 of photophobia or phonophobia

[a]Options are less than 1, 1 to 14, and greater than 14.

From Vincent M, Wang S. Headache Classification Committee of the International Headache Society (IHS) The International Classification of Headache Disorders, 3rd edition. Cephalalgia. 2018;38(1):1-211. https://doi.org/10.1177/0333102417738202; with permission.

survey.[6] This screening tool uses 6 questions to assess the level of disability at school, home, and activities for the prior 3 months. The PedMIDAS may, however, underrepresent disability during the summer months and holiday breaks when adolescents are out of school (**Box 2**).

New Daily Persistent Headache

NDPH is more common in children and adolescents than adults.[7] NDPH is defined as a clearly recalled, new-onset persistent headache, lasting at least 3 months, in patients without a notable prior headache history (**Box 3**). The onset of headache may be preceded by illness such as Epstein-Barr virus, Valsalva,[8] or a stressful event. A retrospective NDPH study of school-aged children found that 39% of cases began in either September or January, correlating with school onset.[9] Headache characteristics of this disorder commonly overlap with migraine features and may be quite refractory to treatment.[10]

Trigeminal Autonomic Cephalagias

TACs such as cluster headache and hemicrania continua are rarely encountered in adolescents, but when they are, consideration for secondary intracranial pathology must be excluded. A recent review of 1788 pediatric, primary TAC publications found 86 studies that met their basic inclusion criteria.[11] Fifty-six of those studies focused on cluster headache. For pediatric cluster headache, the review found they can typically fulfill the adult criteria except for maximum of 6 instead of 8 attacks per day. Also, cranial autonomic features, number of attacks, and restlessness occurred at lower rates than in adults.

ABORTIVE THERAPIES

During a severe migraine attack, the goal of short-term treatment is to provide rapid relief of symptoms with minimal side effects. Adolescents should be advised to take their rescue medications earlier in the migraine attack, because short-term migraine

---

Box 2
Pediatric Migraine Without Aura Diagnostic Criteria

A. At least 5 attacks fulfilling criteria B to D

B. Headache attacks lasting 2 (instead of 4) to 72 hours (when untreated or unsuccessfully treated)

C. Headache has at least 2 of the following 4 characteristics:
   1. Bilateral (instead of unilateral) location
   2. Pulsating quality
   3. Moderate or severe pain intensity
   4. Aggravation by or causing avoidance of routine physical activity (eg, walking or climbing stairs)

D. During headache at least 1 of the following:
   1. Nausea and/or vomiting
   2. Photophobia and phonophobia

E. Not better accounted for by another International Classification of Headache Disorders (ICHD)-3 diagnosis.

From Vincent M, Wang S. Headache Classification Committee of the International Headache Society (IHS) The International Classification of Headache Disorders, 3rd edition. Cephalalgia. 2018;38(1):1-211. https://doi.org/10.1177/0333102417738202; with permission.

> **Box 3**
> **New Daily Persistent Headache Diagnostic Criteria**
>
> A. Persistent headache fulfilling criteria B and C
>
> B. Distinct and clearly remembered onset, with pain becoming continuous and unremitting within 24 hours
>
> C. Present for greater than 3 months
>
> D. Not better accounted for by another ICHD-3 diagnosis
>
> *From* Vincent M, Wang S. Headache Classification Committee of the International Headache Society (IHS) The International Classification of Headache Disorders, 3rd edition. Cephalalgia. 2018;38(1):1-211. https://doi.org/10.1177/0333102417738202; with permission.

treatments are more effective when the pain is still mild. The American Academy of Neurology provided updated guidelines in 2019 on short-term treatment of migraine in children and adolescents, which found that ibuprofen, acetaminophen, almotriptan, rizatriptan, sumatriptan/naproxen, sumatriptan, and zolmitriptan nasal sprays exhibited pain improvement or 2-hour pain freedom in placebo-controlled pediatric trials.[12] Other major treatment recommendations include coupling triptans with ibuprofen or naproxen if a migraine is incompletely responsive, administering a second dose of a short-term migraine medication within a 24-hour period, treating migraine-associated nausea, and avoiding medication overuse by limiting use of ibuprofen or acetaminophen to 14 or fewer days per month, and triptans to 9 or fewer days per month.[13] The ensuing discussion on short-term treatments will focus on the most commonly studied classes of medications for acute migraine treatment: over-the-counter analgesics, triptans, and dopamine receptor antagonists.

Over-the-Counter Analgesics

Most individuals with migraine use over-the-counter analgesics, including acetaminophen, ibuprofen, naproxen, and combination containing analgesics, as first-line therapy. Nonsteroidal anti-inflammatory drugs (NSAIDs) are typical mainstays of therapy, and there is limited evidence in the pediatric and adolescent population showing superiority of ibuprofen over acetaminophen and placebo.[14] Longer-acting NSAIDs such as naproxen can also be considered as first-line short-term treatment, especially if other over-the-counter analgesics have been ineffective. Other NSAIDs include diclofenac and etodolac, and more recently a liquid formulation of celecoxib has shown effectiveness in adults for short-term treatment of episodic migraine.[15] There is evidence in adults with chronic migraine that when naproxen is used frequently over a period of 3 months it can lead to a substantial reduction in migraine frequency, providing a prophylactic benefit.[16] It is the authors' experience that twice daily naproxen can be used for a few days up to 1 month as "bridging therapy" when migraine frequency is high. For example, it can be used in this manner concurrent with initiation of a new migraine preventive, viral illness, perimenstrually, with mild head injury, or during final examination time. Patients can be advised to take naproxen with food to prevent stomach upset, and revert to using it fewer than 15 days per month after the bridging period has ended to prevent medication side effects and concern for medication-overuse headache with frequent long-term use.

Triptans

Triptans are 5-hydroxytryptamine (5-HT$_{1B/1D}$) receptor agonists and were the first medication class designed specifically for acute migraine management. Since

sumatriptan's US Food and Drug Administration (FDA) approval in 1991, 6 more triptans with varying routes of administration have been developed. There are 3 triptans
and 1 triptan/NSAID combination currently approved by the FDA for use in the pediatric and adolescent populations. These medications include rizatriptan for ages 6
to 17 years, and almotriptan, zolmitriptan nasal spray, and sumatriptan/naproxen sodium for ages 12 to 17 years (**Table 1**).

Triptans are generally well tolerated, and are more effective if taken when the pain is
still mild. Although they may not shorten visual or sensory aura duration, in one-third of
people triptans are effective in aborting a migraine attack within 2 hours of administration.[17] If triptan side effects occur, which include fatigue, dizziness, nausea, sensation
of feeling hot, or chest or jaw tightness, consideration can be given to switching to a
triptan with a lower side effect profile (ie, frovatriptan or naratriptan). Triptan contraindications include cardiovascular disease, uncontrolled hypertension, stroke, and
pregnancy, which are not usual health concerns in the adolescent population.
Although the FDA has not yet updated its guidelines advising against use of triptans
in hemiplegic migraine or migraine with brainstem aura, triptans continue to be used
with caution in adolescents with these aura symptoms if symptoms are instead due
to stroke.

When choosing a triptan the provider can consider FDA approval status in the
adolescent population, which may be more easily covered by insurance. If the
pain escalates quickly or there are associated symptoms of nausea or emesis, a
nasal spray formulation (sumatriptan, zolmitriptan) or injection (sumatriptan) can
be considered. Providers should also take into consideration prescribing an appropriate initial dose, especially if the patient has previously required repeat dosing after
2 hours. Other considerations include combining the triptan with an NSAID for
improved effect, in addition to avoiding use of triptans and dihydroergotamine within
24 hours of each other.

Table 1
Triptans

Medication	Route of Administration	Weight ≤ 40 kg (mg)	Weight ≥ 40 kg (mg)
Almotriptan[b]	Oral	6.25	12.5
Eletriptan	Oral	20	40–80
Rizatriptan[a]	Oral	5	10
	ODT	5	10
Sumatriptan	Oral	25	50–100
	Nasal	5	20
	Subcutaneous	0.06 mg/kg	4,6
Sumatriptan/naproxen sodium[b]	Oral	N/A	10/60 85/500
Zolmitriptan[b]	Oral	2.5	5
	Nasal	N/A	5
Naratriptan	Oral	1	2.5
Frovatriptan	Oral	1.25	2.5

Abbreviations: N/A, not applicable; ODT, oral disintegrating tablet.
[a] FDA approved in children aged 6 to 17 years.
[b] FDA approved in children aged 12 to 17 years.

Dopamine Receptor Antagonists

Dopamine receptor antagonists are often used as migraine abortive therapy in emergency centers in intravenous (IV) form; however, they can also be prescribed for home use in the oral form. Dopamine receptor agonists can be considered as a rescue therapy in those in whom triptans have either not worked or are contraindicated and provide a good option before sending patients to the emergency room for IV therapy. Various prospective and retrospective trials in the pediatric and adolescent population have found that the phenothiazines, prochlorperazine and chlorpromazine in IV form, are effective in either reducing headache intensity by 50% or more[18–20] or preventing the need for further rescue therapy, hospitalization, or return within 48 hours.[21,22] A more recent randomized, double-blind controlled trial in adults found that both IV prochlorperazine and IV chlorpromazine reduced headache severity scores, without superiority in efficacy of one agent over the other.[23] Metoclopramide is also used for acute migraine treatment, and antagonizes both dopamine and 5-HT$_3$ receptors. In adults metoclopramide has level B evidence that it is probably effective for acute migraine treatment[24]; however, in adult studies have shown inferiority to prochlorperazine at comparable doses.[25,26]

Extrapyramidal side effects such as akathisia and a dystonic reaction can occur with this class of medication and can be mitigated in some individuals with diphenhydramine premedication. Chlorpromazine can cause worsening of hypotension, and this medication class as a whole can cause sedation. Caution should also be used with patients taking other QTc prolonging medications such as some antipsychotics.

Ditans and Gepants

Ditans are a newer class of medications developed for acute migraine treatment that cross the blood-brain barrier and target the 5-HT$_{1F}$ receptors found in the peripheral and central trigeminovascular system. Ditans do not cause the vasoconstriction that triptans do and may be a suitable alternative in those with cardiac or vascular disease. Lasmiditan was FDA approved in October 2019 for use in ages 18 and more based on phase 3 trial results showing superiority over placebo in achieving 2-hour pain freedom (200 mg dosing: 38.8% vs 21.3%; odds ratio [OR], 2.3; 95% confidence interval [CI] 1.8–3.1; $P<.001$).[27] Side effects can include dizziness, somnolence, nausea, and paresthesias, and patients should avoid driving for 8 hours following administration.

Gepants are another class of small molecule calcitonin gene related peptide (CGRP) antagonists that cross the blood-brain barrier and are FDA approved in those aged 18 years and older for short-term and/or preventive therapies. Rimegepant is the only drug in this class showing efficacy as both short-term and preventive therapy, and in February 2020 it was approved by the FDA for short-term use in those aged 18 years and older based on multicenter, randomized, double-blind placebo-controlled trial findings that pain freedom with rimegepant 75 mg oral disintegrating tablet occurred in 21% of patients compared with 11% placebo ($P<.0001$).[28] Ubrogepant is another medication in this class approved by the FDA in December 2019 for acute migraine use in those aged 18 years and more, following results of a phase 3, randomized, placebo-controlled trial revealing pain freedom for the 100 mg dose (21.2%, $P = .002$), 50 mg dose (19.2%, $P<.001$), and placebo (11.8%).[29] Zavegepant is the first third-generation gepant being studied in oral, subcutaneous, and intranasal formulations and has shown efficacy with the intranasal formulation. Although gepants are not approved for use in adolescents younger than 18 years, there are phase 3 randomized controlled trials in the pediatric and adolescent populations currently underway.

LIFESTYLE FACTORS

Addressing lifestyle factors that may be contributing to headache burden are an important part of headache education and management. These factors include sleep, diet, hydration, physical activity, caffeine, and mood. When discussing these healthy habits, expectations should be relayed to the patient that although these interventions support general health and may lead to a reduction in headache burden, there is no guarantee that this will happen. In addition, there may be external or internal circumstances making it difficult for adolescents to follow a routine, and blaming the patient may lead to further internalized stigma.

Sleep

The American Academy of Sleep Medicine (AASM) recommends that adolescents get 8 to 10 hours of sleep per night.[30] Teenagers have a physiologically delayed sleep phase that predisposes them to go to bed later and wake up later,[31] which can lead to shorter overall sleep duration during the school week. In addition to physiology, use of electronic devices often interferes with sleep schedules. In one study, most adolescents reported using 1 or more electronic devices in the hour before bedtime. A dose-response relationship was observed between sleep duration and use of electronic devices, such that a total screen time greater than 4 hours was associated with an increased risk of less than 5 hours of sleep (OR, 3.64; 95% CI, 3.06–4.33).[32] In addition to electronic content contributing to mental and bodily arousal, light exposure from electronic devices can affect circadian rhythms by reducing or delaying the release of the sleep-potentiating hormone melatonin from the pineal gland.[33]

Addressing sleep disruption has the potential to improve headache symptoms. Counseling can include putting away electronic devices at least 30 minutes to 1 hour before bedtime. If that is not possible due to academic or psychosocial factors, families can consider the use of blue blocking glasses to minimize the impact of blue light interference with sleep. Families can be informed that there are differences in the quality of blue-blocking glasses, and those with specific FL-41 tint filters can also be helpful for individuals who have light and screen sensitivity. Natural sleep-promoting therapies can also include herbal teas, cherry juice,[34] mindfulness exercises, and melatonin. If headache burden is high and interfering with high school or college performance, accommodations can be sought to adjust the patient's academic schedule accordingly.

Diet

Counseling on eating regular, healthy meals with snacks is a typical part of a headache visit. Although this practice stems from a belief that disruptions in routine can be a trigger for migraine attacks, it is unclear whether and to what degree skipping meals may contribute to migraine frequency. In addition, comorbid symptoms such as nausea or delayed gastric emptying may interfere with eating regular meals. Studies in the adult and adolescent populations have found that skipping meals, breakfast in particular, is common in individuals with migraine[35–37]; however, the association between skipping a meal and triggering a migraine attack has not been as consistently made.

Patients with migraine often ask about migraine food triggers. In the hours before the headache phase of migraine, there is a premonitory phase involving hypothalamic changes, which can cause symptoms of increased yawning, irritability, fatigue, neck pain, increased urination, and also food cravings.[38–40] If an individual craves a certain food such as chocolate or a carbohydrate-rich snack during this time, they may associate that food with triggering a migraine attack, when in fact migraine-related brain changes result in the food craving. Providers can encourage the adolescent to eat regular healthy meals as a good practice for overall health and explain that certain identified food triggers may actually be hypothalamic-driven food cravings attributed to the premonitory phase of migraine.

Hydration and Physical Activity

Dehydration can exacerbate various headache disorders and is multifactorial.[41] The mechanisms by which this provocation occurs can include fasting from both food and water, in addition to activation of central nervous system pain networks and reduced pain threshold.[42] Most children and adolescents are mildly dehydrated,[43] and increasing water intake in adults can lead to decreased hours of headache, migraine quality of life, and reduction in headache days.[44,45] The Institute of Medicine provides recommendations for adequate daily water intake based on age and sex, which in 14- to 18-year-old adolescents ranges between 64 oz (girls) and 88 oz (boys) of water per day. Both caffeinated and noncaffeinated beverages are thought to contribute to total water intake.[46] These recommendations are not absolute, and consideration should be given to comorbid conditions such as orthostatic intolerance and renal or cardiac disease, which alter these daily allowances.

Multiple studies have shown that routine physical activity can have a positive impact on headache frequency, quality of life, and mood.[47] Conversely, low levels of physical activity and being overweight are associated with recurrent headaches in adolescents.[48] Obesity is also a known risk factor for progression from episodic to chronic migraine,[49] emphasizing the potential influence of diet and physical activity on preventing escalation of headache burden. Studies have also shown that exercise may be as effective as a daily migraine preventive. More specifically, migraine frequency in individuals with episodic migraine decreased in all participants in a randomized trial comparing topiramate alone, a relaxation program, or aerobic exercise 3 times per week.[50] Another study in individuals with chronic migraine randomized participants to take amitriptyline 25 mg alone versus amitriptyline plus exercise involving fast walking 3 times per week for 12 weeks. Although there was a substantial decrease in both groups, the combined medication and exercise group experienced a greater reduction, with a therapeutic gain of approximately 6 days.[51]

Adolescent patients can be given suggested water intake goals and encouraged to drink water regularly throughout the day. They can also be encouraged to engage in some form of exercise 3 days/wk. If aerobic exercise is a migraine trigger, lower-intensity physical activity can be suggested in its place. Because there are sometimes practical barriers to hydration such as school rules preventing drinks in the class or limiting bathroom use, providing the patient with a school accommodation letter can be a simple way to improve adherence.

PREVENTIVE THERAPIES

Adolescents with chronic and bothersome recurring headaches most commonly have migraine. Thus, the following discussion focuses on pharmacologic and nonpharmacologic measures for migraine prevention. When the frequency of moderate to severe headache reaches at least a weekly basis, consideration should be given for initiation of a preventive treatment. Because FDA-approved headache treatments are rare in adolescents, medications should be chosen based on side effect profiles, prior medication tolerability, adherence, and medical history. Common coexisting medical conditions that may also influence medication options include depression, anxiety, asthma, heart/vascular disease, and postural orthostatic tachycardia syndrome. Patients should be counseled on the time required for headache treatments to see benefit, which is typically a minimum of 8 weeks. The level of benefit in the short and long term should be discussed to provide realistic expectations; a typical goal is to achieve at least a 50% reduction in the headache pattern. Adjunctive therapies may be required for refractory cases, but increased caution should be used to assess for medication interactions. Duration of preventive treatment depends on the duration and severity of the headache presentation. A reasonable goal is 3 to 6 months of good headache control before discussion of weaning preventive modalities.

The American Academy of Neurology in conjunction with the Child Neurology Society updated their 2004 pediatric migraine treatment guidelines in August 2019.[52] The update involved a comprehensive literature search of nearly 2000 abstracts from 2003 through 2017. Inclusion criteria were trials of preventive therapy, with at least 90% of participants aged 3 to 18 years, with a diagnosis of migraine, and treatment was compared with placebo. Studies that had fewer than 20 participants were excluded. Using these criteria, only 16 articles remained.

Anticonvulsants have long been used for migraine prevention. When looking at topiramate the guidelines concluded with moderate confidence that patients on topiramate were probably more likely than those taking placebo to have a reduction in the frequency of migraine or headache days. Topiramate is the only FDA-approved medication for migraine prevention in those aged 12 to 17 years. For extended-release divalproex sodium, the guidelines concluded, with very low confidence, that there was insufficient evidence to determine if it is more or less likely than placebo to reduce headache frequency.

For antidepressants, only amitriptyline was discussed. The guidelines concluded, with very low confidence, that there was insufficient evidence to determine if it is more or less likely than placebo to reduce headache frequency or migraine disability. However, there was high confidence to support amitriptyline use with cognitive behavioral therapy (CBT) to reduce headache frequency and possibly disability.

Antihypertensives were also reviewed. For the beta-blocker propranolol, the guidelines concluded, with low confidence, that it is more likely than placebo to have at least a 50% reduction in headache frequency. There was insufficient evidence for use of the calcium channel blocker flunarizine, which is not available in the United States, or nimodipine.

The CHAMP trial was a landmark multicenter pediatric and adolescent migraine study that was included in the aforementioned guideline data.[53] This study consisted of 3 arms including treatment with topiramate, amitriptyline, and placebo. The trial was stopped early due to futility because the intervention arms did not show benefit over placebo and had increased adverse effects. Notably the placebo response rate was 61%. In light of these results, nonpharmacologic interventions and nutraceutical recommendations can strongly be considered as first-line treatment. Nutraceutical options with some evidence of migraine benefit include riboflavin,[54] melatonin,[55,56] coenzyme Q10,[57] and possibly magnesium[58] (**Table 2**). There is evidence to suggest that treatments such as coenzyme Q10 and magnesium are more likely to have benefit if there is associated deficiency.[57,58]

Not discussed in the 2019 guidelines are the newer anti-CGRP monoclonal antibodies (mAbs), which include erenumab, galcanezumab, fremanezumab, and eptinezumab. These mAbs are not currently FDA approved for the treatment of migraine in patients younger than 18 years. Expert opinion suggests that these agents may be considered in adolescents with refractory migraine.[59] Patient characteristics such as age, weight, pubertal status, and medical comorbidities should be considered,

Table 2
Nutraceuticals for migraine prevention

Nutraceutical	Dosing (if At Least 40 kg)
Riboflavin	200 mg BID
Melatonin	3 mg 30 min before bedtime
Coenzyme Q10	1–3 mg/kg/d divided BID or 100 mg BID
Magnesium oxide	9 mg/kg/d divided BID to TID (maximum 600 mg/d)

Abbreviations: BID, twice daily; TID, 3 times per day.

and close follow-up is recommended. More specifically, adolescents with refractory chronic primary headache, with significant headache disability, weighing at least 40 kg, are postpubertal, without significant bone disease, not pregnant or breastfeeding, and without disrupted blood-brain barrier may be good candidates. A recent multicenter retrospective study of CGRP mAbs in adolescents with refractory chronic migraine, NDPH, or persistent PTH has shown at least some benefit in more than two-thirds of patients treated.[60] The side effect profile was similar to that of adult studies of mAbs with only 5 of 112 patients discontinuing due to adverse effects.

ALTERNATIVE THERAPIES
Neuromodulation Therapies

Neuromodulatory devices modulate head pain by providing nonpharmacologic electric current or magnetic stimulation to the central or peripheral nervous system, and can be used as either individual or add-on therapies. There are 4 devices currently approved by the FDA for acute (remote electrical neuromodulation [REN])[61] or concurrent short-term and preventive use (external trigeminal nerve stimulation [eTNS],[62] noninvasive vagal nerve stimulation,[63] single-pulse transcranial magnetic stimulation [sTMS][64]) in adolescents ages 12 years and greater. The REN device delivers transcutaneous electrical stimulation to the upper arm, which uses conditioned pain modulation to activate pain inhibitory centers and exert a generalized analgesic effect.[65] The eTNS device is now available online without a prescription, whereas the other devices require a prescription. The noninvasive vagus nerve stimulation is also approved by the FDA for short-term and preventive treatment of cluster headache. These devices are generally well tolerated, and can be beneficial for those who are either on multiple medications or have frequent attacks placing them at risk of developing medication overuse headache.

Behavioral Therapies

Biobehavioral therapies have become very important therapies in teaching pain coping mechanisms and regulation of autonomic arousal due to migraine. CBT, biofeedback, and relaxation therapies have grade A evidence for use as preventive therapies for migraine, and are increasingly being studied for short-term use.[66] In the adolescent population, CBT with a trained therapist can be extremely valuable in helping patients acquire skills to make healthy changes in thoughts, feelings, physical sensations, and behaviors, with the goal of improving pain and functioning.[67] CBT was studied in a 20-week-long randomized controlled trial of 135 pediatric and adolescent patients with chronic migraine concurrently taking amitriptyline, and it was found that 10 sessions of 1-hour individual CBT was more effective than 10 headache education sessions.[68] This benefit was also sustained 12 months out,[69] suggesting ongoing benefits of this behavioral therapy especially when combined with pharmacotherapy.

Although biobehavioral therapies have traditionally been delivered in person, smartphone application formats have been developed for the adolescent[70] and adult population[71] and can increase access to these beneficial therapies.

Procedures

For adolescent migraine, greater occipital nerve (GON) blocks are relatively well studied and generally well tolerated. There is significant provider variation whether the blocks are done unilaterally or bilaterally; there are also variations in anesthetic agents chosen such as lidocaine or bupivacaine as well as whether to add a steroid such as methylprednisolone or dexamethasone.[72] In a retrospective study of 40 patients younger than 18 years with a chronic primary headache disorder, 53% found at least some benefit from a unilateral GON block with methylprednisolone acetate and 2% lidocaine.[73] There were no serious adverse effects in this study, although common reactions include injection site pain and potential for localized infection. Adults can usually easily tolerate 3 mL volume at an injection site. It is the authors' recommendation that if there is a minimal amount of subcutaneous tissue at the GON site, one should consider using less volume such as 2 mL to avoid tissue injury.

Sphenopalatine ganglion (SPG) blocks have been used for decades for short-term management of migraine and cluster headache, and newer intranasal devices can offer higher tolerability.[74] The anesthetics used include 2% lidocaine or 0.5% bupivacaine, which are injected via each nare into the pterygopalatine fossa while the patient is laying supine with cervical spine extension. A double-blind, placebo-controlled study of weekly SPG blocks over 6 weeks for short-term treatment of chronic migraine in adults revealed significant reduction in numeric pain scores through 24 hours postprocedure.[75] The procedure is overall safe and well-tolerated,[76] with a recent retrospective study in the pediatric and adolescent population demonstrating statistically significant reduction in pain scores immediately postprocedure.[77] A small prospective case series of adolescents with chronic headache disorders unresponsive to standard therapies found reduction in depressive symptoms and improvement in global impression of change scores following repetitive SPG blockade.[78] Future studies are needed to elucidate the long-term benefit of this procedure.

Using botulinum toxin injections for chronic migraine in adults has long been approved by the FDA but still not approved in those younger than 18 years. Most providers use the standard 31 injections distributing 155 units of onabotulinumtoxin A (BOTOX) with an interval of 3 months; this requires selecting patients who can tolerate this regimen. High-quality evidence for BOTOX in the adolescent chronic migraine population remains quite scant per a literature review,[79] although 2 recent retrospective studies and 1 small placebo-controlled study have shown benefit in this population.[80–82] One study found that poorly controlled generalized anxiety disorder may be a risk factor for lack of response to BOTOX therapy in adolescents.[83]

SUMMARY

Adolescents may be strongly impacted by chronic headache disorders resulting in disability at home, school, and in maintaining peer relationships. Their headache characteristics may share some but not all features of the same adult headache disorder. Some headache disorders such as NDPH are more common in adolescents, whereas others such as TACs are less prevalent.

Abortive therapy for adolescents with migraine has expanded to include the ditans, gepants, minor procedures, as well as neuromodulation. Preventive therapy may initially rely on treatments with low risk for adverse effects such as CBT and nutraceuticals. For refractory adolescent migraine, monoclonal antibodies against CGRP are starting to be used, but further high-quality evidence in adolescents is needed to gain FDA approval.

CLINICS CARE POINTS

- Migraine in children and adolescents can be of shorter duration and bilateral location compared to adults, and is distinguishable from tension type headache by severity, movement sensitivity, photophobia and phonophobia, and/or nausea.

- Triptans are effective abortive medications to use in adolescents, and can have improved effect when coupled with NSAID medications.

- Treating migraine-associated nausea is important, and is part of the American Academy of Neurology guidelines for short-term treatment of migraine in children and adolescents.

- Non-pharmacologic lifestyle and behavioral interventions, nutraceutical medications, and neuromodulation devices can be considered as first-line therapies for migraine prevention in children and adolescents prior to prescription migraine preventive medications.

DISCLOSURE

Dr I. Patniyot has received institutional research support from Teva and Theranica Bio-Electronics for multicenter trial participation. Dr W. Qubty has nothing to disclose.

REFERENCES

1. Burch RC, Buse DC, Lipton RB. Migraine: Epidemiology, Burden, and Comorbidity. Neurol Clin 2019;37(4):631–49.
2. Lewis DW. Pediatric Migraine. Neurol Clin 2009;27(2):481–501.
3. Vos T, Abajobir AA, Abbafati C, et al. Global, regional, and national incidence, prevalence, and years lived with disability for 328 diseases and injuries for 195 countries, 1990-2016: A systematic analysis for the Global Burden of Disease Study 2016. Lancet 2017;390(10100):1211–59.
4. Steiner TJ, Stovner LJ, Vos T, et al. Migraine is first cause of disability in under 50s: will health politicians now take notice? J Headache Pain 2018. https://doi.org/10.1186/s10194-018-0846-2.
5. Allain-Regnault M, Bwibo NO, Chigier E. Young people's health - A challenge for society. World Heal Organ - Tech Rep Ser 1986;731:1–117.
6. Hershey AD, Powers SW, Vockell ALB, et al. Development of a patient-based grading scale for PedMIDAS. Cephalalgia 2004;24(10):844–9.
7. Yamani N, Olesen J. New daily persistent headache: A systematic review on an enigmatic disorder. J Headache Pain 2019. https://doi.org/10.1186/s10194-019-1022-z.
8. Rozen TD. New daily persistent headache (NDPH) triggered by a single Valsalva event: A case series. Cephalalgia 2019;39(6):785–91.
9. Grengs LR, Mack KJ. New Daily Persistent Headache Is Most Likely to Begin at the Start of School. J Child Neurol 2016;31(7):864–8.
10. Strong E, Pierce EL, Langdon R, et al. New Daily Persistent Headache in a Pediatric Population. J Child Neurol 2021;36(10):888–93.
11. Ghosh A, Silva E, Burish MJ. Pediatric-onset trigeminal autonomic cephalalgias: A systematic review and meta-analysis. Cephalalgia 2021;41(13):1382–95.

12. Oskoui M, Pringsheim T, Holler-Managan Y, et al. Practice guideline update summary: Acute treatment of migraine in children and adolescents: Report of the Guideline Development, Dissemination, and Implementation Subcommittee of the American Academy of Neurology and the American Headache Society. Neurology 2019;93(11):487–99.
13. Patniyot I, Qubty W. Short-term treatment of Migraine in Children and Adolescents. JAMA 2020;174(8):789–90.
14. Hämäläinen ML, Hoppu K, Valkeila E, et al. Ibuprofen or acetaminophen for the acute treatment of migraine in children: A double-blind, randomized, placebo-controlled, crossover study. Neurology 1997;48(1):103–7.
15. Lipton RB, Munjal S, Brand-Schieber E, et al. Efficacy, Tolerability, and Safety of DFN-15 (Celecoxib Oral Solution, 25 mg/mL) in the Acute Treatment of Episodic Migraine: A Randomized, Double-Blind, Placebo-Controlled Study. Headache 2020;60(1):58–70.
16. Cady R, Nett R, Dexter K, et al. Treatment of chronic migraine: A 3-month comparator study of naproxen sodium vs SumaRT/Nap. Headache 2014;54(1):80–93.
17. Ferrari MD, Roon KI, Lipton RB, et al. Oral triptans (serotonin 5-HT1B/1D agonists) in acute migraine treatment: A meta-analysis of 53 trials. Lancet 2001; 358(9294):1668–75.
18. Kabbouche MA, Vockell AL, LeCates SL, et al. Tolerability and effectiveness of prochlorperazine for intractable migraine in children. Pediatrics 2001;107(4). https://doi.org/10.1542/peds.107.4.e62.
19. Trottier ED, Bailey B, Lucas N, et al. Prochlorperazine in children with migraine: A look at its effectiveness and rate of akathisia. Am J Emerg Med 2012;30(3): 456–63.
20. Brousseau DC, Duffy SJ, Anderson AC, et al. Treatment of Pediatric Migraine Headaches: A Randomized, Double-Blind Trial of Prochlorperazine Versus Ketorolac. Ann Emerg Med 2004;43(2):256–62.
21. Trottier ED, Bailey B, Dauphin-Pierre S, et al. Clinical outcomes of children treated with intravenous prochlorperazine for migraine in a pediatric emergency department. J Emerg Med 2010;39(2):166–73.
22. Kanis JM, Timm NL. Chlorpromazine for the treatment of migraine in a pediatric emergency department. Headache 2014;54(2):335–42.
23. Hodgson SE, Harding AM, Bourke EM, et al. A prospective, randomized, double-blind trial of intravenous chlorpromazine versus intravenous prochlorperazine for the treatment of acute migraine in adults presenting to the emergency department. Headache 2021;61(4):603–11.
24. Marmura MJ, Silberstein SD, Schwedt TJ. The acute treatment of migraine in adults: The american headache society evidence assessment of migraine pharmacotherapies. Headache 2015;55(1):3–20.
25. Jones J, Pack S, Chun E. Intramuscular prochlorperazine versus metoclopramide as single-agent therapy for the treatment of acute migraine headache. Am J Emerg Med 1996;14(3):262–4.
26. Friedman BW, Esses D, Solorzano C, et al. A Randomized Controlled Trial of Prochlorperazine Versus Metoclopramide for Treatment of Acute Migraine. Ann Emerg Med 2008;52(4):399–406.
27. Goadsby PJ, Wietecha LA, Dennehy EB, et al. Phase 3 randomized, placebo-controlled, double-blind study of lasmiditan for acute treatment of migraine. Brain 2019;142(7):1894–904.
28. Croop R, Goadsby PJ, Stock DA, et al. Efficacy, safety, and tolerability of rimegepant orally disintegrating tablet for the acute treatment of migraine: a

randomised, phase 3, double-blind, placebo-controlled trial. Lancet 2019; 394(10200):737–45.

29. Dodick DW, Lipton RB, Ailani J, et al. Ubrogepant for the Treatment of Migraine. N Engl J Med 2019;381(23):2230–41.

30. Paruthi S, Brooks LJ, D'Ambrosio C, et al. Consensus Statement of the American Academy of Sleep Medicine on the Recommended Amount of Sleep for Healthy Children: Methodology and Discussion. J Clin Sleep Med 2016;12(11):1549–61.

31. Carskadon MA, Tarokh L. Developmental changes in sleep biology and potential effects on adolescent behavior and caffeine use. Nutr Rev 2014;72(S1):60–4.

32. Hysing M, Pallesen S, Stormark KM, et al. Sleep and use of electronic devices in adolescence: Results from a large population-based study. BMJ Open 2015; 5(1):1–7.

33. Cajochen C, Frey S, Anders D, et al. Evening exposure to a light-emitting diodes (LED)-backlit computer screen affects circadian physiology and cognitive performance. J Appl Physiol 2011;110(5):1432–8.

34. Howatson G, Bell PG, Tallent J, et al. Effect of tart cherry juice (Prunus cerasus) on melatonin levels and enhanced sleep quality. Eur J Nutr 2012;51(8):909–16.

35. Bektaş Ö, Uğur C, Gençtürk ZB, et al. Relationship of childhood headaches with preferences in leisure time activities, depression, anxiety and eating habits: A population-based, cross-sectional study. Cephalalgia 2015;35(6):527–37.

36. Peris F, Donoghue S, Torres F, et al. Towards improved migraine management: Determining potential trigger factors in individual patients. Cephalalgia 2017; 37(5):452–63.

37. Gelfand Amy A, Pavitt Sara, Greene Kaitlin, et al. High School Start Time and Migraine Frequency in High School Students. Headache 2019;59(7):1024–31.

38. Goadsby PJ, Holland PR, Martins-Oliveira M, et al. Pathophysiology of Migraine: A Disorder of Sensory Processing. Physiol Rev 2017;97(2):553–622.

39. Cuvellier JC, Mars A, Vallée L. The prevalence of premonitory symptoms in paediatric migraine: A questionnaire study in 103 children and adolescents. Cephalalgia 2009;29(11):1197–201.

40. Karsan N, Bose P, Goadsby PJ. The Migraine Premonitory Phase. Contin Lifelong Learn Neurol 2018;24(4-Headache):996–1008.

41. Arca KN, Halker Singh RB. Dehydration and Headache. Curr Pain Headache Rep 2021;25(8):4–9.

42. Perry BG, Bear TLK, Lucas SJE, et al. Mild dehydration modifies the cerebrovascular response to the cold pressor test. Exp Physiol 2016;101(1):135–42.

43. Kenney EL, Long MW, Cradock AL, et al. Prevalence of inadequate hydration among US children and disparities by gender and race/ethnicity: National Health and Nutrition Examination Survey, 2009-2012. Am J Public Health 2015;105(8): e113–8.

44. Spigt M, Weerkamp N, Troost J, et al. A randomized trial on the effects of regular water intake in patients with recurrent headaches. Fam Pract 2012;29(4):370–5.

45. Khorsha F, Mirzababaei A, Togha M, et al. Association of drinking water and migraine headache severity. J Clin Neurosci 2020;77:81–4.

46. Medicine I of. Dietary Reference Intakes for Water, Potassium, Sodium, Chloride, and Sulfate.; 2005. doi:10.17226/10925.

47. Amin FM, Aristeidou S, Baraldi C, et al. The association between migraine and physical exercise. J Headache Pain 2018;19(1):83.

48. Robberstad L, Dyb G, Hagen K, et al. An unfavorable lifestyle and recurrent headaches among adolescents: The HUNT Study. Neurology 2010;75(8):712–7.

49. Bigal ME, Liberman JN, Lipton RB. Obesity and migraine: A population study. Neurology 2006;66(4):545–50.
50. Varkey E, Cider Å, Carlsson J, et al. Exercise as migraine prophylaxis: A randomized study using relaxation and topiramate as controls. Cephalalgia 2011;31(14): 1428–38.
51. Santiago MDS, Carvalho D de S, Gabbai AA, et al. Amitriptyline and aerobic exercise or amitriptyline alone in the treatment of chronic migraine: A randomized comparative study. Arq Neuropsiquiatr 2014;72(11):851–5.
52. Oskoui M, Pringsheim T, Billinghurst L, et al. Practice guideline update summary: Pharmacologic treatment for pediatric migraine prevention. Neurology 2019. https://doi.org/10.1212/wnl.0000000000008105.
53. Powers SW, Coffey CS, Chamberlin LA, et al. Trial of amitriptyline, topiramate, and placebo for pediatric migraine. N Engl J Med 2017. https://doi.org/10.1056/NEJMoa1610384.
54. Das R, Qubty W. Retrospective Observational Study on Riboflavin Prophylaxis in Child and Adolescent Migraine. Pediatr Neurol 2021;114. https://doi.org/10.1016/j.pediatrneurol.2020.09.009.
55. Ebrahimi-Monfared M, Sharafkhah M, Abdolrazaghnejad A, et al. Use of melatonin versus valproic acid in prophylaxis of migraine patients: A double-blind randomized clinical trial. Restor Neurol Neurosci 2017;35(4):385–93.
56. Gonçalves AL, Ferreira AM, Ribeiro RT, et al. Research paper: Randomised clinical trial comparing melatonin 3 mg, amitriptyline 25 mg and placebo for migraine prevention. J Neurol Neurosurg Psychiatry 2016;87(10):1127.
57. Sazali S, Badrin S, Norhayati MN, et al. Coenzyme Q10 supplementation for prophylaxis in adult patients with migraine-a meta-analysis. BMJ Open 2021;11(1). https://doi.org/10.1136/BMJOPEN-2020-039358.
58. von Luckner A, Riederer F. Magnesium in Migraine Prophylaxis—Is There an Evidence-Based Rationale? A Systematic Review. Headache J Head Face Pain 2018;58(2):199–209.
59. Szperka CL, VanderPluym J, Orr SL, et al. Recommendations on the Use of Anti-CGRP Monoclonal Antibodies in Children and Adolescents. Headache 2018; 58(10). https://doi.org/10.1111/head.13414.
60. Greene KA, Gentile CP, Szperka CL, et al. CGRP Monoclonal Antibody use for the Preventive Treatment of Refractory Headache Disorders in Adolescents. Pediatr Neurol 2021;114:62.
61. Hershey AD, Lin T, Gruper Y, et al. Remote electrical neuromodulation for acute treatment of migraine in adolescents. Headache 2021;61(2):310–7.
62. Chou DE, Shnayderman Yugrakh M, Winegarner D, et al. Acute migraine therapy with external trigeminal neurostimulation (ACME): A randomized controlled trial. Cephalalgia 2019;39(1):3–14.
63. Grazzi L, Egeo G, Liebler E, et al. No Title. Neurol Sci 2017;38(Suppl 1):S197–9.
64. Irwin SL, Qubty W, Allen IE, et al. Transcranial Magnetic Stimulation for Migraine Prevention in Adolescents: A Pilot Open-Label Study. Headache 2018;58(5):724–31.
65. Yarnitsky D, Volokh L, Ironi A, et al. Nonpainful remote electrical stimulation alleviates episodic migraine pain. Neurology 2017;88(13):1250–5.
66. Ailani J, Burch RC, Robbins MS. The American Headache Society Consensus Statement: Update on integrating new migraine treatments into clinical practice. Headache 2021;61(7):1021–39.
67. Ernst MM, O'Brien HL, Powers SW. Cognitive-behavioral therapy: How medical providers can increase patient and family openness and access to evidence-based multimodal therapy for pediatric migraine. Headache 2015;55(10):1382–96.

68. Power SW, Kashikar-Zuck SM, Allen JR, et al. Cognitive behavioral therapy plus amitriptyline for chronic migraine in children and adolescents: A randomized clinical trial. JAMA 2013;310(24):2622–30.
69. Kroner JW, Hershey AD, Kashikar-Zuck SM, et al. Cognitive Behavioral Therapy plus Amitriptyline for Children and Adolescents with Chronic Migraine Reduces Headache Days to ≤4 per Month. Headache 2016;56(4):711–6.
70. Stubberud A, Tronvik E, Olsen A, et al. Biofeedback Treatment App for Pediatric Migraine: Development and Usability Study. Headache 2020;60(5):889–901.
71. Minen MT, Adhikari S, Padikkala J, et al. Smartphone-Delivered Progressive Muscle Relaxation for the Treatment of Migraine in Primary Care: A Randomized Controlled Trial. Headache 2020;60(10):2232–46.
72. Szperka CL, Gelfand AA, Hershey AD. Patterns of Use of Peripheral Nerve Blocks and Trigger Point Injections for Pediatric Headache: Results of a Survey of the American Headache Society Pediatric and Adolescent Section. Headache 2016;56(10):1597–607.
73. Gelfand AA, Reider AC, Goadsby PJ. Outcomes of greater occipital nerve injections in pediatric patients with chronic primary headache disorders. Pediatr Neurol 2014;50(2):135–9.
74. Robbins MS, Robertson CE, Kaplan E, et al. The Sphenopalatine Ganglion: Anatomy, Pathophysiology, and Therapeutic Targeting in Headache. Headache 2016;56(2):240–58.
75. Cady R, Saper J, Dexter K, et al. A double-blind, placebo-controlled study of repetitive transnasal sphenopalatine ganglion blockade with Tx360® as acute treatment for chronic migraine. Headache 2015;55(1):101–16.
76. Binfalah M, Alghawi E, Shosha E, et al. Sphenopalatine Ganglion Block for the Treatment of Acute Migraine Headache. Pain Res Treat 2018;2018. https://doi.org/10.1155/2018/2516953.
77. Mousa MA, Aria DJ, Mousa AA, et al. Sphenopalatine ganglion nerve block for the treatment of migraine headaches in the pediatric population. Pain Physician 2021;24(1):E111–6.
78. Kouri M, Somaini M, Cárdenas VHG, et al. Transnasal sphenopalatine ganglion block for the preventive treatment of chronic daily headache in adolescents. Children 2021;8(7):1–8.
79. Marcelo R, Freund B. The Efficacy of Botulinum Toxin in Pediatric Chronic Migraine: A Literature Review. J Child Neurol 2020;35(12):844–51.
80. Goenka A, Yu SG, George M, et al. Is Botox right for me: When to assess the efficacy of the Botox injection for chronic migraine in pediatric population. Neuropediatrics 2022. https://doi.org/10.1055/A-1832-9168.
81. Ali SS, Bragin I, Rende E, et al. Further Evidence that Onabotulinum Toxin is a Viable Treatment Option for Pediatric Chronic Migraine Patients. Cureus 2019;11(3). https://doi.org/10.7759/CUREUS.4343.
82. Shah S, Calderon MD, Crain N, et al. Effectiveness of onabotulinumtoxinA (BOTOX) in pediatric patients experiencing migraines: a randomized, double-blinded, placebo-controlled crossover study in the pediatric pain population. Reg Anesth Pain Med 2021;46(1):41–8.
83. Goenka A, Grace Yu S, Chikkannaiah M, et al. Generalized Anxiety Disorder: A Predictor for Poor Responsiveness to Botulinum Toxin Type A Therapy for Pediatric Migraine. Pediatr Neurol 2022;130:21–7.

Dysautonomia
Diagnosis and Management

Alexandra Hovaguimian, MD

KEYWORDS

- Autonomic nervous system • Dysautonomia • Autonomic dysfunction
- Autonomic testing • Tilt table testing • Neurogenic orthostatic hypotension
- Postural orthostatic tachycardia syndrome • Autonomic neuropathy

KEY POINTS

- Dysautonomias are a heterogenous group of disorders that can cause variable symptoms ranging from isolated impairment of one autonomic function to multisystem failure.
- Not all symptoms of orthostatic intolerance are associated with autonomic impairment, such as neurogenic orthostatic hypotension or postural orthostatic tachycardia syndrome.
- Dysautonomias can be due to central or peripheral autonomic impairment, and the latter is often secondary to other disorders causing autonomic neuropathies.
- Identifying and treating any underlying disease that causes or exacerbates the condition is central to clinical care.
- Treatment should be patient centered with the goal of improving quality of life and functioning.

INTRODUCTION

The term dysautonomia is used broadly to describe a wide range of autonomic impairments ranging from hyperhidrosis to multiple system atrophy (MSA). In this review, the author explores a practical, clinically oriented approach to dysautonomias. The article focuses on key features of a patient's history and examination that allow clinicians to generate an appropriate differential diagnosis and initial assessment. The author then explores the first-line evaluation, including different types of autonomic testing and interpretation of these results. Nonpharmacologic and pharmacologic management of 2 common clinical phenotypes: neurogenic orthostatic hypotension (NOH) and postural orthostatic tachycardia syndrome (POTS) will then be reviewed. In recent years, there has also been growing interest in dysautonomia associated with so-called long-COVID patients. A detailed exploration of this topic exceeds the scope of this article, but the author explores a few issues that clinicians should consider when evaluating patients with autonomic symptoms after a COVID-19 infection.

Beth Israel Deaconess Medical Center, Harvard Medical School, 330 Brookline Avenue, KS 432, Boston, MA 02215, USA
E-mail address: ahovagui@bidmc.harvard.edu

Neurol Clin 41 (2023) 193–213
https://doi.org/10.1016/j.ncl.2022.08.002
0733-8619/23/© 2022 Elsevier Inc. All rights reserved.

DEFINITION

A dysautonomia is a disorder of the autonomic nervous system (ANS). The ANS controls a broad range of involuntary bodily functions ranging from blood pressure regulation to sweating, and dysautonomias can be disorders of one of these functions or, alternatively, of the ANS more pervasively. This means that patients may have diverse presentations, ranging from isolated enteric symptoms[1] to extensive autonomic failure, as is seen in MSA.[2] Because the ANS is so widely involved in end-organ functions, patients with multiple symptoms involving different systems may be characterized as having a dysautonomia without careful examination of the evidence for this diagnosis or the other comorbidities that may impact clinical interpretation. Most true dysautonomias are difficult to treat, and actual disease-modifying therapies are often lacking. It is therefore essential that clinicians be meticulous in their diagnosis, excluding treatable mimics and secondary causes of autonomic impairment that, if identified and treated, could improve patient outcomes.

One of the most common presenting constellations of symptoms for patients with dysautonomias is orthostatic intolerance (OI). OI refers to symptoms of lightheadedness with postural changes, non–vertiginous dizziness, and/or palpitations.[3–5] For some autonomic disorders, such as POTS, symptoms of OI are required for the diagnosis, as there are patients with postural tachycardias who are asymptomatic.[4,5]

The vital sign findings in dysautonomias, such as a postural tachycardia or orthostatic hypotension (OH), are symptoms of the underlying disorder, comparable to fever. This can be a source of confusion, especially when it comes to the diagnosis of POTS. Just as fever is an important vital sign abnormality that indicates the need to evaluate for an underlying cause, in dysautonomias, patients can have NOH or a postural tachycardia, and these vital sign abnormalities are signs of an underlying disorder. Clinicians must therefore investigate the cause of the vital sign abnormality while simultaneously counseling the patient and/or their caregivers about the vital sign findings, how they relate to symptoms, and underlying disease or diseases. Early education on symptom management versus disease modification helps to establish realistic patient expectations for treatment and prognosis.

It is equally important to recognize that vasovagal syncope is not a disease but rather an autonomic variant.[5,6] Patient education around this topic is also necessary, as patients may presume that the diagnosis of vasovagal syncope is a form of dysautonomia with a comparable prognosis as neurodegenerative disorders, such as MSA or autonomic neuropathies.

PREVALENCE

Depending on the cause, dysautonomias can be extremely rare or quite common. Diabetic autonomic neuropathies, for example, occur commonly in patients with type I and type II diabetes and are likely underdiagnosed. The actual reported prevalence however varies depending on how the condition is defined, and estimates range up to a 90% prevalence in patients with diabetes.[7,8] By contrast, familial dysautonomia (also known as hereditary sensory and autonomic neuropathy type 3 or Riley-Day syndrome) is a rare genetic disease only occurring in 1:3700 live births of Ashkenazis.[9] Many dysautonomias are due to primary disorders, such as autoimmune diseases, a phenomenon called an autonomic neuropathy, but notably not all of these primary disorders cause or manifest with autonomic disfunction. Therefore, estimating the true prevalence of dysautonomias is challenging given the heterogenicity of clinical presentations.

DIAGNOSIS

The diagnostic approach to a dysautonomia is the same framework that neurologists use for other neurologic disorders. The ANS has central and peripheral components. Disorders of the autonomic nerve systems can be therefore classified as central, peripheral, or both. Similarly, a dysautonomia can be a primary disorder (owing to a disease of the autonomic systems in the central nervous system or peripheral nervous system), or a secondary disorder (owing to a disease that secondarily damages the central and/or peripheral ANS). The causes of dysautonomias parallel other neurologic diseases and can be genetic, neurodegenerative, toxic, infectious, metabolic, autoimmune, neoplastic, and so forth.

Peripheral dysautonomias are often due to small fiber autonomic neuropathies.[10] The small nerve fibers are unmyelinated C-fibers and myelinated Aδ fibers and are responsible for sensory functions, including pain and temperature as well as itch. These fibers are also involved in peripheral autonomic function.[10] Disorders that cause small fiber neuropathies (SFN) therefore can manifest with autonomic symptoms and are then referred to as autonomic neuropathies.[11–16] Just as with other peripheral nerve disorders, autonomic neuropathies can be acute, subacute, or chronic and have diverse causes with variability in the types and severity of autonomic symptoms.[11–13] They can even affect the ganglion, in a condition known as an autoimmune autonomic ganglionopathy. **Table 1** includes a list of established causes of central autonomic failure and peripheral autonomic neuropathies. There is some evidence that COVID-19 can cause a secondary dysautonomia,[14] although patients may also have symptoms of OI without objective findings on autonomic testing.[17]

EVALUATION

As with all neurologic conditions, assessment of a dysautonomia starts at the bedside with a detailed history and neurologic examination. Long-standing NOH is often well tolerated because of cerebral autoregulatory adaptation. It may therefore be underreported. It is therefore important to recognize high-risk populations, such as patients with long-standing diabetes[18] and Parkinson disease.[19]

When interpreting a patient's clinical history, clinicians should consider if the autonomic system is hyperactive or hypoactive. Similarly, the time course of the disease should be mapped (ie, are the symptoms acute/subacute, chronic progressive, static, or episodic/paroxysmal). It is critical that the examiner complete a careful review of systems to ascertain if there are signs of isolated autonomic impairment or more pervasive autonomic dysfunction and/or other associated neurologic and systemic symptoms. **Fig. 1** includes an example of an autonomic review of systems.

Similarly, a detailed review of medications, including over-the-counter treatments and herbal remedies, should be included. Current and prior substance and alcohol use history should also be explicitly elucidated, as alcohol use disorders, even if currently in remission, can cause autonomic neuropathies and acute ingestion, or withdrawal from some substances can cause autonomic disturbances. Family histories are also important, as some autonomic conditions are inherited. Patients should also be screened for cardiovascular conditioning, including their weekly exercise habits, volume, sodium and caffeine intake, as this will provide information about their baseline function, and valuable data for later treatment counseling.

The neurologic examination should start with orthostatic vital sign measurements (**Fig. 2**).[5]

Table 1
Causes of central and peripheral dysautonomias

Peripheral causes

Endocrinologic	• Diabetes	• Impaired glucose intolerance	• Abnormal thyroid function
Autoimmune	• Rheumatoid arthritis • Systemic lupus erythematosus	• Sjogren syndrome • Ankylosing spondylitis	• Scleroderma • Connective tissue disorders	• Psoriatic arthritis • Sarcoidosis
Genetic	• Acute autonomic and sensory neuropathy • Amyloidosis	• Ehlers-Danlos syndrome • Fabry disease	• Wilson disease • Charcot-Marie-Tooth disease	• Familial amyloidosis • Pompe
Infectious	• Human immunodeficiency virus	• Hepatitis C • Chagas disease	• COVID-19 • Botulism	• Leprosy • Lyme disease
Vitamin deficiencies	• Vitamin B12 deficiency	• Vitamin E deficiency	• Copper deficiency	
Neuroimmunologic	• Autoimmune autonomic ganglionopathy	• Autonomic neuropathies • Guillian-Barré syndrome	• Antiganglionic nicotinic acetylcholine receptor	• Chronic inflammatory demyelinating polyneuropathy
Neoplastic	• Primary systemic amyloidosis	• Anti-CRMP5 (CV-2) • Anti-Hu (ANNA-1)	• Lambert-Eaton myasthenic syndrome • Paraneoplastic autonomic neuropathies	• Disorders with voltage-gated potassium channel complex antibodies
Gastrointestinal	• Ulcerative colitis	• Crohn disease	• Celiac disease	• Idiopathic gastrointestinal dysmotility
Other	• Autonomic seizures • Alcohol	• Chemotherapy • Neurotoxic drugs	• Monoclonal gammopathy • Fibromyalgia	• Mast cell activation disorders • Idiopathic anhidrosis • Cholinergic neuropathy

Central causes

Neurodegenerative	• Parkinson disease	• Multiple system atrophy	• Lewy body dementia	• Pure autonomic failure
Traumatic/vascular	• Subarachnoid hemorrhage	• Insular stroke	• Traumatic brain injury	• Cervical spinal cord transection at or above T6
Neuroimmunologic	• Multiple sclerosis			

Data from Refs.[11–14,16–18]

Vasomotor: hypo and hyperhidrosis, goose flesh, cold hands and/or feet
Cardiovascular: Postural lightheadedness, tachycardia, Coat hanger headache (neck/shoulder pain)
Pupillary dysfunction: blurry vision with bright or dim light
SICCA complex: dry eyes or dry mouth
Sleep: acting out dreams
Movement: tremor, postural instability, falls, ataxia
Cognition: cognitive impairment
Smell: Anosmia
GI: gastroparesis, constipation, diarrhea, early satiety, bloating
GU: neurogenic bladder, Erectile dysfunction

Fig. 1. Autonomic review of systems.

This should be followed by a standard neurologic examination with attention to the patient's coordination and a detailed small fiber sensory examination. Clinicians should also include the following general medical examination components:

- Cardiac examination: Evaluating for evidence of arrhythmias, tachycardia, murmurs, and heart failure
- Dermatologic screening: Assessing vasomotor changes, Raynaud phenomenon, dermatographia, and anhidrosis
- Musculoskeletal examination: Examining for hypermobility

The differential diagnosis for a potential dysautonomia should emerge based on the findings from a patient's history (system/organ involvement, temporal characteristics, comorbidities), the neurologic examination findings, and localization. A full description of all the history and examination findings of central and peripheral dysautonomias exceeds the scope of this discussion, but patterns and features on history and examination to suggest central or peripheral dysautonomias are included in **Table 2:**[10]

Understanding the clinical features of different types of dysautonomias is important, as diseases that adversely impact the ANS are difficult to treat, and clinicians should focus on identifying any reversible or treatable conditions to prevent progressive autonomic impairment.

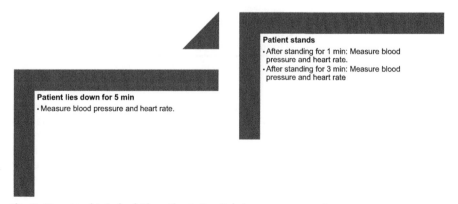

Patient stands
- After standing for 1 min: Measure blood pressure and heart rate.
- After standing for 3 min: Measure blood pressure and heart rate

Patient lies down for 5 min
- Measure blood pressure and heart rate.

Fig. 2. How to obtain bedside orthostatic vital sign measurements.

Table 2
Features of central and peripheral dysautonomias

Pathology	Clinical Features	Timing/Progression
Central dysautonomias		
Neurodegenerative (α-synucleinopathies)		
• MSA • Lewy body dementia • Parkinson disease • Pure autonomic failure	• Cognitive impairment • Anosmia • REM behavior disorder • Movement disorder	Subacute Progressive Later Age
Neurovascular		
• Subarachnoid hemorrhage • Insular stroke	• Other focal neurologic features on history, examination, and imaging	Acute onset
Traumatic		
• T6 or above spinal cord injury • Traumatic brain injury	• Other focal neurologic features on history and examination, and imaging	Acute onset
Multiple sclerosis	• Progressive without treatment • Other focal neurologic features on history and examination, and imaging	Acute/subacute
Peripheral dysautonomias		
Guillain-Barré	• Based on history and sensory and reflex findings neurologic findings on examination	Acute/subacute
Autoimmune autonomic ganglionopathy	• Other focal neurologic features on history and examination	Acute/subacute/progressive
Autonomic neuropathies secondary to systematic causes	• Infectious • Rheumatologic • Gastroenterologic • Malignancy and paraneoplastic • Endocrinologic • Genetic • Toxic/nutritional	All associated with systemic features on history, examination, additional testing, ± family history, ± exposure history

WORKUP AND TESTING

Clinicians should refer patients for additional hypothesis-driven diagnostic testing based on the differential diagnoses. Primary or comorbid cardiovascular diseases are common, especially in patients with diabetes and with growing age. There are also well-established guidelines for evaluation of syncope.[20] When indicated based on the patient's history, examination, and/or comorbidities, clinicians should carefully screen for cardiac causes or comorbidities with additional testing, including an electrocardiogram, echocardiogram, Holter monitoring, Zio patch, 24-hour ambulatory blood pressure monitoring, and/or cardiac nuclear testing, as appropriate.[21]

If neurologic findings are present on history or examination, clinicians should follow the appropriate workup of these findings. If there are central features to suggest a neurogenerative cause, such as Parkinsonism, Lewy body dementia, MSA, or a cerebellar disorder, clinicians should follow the standard neurologic workup for alpha-synucleinopathies,[22] and imaging may be considered, although many of these disorders are still clinical diagnoses. If symptoms and/or findings localize to spinal cord pathologic condition, particularly at or above T6, further imaging is warranted to assess for cord lesions causing autonomic dysreflexia,[23] although it is very rare to have this phenotype without a known cord lesion based on prior history. Subarachnoid hemorrhage (SAH)[24] and insular strokes[25] will both present with acute onset syndromes that may have autonomic features. The workup for both conditions should include standard neuroimaging and additional vascular neurology assessments for the causes of stroke and SAH as well as secondary prevention. Autonomic seizures are rare,[15] but autonomic findings, such as tachycardias and arrhythmias, are not uncommon with seizures in general and have been implicated in sudden unexpected death from epilepsy.[16] If there is concern for autonomic involvement from seizures/epilepsy, additional electroencephalogram assessment is warranted.

When the neurologic examination reveals sensory abnormalities suggestive of a SFN, screening laboratory tests for reversible causes of small fiber and autonomic neuropathies should be sent. **Table 1** includes a list of systemic disorders that are known to cause autonomic neuropathies. Clinicians should practice high-value care and not order all laboratory tests, but rather use clinical judgment to screen for the most likely causes based on a patient's history, examination, and risk factors. If large fiber neuropathy is also identified, an electromyography may also be considered, and when concern for Guillain-Barré syndrome is present, appropriate workup with lumbar puncture should be initiated.[26]

AUTONOMIC-SPECIFIC TESTING

Testing of the ANS can be divided into those tests that assess structure and those that evaluate function. There are also numerous tests used for research purposes and/or those used by autonomic centers because of their specialized testing requirements and/or narrow clinical applicability. Discussion of those tests exceeds the scope of this review. The author focuses on autonomic tests that are more widely available in clinical practice and commonly used for diagnostic purposes. The physiologic mechanisms of these tests is not discussed, but their clinical applications and an overview of what patients experience during evaluation are reviewed.

Tests of Autonomic Structure

Skin biopsy for intraepidermal nerve fiber density

This test quantifies the number of unmyelinated C nerve fibers and thin myelinated Aδ fibers in the skin. Three-millimeter punch biopsies are typically obtained at standard sites at the distal calf (10 cm above the lateral malleus) and sometimes at other locations. The biopsies are stained with protein gene product-9.5 with immunocytochemistry. The intraepidermal nerve fiber density is then quantified and compared with normative data based on age and sex.[27–30]

Patients with SFN may have autonomic neuropathies and vice versa, but the 2 conditions may exist separately as well. There is growing interest in use of special staining of the intraepidermal nerve fiber to assess for evidence of specific pathologic conditions, such as α-synucleinopathies,[31,32] and other conditions, such as fibromyalgia.[33] In the last 2 years, there has also been evidence of the development of SFN in patients post–COVID-19[34] and a case report of a patient developing an SFN after receiving COVID-

19 vaccination.[35] Clinicians should use the history and physical examination findings, including pinprick and temperature testing to help guide if a skin biopsy will be helpful as a diagnostic tool, remembering that patients with SNF may also have hypoesthesia or hyperesthesia and/or allodynia.[28,36] Biopsy should be obtained when objective confirmation of an SFN is needed, such as to corroborate subjective symptoms and/or to monitor objective response to treatment.[36]

Tests of Function

Tilt table testing, also known as head up tilt

During the tilt table testing (TTT) (or head up tilt [HUT]), the patient starts testing in the supine position, at rest for 20 minutes while baseline measurements are recorded, and blood pressure and heart rate equilibrium is established. Supine hypertension can be detected with this monitoring. The patient is then rapidly tilted, with the head up and the feet down, on a supported platform, to 60° to 80° in the reverse Trendelenburg position. For safety, the patient's lower extremities and torso are secured as are the blood pressure and heart rate monitoring equipment.

The patient is continuously monitored, and the duration of the testing varies from medical centers, often only running for 10 minutes. This can be too brief to detect delayed orthostatic hypotension (DOH) or vasovagal syncope, however. Therefore, when referring a patient for TTT testing, clinicians should be aware of the testing center's protocol and, if necessary, request a longer TTT as appropriate based, on the indications for testing.

The testing is terminated based on the following:

- Patient preference/discomfort
- Syncope or presyncope, even if there is no hemodynamic correlate (ie, pseudosyncope)
- Sustained hypotension
- Blood pressure and heart rate response consistent with vasovagal syncope

If syncope occurs, patients should be monitored for bradycardia and asystole and placed in the Trendelenburg position if needed. A physician and code cart should be on hand. There are no direct contraindications for TTT, but if a patient cannot stand for the testing, they may not be able to participate. There are also weight limits to tilt tables, and clinicians should be familiar with the limit restrictions when referring patients to testing centers.

This test measures both sympathetic adrenergic and parasympathetic function. The heart rate response to the tilt is a measure of parasympathetic function, whereas the blood pressure response measures sympathetic adrenergic function. This test can detect OH, DOH, POTS, and vasovagal syncope.

Active standing

During this test, the patient is initially placed in the supine position at rest for at least 5 minutes. Baseline blood pressure and heart rate measurements are recorded, and supine hypertension can be detected with this monitoring. The patient then transitions to standing as quickly as possible (optimally within 3 seconds), but safety must be ensured. The patient then stands still, without support, for 5 minutes. The heart rate is monitored continuously (see later discussion), and the blood pressure is monitored at minutes 1, 3, and 5.

This is a test of both sympathetic adrenergic and parasympathetic function. The blood pressure change from the supine baseline to standing is a measure of sympathetic adrenergic function. The heart rate response during active standing, measured by the 30:15 ratio (the ratio of the slowest standing heart rate after 30 seconds divided by the fastest heart rate at 15 seconds), is a parasympathetic measure. A higher 30:15 ratio reflects preserved parasympathetic function.[37] This test can detect OH or POTS.

Valsalva maneuver
During this test, the patient breathes against resistance for 15 seconds in a standardized technique while the blood pressure and heart rate are monitored. An adequate respiratory effort is required for the test to be interpretable. This test should not be performed in patients with untreated glaucoma, diabetic retinopathy, or eye surgery in the last 3 months.

There are 4 phases of the maneuver, and the blood pressure response during testing is a measure of sympathetic adrenergic function, whereas the heart rate response is a measure of parasympathetic function. Patients can have isolated sympathetic adrenergic failure or parasympathetic failure or both.

Heart rate variability to paced breathing
During this test, the patient is asked to practice metronomic breathing over 9 cycles of inhalation over 5 seconds and exhalation over 5 seconds. The patient's effort impacts the interpretation of the results. This test of respiratory sinus arrhythmia is a measure of parasympathetic function. Results are interpreted based on normative data for age and sex, and impaired functioning can reflect isolated parasympathetic dysfunction or be part of pervasive autonomic failure.

Gastric-emptying study
During a gastric-emptying study, a patient consumes a standardized meal with a tracer. Scintigraphy is obtained at hours 0, 1, 2, and 4 hours, and if food is retained beyond the standard measurements, the patient may have delayed gastric emptying (ie, gastroparesis) if there is no obstructive cause identified. If the food transits quickly, the patient may have rapid gastric emptying. Patients can have isolated gastrointestinal autonomic dysfunction, or gastrointestinal dysfunction can be part of more pervasive autonomic failure.[38] This test should be used to assess for symptoms of gastroparesis[39] if the testing will change management. It should be noted that gastrointestinal symptom severity does not correlate well with the degree of delayed gastric emptying.[38]

Urodynamics
Urodynamics encompass a group of tests of that are designed to evaluate micturition voiding and storage functions. Standard urodynamic testing includes tests that are invasive (cystometry, sphincter electromyography, pressure-flow study, and urethral pressure profile), and tests that are noninvasive (uroflowmetry). Detailed description of the procedures for the testing exceeds the scope of this review. An active urinary tract infection is a contraindication to urodynamic testing. It should be noted that patients with spinal cord injuries above T6 are at risk for developing autonomic dysreflexia during urodynamic testing. Patients and testing centers should be advised of this risk before performing the test and be prepared to manage severe hypertension and/or bradycardia.[40] From an autonomic perspective, urodynamic testing can be used to identify neurogenic bladder dysfunction (detrusor over or underactivity), detrusor sphincter dyssynergia, and other comorbid structural/nonneurogenic causes of urinary dysfunction.[41]

Choosing the Right Tests
One of the challenges in the care of patients with dysautonomias is the perception that patients must have autonomic testing, and specifically, the TTT/HUT. The equipment

required to perform this testing and the staffing to interpret the testing are not widely available, which may result in delayed diagnosis and care.[37] Understanding what information is gathered from more common autonomic tests will aid clinicians in deciding both what testing is needed and how to interpret the results.

In addition, it is helpful to note that many autonomic testing centers will combine the TTT/HUT with the Valsalva and heart rate variability, sometimes in combination with other tests, including cerebral blood flow,[42] to provide a more comprehensive assessment of a patient's autonomic function. Understanding what components of the ANS the tests evaluate will aid referring clinicians in interpreting how the results, in combination with the clinical picture, provide a diagnosis. Clinicians should only refer patients for testing if it will change management of the patient, such as provide diagnostic confirmation, offer insight into the differential diagnosis, and/or allow for treatment planning/monitoring.

Many medications influence autonomic test results, particularly the TTT/HUT. Referring clinicians must therefore decide if it is important to hold medications to assess a patient's autonomic function without medication confounders, or alternatively, to assess a patient's autonomic functioning in the context of their polypharmacy, as the latter reflects their clinical context. In addition, many medications are used for specific indications in which rapid withdrawal is not advisable. When tapering a medication, clinicians must consider the half-life of the drug and that some medications also have withdrawal effects with autonomic implications.[37]

The COVID-19 pandemic has created substantial challenges on the health care system, and providing safe medical testing environments is one such factor. In 2020, the American Autonomic Society published a position statement with clear guidelines on how to refer and perform testing safely, however.[43] When safety guidelines are adhered to appropriately, there should not be a barrier to care.

COMMON AUTONOMIC TEST RESULTS AND HOW TO INTERPRET THEM

The purpose of autonomic testing is to aid in clinical diagnosis and management. One of the most common sources of confusion is how to interpret blood pressure and heart rate when evaluating orthostatic vital signs.

The key points to remember are the following:

1. A clinically significant drop in blood pressure is a drop upon standing of the systolic blood pressure (SBP) greater than 20 and/or diastolic blood pressure (DBP) greater than 10; this is called OH.[21,44]
2. The diagnosis of OH is not influenced by the heart rate response. The heart rate response to OH does tell clinicians about the overall autonomic functioning, however.[44]
3. OH identified on autonomic testing does not differentiate NOH from other causes. When OH is identified, clinicians must carefully rule out other causes before interpreting OH as due to an autonomic disorder.
4. POTS is defined only by a sustained increased in the heart rate by greater than 30 bpm or 120 bpm within 10 minutes of standing and occurs without any clinically significant blood pressure change.[44]
5. Patients may have OH or a postural tachycardia and be asymptomatic. Similarly, patients may experience symptoms of lightheadedness with standing or postural changes without any hemodynamic correlate. It is therefore important to document if there are symptoms of OI and, if present, if these are associated with a hemodynamic correlate.

Five common autonomic phenotypes are listed that can be recognized from the TTT/HUT and/or active standing. It should be noted that syncope can occur with OH if the blood pressure is so low that it is insufficient to sustain cerebral perfusion.

- *OH,* also called *classical OH,* is defined as a sustained reduction of at least 20 mm Hg of SBP or 10 mm Hg of DBP within 3 minutes of standing or head-up TTT. In patients with more preserved autonomic function, there may be a compensatory tachycardia. With more severe autonomic impairment, however, this response may decrease or extinguish.

There are a few features on testing that can help clinicians distinguish between NOH and non-NOH. These include a greater decrease in orthostatic SBP and a lesser increase in heart rate. These findings are due to impaired sympathetic cardiac innervation limiting compensatory tachycardia.

- OH can manifest in 3 different patterns, as follows:
  - *Classic OH* as described above
  - *DOH*: DOH is OH that occurs only after 3 minutes of standing/upright tilt. Clinically, patients with DOH may have milder autonomic impairment, and their OH may not be detected during classic orthostatic vital sign testing. For patients who report symptoms that only occur after prolonged standing (such as waiting at the grocery store in line, and so forth), formal autonomic testing may be warranted if bedside orthostatic vital signs are normal as detection may be challenging if the time to blood pressure drop is prolonged.
  - *Initial OH:* In this context, the SBP with standing will drop greater than 40 mm Hg and/or the DBP will drop 20 mm Hg within the first 15 seconds of standing transiently. Different from classic OH, the blood pressure then corrects. This more dramatic blood pressure drop may not be elicited by the TTT but instead by being identified with active standing or with bedside measurements. This finding is not inherently associated with autonomic failure[21] but can cause symptoms and may be associated with an increased fall risk in the elderly.[45]
- POTS: POTS is a heterogenous disorder in which patients experience symptoms of OI and rarely syncope. They often have numerous other symptoms, including cognitive impairment, fatigue, and nausea.[4] Based on the current diagnostic criteria, a patient must have all of the following to have POTS[4,46,47]:
  - A sustained heart rate increased of ≥30 bpm upon standing/tilt within the first 10 minutes without OH. It should be noted that the criteria for POTS are different in children and adolescents.
  - At least 6 months of symptoms of OI. This is because many patients have transient symptoms of OI after illnesses, which are not sustained, and therefore do not meet criteria over time.
  - There is no other overt cause of sinus tachycardia or symptoms that are identified (medications, comorbidities, injections, stressors, and such).

Syncope is less common with POTS but may occur, especially in patients who have both POTS and vasovagal syncope (described in the next section).

- Vasovagal syncope (also known as neurally mediated syncope [NMS] or neurocardiogenic syncope) is a form of reflex syncope that is caused by a rapid change in autonomic activity, which triggers transient hypotension and/or bradycardia with subsequent cerebral hypoperfusion. Because it is a reflex, this phenomenon has an afferent and efferent component, and the episodes are often triggered by stimuli, such as pain or emotions (fear). Prolonged orthostatic stress can be a trigger for some, but in many patients, no trigger is identified. As the afferent arm of the reflex is triggered, most patients report prodromal symptoms of OI, nausea, diaphoresis, pallor, and even tunnel vision before the syncopal event. During the event, the patient may have hypotension ± bradycardia and even asystole in some cases. As with all reflexes, the episode will terminate once the reflex arc is complete, but patients may not feel immediately back to baseline depending on how severely symptomatic they were during the event and may report fatigue after the event.[5] Patients with vasovagal syncope may only have presyncope, especially if they are able to recognize the prodromal symptoms and are able to get into the recumbent position to avoid significant hypotension.[4,48]

There are well-established guidelines on how to distinguish vasovagal syncope from other causes of syncope/transient loss of consciousness, and recommendations on appropriate workup for cardiogenic causes if the history is not clear.[4,20,44]

When more advanced autonomic testing is not available, clinicians can still obtain very valuable information about a patient's autonomic functioning from bedside vital sign testing using the following approach:

1. Measuring the patient's blood pressure first after the patient has been supine at rest for at least 5 minutes, supine hypertension can be detected.
2. Then, with active standing, initial OH, classic OH, and early signs of POTS can be identified. The heart rate response to orthostatic challenge can also be examined, although more detailed information from the 30:15 ratio will not be available. DOH, POTS that occurs after 5 minutes, and NMS may be missed, however.

TREATMENT

Initial treatment of dysautonomia should be focused on a 3-fold approach, as follows:

1. Identifying and treating any underlying disease that causes or exacerbates the condition: The workup for secondary causes of autonomic neuropathies and comorbidities is outlined[3] in **Table 1**. If a peripheral autoimmune autonomic disorder, such as an autoimmune autonomic ganglionopathy, is suggested based on history and examination, additional workup with autoimmune antibody is recommended, although not all autoantibody testing may be positive. In these cases, immune modulation should be considered a disease-modifying treatment.[49]
2. Removing polypharmacy that exacerbates the autonomic problem when possible: This requires a careful review of all the medications a patient is taking, including prescriptions, over-the-counter treatments, and herbal remedies, to assess for autonomic side effects. There is an extensive list of medications known to cause OH ranging from diuretics and antihypertensives to some muscle relaxants, psychiatric medications, and medications for benign prostatic hyperplasia.[3,50] These medications should not necessarily be discontinued, but rather, the patient should have interdisciplinary coordinated care in which a discussion should be had with the prescriber about either lowering the dose, switching to an alternative treatment with less autonomic impact, or reducing polypharmacy when appropriate.
3. Optimizing lifestyle modifications: There are several nonpharmacologic approaches to enhance volume status, reduce symptom triggers, and improve cardiovascular conditioning, which can ameliorate symptoms and, in some circumstances, autonomic function.
   a. *Oral volume expansion*: The combination of a high-fluid and -sodium diet results in increased blood volume and can improve symptoms of OI.[3,21,47] *Use these measures with caution in patients with heart failure and/or renal impairment.*

    i. Sodium supplementation: Patients are advised to take in 6 to 10 g of supplemental sodium per day.[3,21,47,51]

    ii. Fluids: Patients are advised to try to ingest 3 L of nonalcoholic/noncaffeinated beverages per day. This is ideally water but can be other fluids if needed and should be done in combination with sodium intake as listed above.[3,21,47,51]

b. *Exercise:* Deconditioning is a common complication of symptoms of OI and chronic illness. Cardiovascular conditioning has been shown to improve symptoms in both POTS[46] and OH, but notably, patients often feel worse when starting treatment.[33,51] Because deconditioning and OI are both limiting factors for exercising tolerance for many patients, starting with recumbent exercises, such as swimming, rowing, or a recumbent bike at mild intensity levels, are recommended, as they may be more tolerable.[33,51]

c. *Physical maneuvers:* Patients should be counseled on physical maneuvers that exacerbate symptoms, which should be avoided, and countermeasures to mitigate symptoms.

    i. Exacerbating maneuvers include the following[51,52]:
        1. Prolonged standing in 1 location
        2. Rapid positional changes
        3. Hot baths/showers

    ii. Alleviating physical maneuvers/countermeasures during symptoms include the following[51,52]:
        1. Gradual changes in position
        2. Static hand-gripping, crossing and contracting the legs, squatting, muscle tensing, elevating the legs, bending at the waist, moving the legs up and down, or walking

d. *External compression:* This technique helps reduce peripheral pooling in lower limbs and splanchnic region. It can be achieved by having patients wear lower-extremity support stockings of 20 to 30 mm Hg or sleeves. The compression stockings are more effective when worn to the waist if tolerated, and increased pressure can be attempted. Putting compression stockings on is a challenge for some patients, and comfort and heat intolerance are additional barriers to their use.[3,4,21,47]

e. *Dietary changes:* Some patients develop postprandial hypotension. In these patients, changing the diet to small, frequent meals may be better tolerated. Patients with gastroparesis may also tolerate this approach better. Lower-carbohydrate, low-fat meals, and alcohol avoidance can also help prevent worsening hypotension.[21]

f. *Sleeping with the head of the bed elevated:* Some patients with NOH have concomitant supine hypertension. This is most common in patients with central autonomic failure. When this occurs, the hypertension when supine can cause pressure diuresis, especially at night when patients are lying flat and supine. This manifests as frequent nocturia on the review of systems, and by morning, patients are volume depleted with worsening NOH. The patient may sleep with the head of the bed elevated, so the entire bed is raised at an angle of 20° to 30° in the reverse Trendelenburg position.[21] This can be achieved by using bricks or other very stable options under the feet of only the head of the bed. Alternatively, bed risers are commercially available and can be easily obtained.

4. *Pharmacologic treatments:* When behavioral approaches are not sufficient, there are several pharmacologic treatments that can be trialed for POTS and OH. **Tables 3** and **4**[3,21,47] outline common first-line treatments for both conditions, including dosing and side effects.

Table 3
Pharmacologic treatment options for postural orthostatic tachycardia syndrome

		Postural Orthostatic Tachycardia Syndrome		
Medication	Dosing	Mechanism of Action	Contraindications/Cautions	Side Effects
Tachycardia-predominant symptoms				
Propranolol	10–2 mg orally up to 4 times daily	Beta-blocker	• Avoid in patients with asthma • Avoid in patients with already very low baseline blood pressure or heart rate	• Hypotension, bradycardia, bronchospasm • May cause/worsen depression
Ivabradine	2.5–7.5 mg orally twice daily	Selective inhibitor of the SA node hyperpolarization-activated cyclic nucleotide-gated channel, which causes reduced heart rate	• Decompensated heart failure • Cardiac conduction abnormalities	• Can cause cardiac arrhythmias including atrial fibrillation and bradycardia • Visual disturbances
Low blood pressure–predominant symptoms				
Midodrine	2.5–10 mg 2–3 times/d	Direct a-1 adrenoreceptor agonist Does not cross the blood-brain barrier and therefore does not cause sympathomimetic side effects (anxiety and tachycardia)	• Avoid in patients with heart failure, severe coronary artery disease, and urinary retention • Last dose must be at least 4 h before going to bed due to supine hypertension	• Scalp itching or tingling (not rash), headache, hypertension

Medication	Dose	Mechanism	Contraindications/Cautions	Side effects
Fludrocortisone	0.05–0.3 mg daily	Mineralocorticoid volume expander Increases sodium reabsorption	• Heart failure • Untreated hypokalemia	• Peripheral edema, hypokalemia • Monitor for supine hypertension • Need to be monitored for volume overload and hypokalemia
Pyridostigmine	30–60 mg 2–3 times/d	Acetylcholinesterase inhibitor Marginal increase in blood pressure	• Use with caution in patients with glaucoma • May cause bradycardia: use with caution in patients with cardiac arrhythmias	• May cause diarrhea and abdominal pain
Desmopressin	0.1–0.2 mg/d as needed	Synthetic vasopressin analogue	• Hyponatremia • Monitor serum sodium when using on an ongoing basis	• Hyponatremia, edema

Hyperadrenergic symptoms: These antihypertensives have been used for the treatment of POTS based on the principle that their mechanism of action decreases central sympathetic nerve activity and peripheral sympathetic norepinephrine release

Medication	Dose	Mechanism	Contraindications/Cautions	Side effects
Methyldopa	125–250 mg qhs-bid	Alpha$_2$-adrenergic agonist antihypertensive	• Active hepatic disease • Concurrent use of monoamine oxidase inhibitors • Start with the lowest dose	• Cardiac arrhythmias • Orthostatic hypotension • Headache • Dizziness • Gastrointestinal (GI) symptoms
Clonidine	0.1–0.2 mg po tid	Alpha$_2$-adrenergic agonist	• Cardiac arrhythmias • Coronary artery disease • Stroke • Start with the lowest dose	• Cardiac arrhythmias • Orthostatic hypotension • Headache • Dizziness • GI symptoms (constipation predominant)

Table 4
Pharmacologic treatment options for neurogenic orthostatic hypotension

| Medication | Dosing | Neurogenic Orthostatic Hypotension | | |
		Mechanism of Action	Contraindications/Cautions	Side Effects
Fludrocortisone	0.05–0.3 mg daily	Mineralocorticoid volume expander Increases sodium reabsorption	• Heart failure • Untreated hypokalemia	• Peripheral edema, hypokalemia • Monitor for supine hypertension • Need to be monitored for volume overload and hypokalemia
Midodrine	2.5–10 mg 2–3 times/d	Direct a-1 adrenoreceptor agonist Does not cross the blood-brain barrier and therefore does not cause sympathomimetic side effects (anxiety and tachycardia)	• Avoid in patients with heart failure, severe coronary artery disease, and urinary retention • Last dose must be at least 4 h before going to bed due to supine hypertension	• Scalp itching or tingling (not rash), headache, hypertension
Pyridostigmine	30–60 mg 2–3 times/d	Acetylcholinesterase inhibitor Marginal increase in blood pressure	• May cause bradycardia: use with caution in patients with cardiac arrhythmias • Use with caution in patients with glaucoma	• May cause diarrhea and abdominal pain
Droxidopa	100–600 mg 3 times/d	Norepinephrine precursor	• May exacerbate underlying cardiac diseases (ischemia, arrhythmia, heart failure)	• Headache • Monitor for supine hypertension

When selecting the right pharmacologic agent, clinicians should consider comorbidities/contraindications, potential drug-drug interactions, and the timing of symptoms. If symptoms occur throughout the day, long-acting medications may be more effective, whereas if symptoms are only most prominent in the mornings or are intermittent and predictable, short-acting medications can be very effective. For patients with POTS, additional consideration to the main cause of disability can help guide pharmacologic therapy. If patients are most troubled by symptoms of palpitations and tachycardia, medications that lower the heart rate can be helpful. If they have significant hyperadrenergic symptoms, there is limited evidence for the use of methyldopa or clonidine.[3]

Selecting the right treatment should be patient-centered with shared decision making, including counseling on medication side effects and, in patients of reproductive age, screening and counseling on pregnancy and teratogenicity. Most of these treatments are not known to be safe in pregnancy or during lactation. Patients must therefore be screened and counseled appropriately during treatment initiation, and monitoring for side effects and adverse reactions should be established. Setting expectations for treatment is also important with the additional emphasis that pharmacologic measures are not a surrogate for the behavioral approaches, particularly cardiovascular conditioning and oral hydration, described above.

Those patients with baseline hypertension and those who are started on pressure support should be monitored for worsening hypertension and supine hypertension. This is especially true for patients with NOH and alpha-synucleinopathies. When supine hypertension is identified, patients should be counseled to sleep in the reverse Trendelenburg position as described above. If this is not sufficient or not tolerated, short-acting antihypertensives, such as captopril, nebivolol, or losartan, may be used at night to help lower nocturnal supine hypertension.[22]

DISCUSSION

Dysautonomias are a diverse group of disorders that can be due to central or peripheral autonomic impairment. The causes are equally heterogeneous, and clinicians should carefully screen patients for causes of secondary dysautonomias based on a patient's history and examination, referring for additional testing as appropriate. Since the onset of the COVID-19 pandemic, there has been growing interest in the impact of immediate COVID-19 infections on the ANS,[34,53,54] COVID-19 vaccinations causing SFN[35] and autonomic symptoms, and more recently, patients with long-COVID having autonomic symptoms.[14,17,55] This is clearly an evolving field, and a detailed exploration of this topic exceeds the scope of this article, but it should be noted that both symptoms of OI and POTS can occur in patients after illness and with deconditioning.[3] Therefore, it is yet to be determined if COVID-19 and long-COVID are directly involved in autonomic impairment, or cause POTS and other symptoms of OI owing to previously identified mechanisms from chronic illness.

SUMMARY

Dysautonomias are a heterogeneous group of disorders with variable clinical presentations. They can cause pervasive autonomic impairment or milder symptoms depending on the systems involved. The causes can vary from central to peripheral autonomic damage either because of primary neurologic conditions or secondary to other diseases that damage the peripheral ANS, known as autonomic neuropathies. Establishing the diagnosis requires a detailed history and examination, which guides the workup. Autonomic testing can aid in confirming the diagnosis, understanding the extent of autonomic impairment, and guiding treatment decision making. The focus of treatment should be to treat any underlying disorders that are reversible or correctable, address polypharmacy that exacerbates symptoms, and optimize lifestyle factors. There are several pharmacologic treatment options for POTS and NOH that can improve symptoms, but these are not disease-modifying therapies. Patient-centered care, including establishing expectations and appropriate counseling, is essential for effective care.

CLINICS CARE POINTS

When evaluating dysautonomias:

- History and neurologic examination are key to making the right diagnosis.
- Screen for comorbidities that contribute to symptoms and causes.
- Beware of treating symptoms without hemodynamic correlate, as not all symptoms of orthostatic intolerance are due to autonomic impairment.
- Optimize oral volume status with fluids and sodium.
- Emphasize cardiovascular conditioning.
- Pharmacologic treatments for neurogenic orthostatic hypotension and postural orthostatic tachycardia syndrome can reduce symptoms but are not disease modifying.

DISCLOSURE

The author has nothing to disclose.

REFERENCES

1. Kornum DS, Terkelsen AJ, Bertoli D, et al. Assessment of Gastrointestinal Autonomic Dysfunction: Present and Future Perspectives. J Clin Med 2021;10(7). https://doi.org/10.3390/jcm10071392.
2. Palma JA, Norcliffe-Kaufmann L, Kaufmann H. Diagnosis of multiple system atrophy. Auton Neurosci Basic Clin 2018;211:15–25.
3. Raj SR, Guzman JC, Harvey P, et al. Canadian Cardiovascular Society Position Statement on Postural Orthostatic Tachycardia Syndrome (POTS) and Related Disorders of Chronic Orthostatic Intolerance. Can J Cardiol 2020;36(3):357–72.
4. Sheldon RS, Grubb BP II, Olshansky B, et al. 2015 Heart Rhythm Society Expert Consensus Statement on the Diagnosis and Treatment of Postural Tachycardia Syndrome, Inappropriate Sinus Tachycardia, and Vasovagal Syncope. Heart Rhythm 2015;12(6):e41–63.
5. Freeman R, Wieling W, Axelrod FB, et al. Consensus statement on the definition of orthostatic hypotension, neurally mediated syncope and the postural tachycardia syndrome. Clin Auton Res 2011;21(2):69–72.
6. Jeanmonod R, Sahni D, Silberman M. Vasovagal Episode. In: StatPearls [Internet]. Treasure Island (FL): StatPearls Publishing; 2022. Available at: https://www.ncbi.nlm.nih.gov/books/NBK470277/.
7. Verrotti A, Prezioso G, Scattoni R, et al. Autonomic Neuropathy in Diabetes Mellitus. Front Endocrinol 2014;5. Available at: https://www.frontiersin.org/article/10.3389/fendo.2014.00205.
8. Vinik AI, Ziegler D. Diabetic Cardiovascular Autonomic Neuropathy. Circulation 2007;115(3):387–97.

9. Axelrod FB. Hereditary sensory and autonomic neuropathies. Familial dysautonomia and other HSANs. Clin Auton Res 2002;12(Suppl 1):I2–14.
10. Kaur D, Tiwana H, Stino A, et al. Autonomic neuropathies. Muscle Nerve 2021; 63(1):10–21.
11. Osztovits J, Horvath E, Tax J, et al. Reversible autonomic dysfunction during antiviral treatment in patients with chronic hepatitis C virus infection: Anti-HCV therapy and autonomic function. Hepat Mon 2011;11(2):114–8.
12. Saperstein DS. Small Fiber Neuropathy. Neurol Clin 2020;38(3):607–18.
13. Raasing LRM, Vogels OJM, Veltkamp M, et al. Current View of Diagnosing Small Fiber Neuropathy. J Neuromuscul Dis 2021;8(2):185–207.
14. Dani M, Dirksen A, Taraborrelli P, et al. Autonomic dysfunction in 'long COVID': rationale, physiology and management strategies. Clin Med 2021;21(1):e63.
15. Baumgartner C, Koren J, Britto-Arias M, et al. Epidemiology and pathophysiology of autonomic seizures: a systematic review. Clin Auton Res 2019;29(2):137–50.
16. Moseley B, Bateman L, Millichap JJ, et al. Autonomic epileptic seizures, autonomic effects of seizures, and SUDEP. Epilepsy Behav 2013;26(3):375–85.
17. Eldokla AM, Ali ST. Autonomic function testing in long-COVID syndrome patients with orthostatic intolerance. Auton Neurosci Basic Clin 2022;241. https://doi.org/10.1016/j.autneu.2022.102997.
18. Wu JS, Yang YC, Lu FH, et al. Population-based study on the prevalence and risk factors of orthostatic hypotension in subjects with pre-diabetes and diabetes. Diabetes Care 2009;32(1):69–74.
19. Mu F, Jiao Q, Du X, et al. Association of orthostatic hypotension with Parkinson's disease: a meta-analysis. Neurol Sci 2020;41(6):1419–26.
20. Brignole M, Moya A, de Lange FJ, et al. 2018 ESC Guidelines for the diagnosis and management of syncope. Eur Heart J 2018;39(21):1883–948.
21. Freeman R, Abuzinadah AR, Gibbons C, et al. Orthostatic Hypotension: JACC State-of-the-Art Review. Spec Focus Issue Blood Press 2018;72(11):1294–309.
22. Mendoza-Velásquez JJ, Flores-Vázquez JF, Barrón-Velázquez E, et al. Autonomic Dysfunction in α-Synucleinopathies. Front Neurol 2019;10. Available at: https://www.frontiersin.org/article/10.3389/fneur.2019.00363.
23. Allen KJ, Leslie SW. Autonomic Dysreflexia. In: StatPearls [Internet]. Treasure Island (FL): StatPearls Publishing; 2022. p. 1–6. Available at: https://www.ncbi.nlm.nih.gov/books/NBK482434/.
24. Wu B, Wang X, Zhang JH. Cardiac Damage After Subarachnoid Hemorrhage. Acta Neurochir Suppl 2011;110/1(Pt 1):215–8.
25. Giammello F, Cosenza D, Casella C, et al. Isolated Insular Stroke: Clinical Presentation. Cerebrovasc Dis 2020;49(1):10–8.
26. Donofrio PD. Guillain-Barré Syndrome. Contin Minneap Minn 2017;23(5): 1295–309. Peripheral Nerve and Motor Neuron Disorders).
27. Myers MI, Peltier AC. Uses of Skin Biopsy for Sensory and Autonomic Nerve Assessment. Curr Neurol Neurosci Rep 2012;13(1):323.
28. Terkelsen AJ, Karlsson P, Lauria G, et al. The diagnostic challenge of small fibre neuropathy: clinical presentations, evaluations, and causes. Lancet Neurol 2017; 16(11):934–44.
29. Joint Task Force of the EFNS and the PNS. European Federation of Neurological Societies/Peripheral Nerve Society Guideline on the use of skin biopsy in the diagnosis of small fiber neuropathy. Report of a joint task force of the European Federation of Neurological Societies and the Peripheral Nerve Society. J Peripher Nerv Syst 2010;15(2):79–92.

30. Collongues N, Samama B, Schmidt-Mutter C, et al. Quantitative and qualitative normative dataset for intraepidermal nerve fibers using skin biopsy. PLoS One 2018;13(1):e0191614.

31. Gibbons CH, Freeman R, Bellaire B, et al. Synuclein-One study: skin biopsy detection of phosphorylated α-synuclein for diagnosis of synucleinopathies. Biomark Med 2022;16(7):499–509.

32. Donadio V. Skin nerve α-synuclein deposits in Parkinson's disease and other synucleinopathies: a review. Clin Auton Res 2019;29(6):577–85.

33. Grayston R, Czanner G, Elhadd K, et al. A systematic review and meta-analysis of the prevalence of small fiber pathology in fibromyalgia: Implications for a new paradigm in fibromyalgia etiopathogenesis. Semin Arthritis Rheum 2019;48(5): 933–40.

34. Abrams RMC, Simpson DM, Navis A, et al. Small fiber neuropathy associated with SARS-CoV-2 infection. Muscle Nerve 2022;65(4):440–3.

35. Waheed W, Carey ME, Tandan SR, et al. Post COVID-19 vaccine small fiber neuropathy. Muscle Nerve 2021;64(1):E1–2.

36. Devigili G, Cazzato D, Lauria G. Clinical diagnosis and management of small fiber neuropathy: an update on best practice. Expert Rev Neurother 2020;20(9): 967–80.

37. Illigens BMW, Gibbons CH. Autonomic testing, methods and techniques. Handb Clin Neurol 2019;160:419–33.

38. Nguyen L, Wilson LA, Miriel L, et al. Autonomic function in gastroparesis and chronic unexplained nausea and vomiting: Relationship with cause, gastric emptying, and symptom severity. Neurogastroenterol Motil 2020;32(8):e13810.

39. Schol J, Wauters L, Dickman R, et al. United European Gastroenterology (UEG) and European Society for Neurogastroenterology and Motility (ESNM) consensus on gastroparesis. Neurogastroenterol Motil 2021;33(8):e14237.

40. Lenherr SM, Clemens JQ. Urodynamics With a Focus on Appropriate Indications. Urol Clin North Am 2013;40(4):545–57.

41. Yao M, Simoes A. Urodynamic testing and interpretation. In: StatPearls [Internet]. Treasure Island (FL): StatPearls Publishing; 2022. p. 1–7. Available at: https://www.ncbi.nlm.nih.gov/books/NBK562310/?report=classic.

42. Norcliffe-Kaufmann L, Galindo-Mendez B, Garcia-Guarniz AL, et al. Transcranial Doppler in autonomic testing: standards and clinical applications. Clin Auton Res Off J Clin Auton Res Soc 2018;28(2):187–202.

43. Figueroa JJ, Cheshire WP, Claydon VE, et al. Autonomic function testing in the COVID-19 pandemic: an American Autonomic Society position statement. Clin Auton Res 2020;30(4):295–7.

44. Thijs RD, Brignole M, Falup-Pecurariu C, et al. Recommendations for tilt table testing and other provocative cardiovascular autonomic tests in conditions that may cause transient loss of consciousness. Clin Auton Res 2021;31(3):369–84.

45. Tran J, Hillebrand SL, Meskers CGM, et al. Prevalence of initial orthostatic hypotension in older adults: a systematic review and meta-analysis. Age Ageing 2021; 50(5):1520–8.

46. Arnold AC, Ng J, Raj SR. Postural tachycardia syndrome – Diagnosis, physiology, and prognosis. Auton Neurosci Basic Clin 2018;215:3–11.

47. Raj SR, Fedorowski A, Sheldon RS. Diagnosis and management of postural orthostatic tachycardia syndrome. Can Med Assoc J 2022;194(10):E378.

48. Buszko K, Kujawski S, Newton JL, et al. Hemodynamic Response to the Head-Up Tilt Test in Patients With Syncope as a Predictor of the Test Outcome: A Meta-Analysis Approach. Front Physiol 2019;10:184.

49. Golden EP, Vernino S. Autoimmune autonomic neuropathies and ganglionopathies: epidemiology, pathophysiology, and therapeutic advances. Clin Auton Res 2019;29(3):277–88.
50. Poon IO, Braun U. High prevalence of orthostatic hypotension and its correlation with potentially causative medications among elderly veterans. J Clin Pharm Ther 2005;30(2):173–8.
51. Fu Q, Levine BD. Exercise and non-pharmacological treatment of POTS. Auton Neurosci Basic Clin 2018;215:20–7.
52. Wieling W, van Dijk N, Thijs RD, et al. Physical countermeasures to increase orthostatic tolerance. J Intern Med 2015;277(1):69–82.
53. Shouman K, Vanichkachorn G, Cheshire WP, et al. Autonomic dysfunction following COVID-19 infection: an early experience. Clin Auton Res 2021;31(3): 385–94.
54. Ghosh R, Roy D, Sengupta S, et al. Autonomic dysfunction heralding acute motor axonal neuropathy in COVID-19. J Neurovirol 2020;26(6):964–6.
55. Stefanou MI, Palaiodimou L, Bakola E, et al. Neurological manifestations of long-COVID syndrome: a narrative review. Ther Adv Chronic Dis 2022;13. 20406223221076890.

Educating Residents and Students in the Clinic

Erin Furr Stimming, MD[a,b,]*, Madhu Soni, MD[c]

KEYWORDS

- Ambulatory care • Medical education • Medical students • Teaching methods
- Residents

KEY POINTS

- Six core competencies are the basis of trainee assessments: patient care, medical knowledge, professionalism, interpersonal and communication skills, practice-based learning and improvement, and systems-based practice.
- Early clinical exposure such as preclerkships increases the confidence and performance of students and is a great opportunity for students to explore their interests.
- A balanced outpatient case mix can improve the range of educational experiences for trainees and ensure training consistency.
- Because of the approachability of peers, near-peer teaching promotes learning and provides a higher sense of safety for learners.
- Active learning involves a higher level of knowledge acquisition, maximizing student engagement by self-directed learning, application of the knowledge, and analysis of the topic.

INTRODUCTION

Neurologic diseases are the leading cause of disability worldwide and impose an increasingly high burden of mortality and morbidity on the health care system. The absolute number of patients with neurological disorders has increased in the past 3 decades and is predicted to rise in the future by population growth and aging.[1] This rate of increase and the consequent mismatch between the need for neurological services and availability of active neurologists have been a growing challenge for public health.[2] The projected estimation of demand for neurologists has shown that the current shortfall is likely to worsen in the future impacting patient access to care.[3] Therefore, it is crucial for health care policymakers to both actively increase the number of

[a] Department of Neurology, McGovern Medical School, The University of Texas Health Science Center at Houston (UTHealth), 6431 Fannin, MSB 7.112, Houston, TX 77030, USA; [b] Huntington's Disease Society of America (HDSA), Center of Excellence at UTHealth, Houston, TX, USA; [c] Clerkship and Advanced Elective Department of Neurological Science, Rush University Medical Center, Professional Building, 1725 West Harrison Street, Suite 1106, Chicago, IL 60612, USA
* Corresponding author.
E-mail address: erin.e.furr@uth.tmc.edu

Neurol Clin 41 (2023) 215–229
https://doi.org/10.1016/j.ncl.2022.08.004   **neurologic.theclinics.com**
0733-8619/23/© 2022 Elsevier Inc. All rights reserved.

neurologists and also ensure that all physicians, regardless of career choice, receive training in neurologic disease. The World Health Organization has identified neurological disorders as an increasing public health problem and has highlighted the importance of teaching neurology at the undergraduate, postgraduate, and continuing education levels.[4] In this context, neurology educators play a vital role in providing content expertise through the delivery of clear, clinically applicable concepts to create a positive learning experience for trainees.

During the 20th century, the focus of neurology training was shifted from outpatient to inpatient training.[5] Although the inpatient setting may offer more complex cases and technologically advanced levels of care, the majority of undergraduate students will need training that prepares them to address common neurology problems.[6,7] This issue can be even more challenging in tertiary care hospitals. For neurology residents, receiving sufficient education in ambulatory care is crucial and this can be overlooked by an imbalanced curriculum design.

The concept of involving medical students in clinical practice is not a novel one. Sir William Osler, among others, advocated for early student involvement in the hospital wards. He likened the hospital to a college. While many physicians may know him as the father of modern medicine for his prowess as a diagnostician, or by the painful red skin nodules that bear his name, few people may know that he was a chairman of medicine who pioneered the role for students in clinical practice and that this apprenticeship later developed into the student clerkship experience.[8] He believed that medicine, as "an old art," should be taught in the wards rather than in lecture halls as the disease is the "student's chief teacher."[8–10] Osler's legacy in the education of medical students, which started at the beginning of the 20th century, has continued to this day in the form of the student clerkship and debates on the education of medical students are still relevant, as it was a century ago.[8]

In the majority of US allopathic medical schools, neurology is a required clerkship and plays a pivotal role in undergraduate medical education. The required experience fosters the development of essential neurologic concepts, knowledge, and clinical skill competency necessary for future medical graduates, irrespective of their specialty choice, to ensure familiarity with the most common neurological problems and emergencies.[11] The clerkship is also an opportunity for students to further explore a potential career interest in the field. A 2012 survey of clerkship directors (CDs) was conducted by a workgroup of the American Academy of Neurology (AAN) Undergraduate Education Subcommittee (UES) and a 2017 survey of all US medical school CDs was conducted by a workgroup of the AAN Consortium of Neurology Clerkship Directors (CNCD) showed that neurology was a required clerkship in 93% and 94% of responding institutions, respectively.[11,12] According to data from the Association of American Medical Colleges (AAMC), of 148 responding US medical schools, 84% had a required neurology clerkship during the 2019–2020 academic year. This is down from 86% for each of the prior 3 academic years. The percentage of schools with a required neurology clerkship is also significantly lower in osteopathic medical schools.[13] These findings raise concerns about the adequacy of neurology education in all medical schools and the competency of graduating medical students in caring for patients with neurologic disease.

For residents, a high-quality clinic training with exposure to a broad range of neurologic diagnoses and number of patients is required to provide a balanced clinical experience.[14] Poorly organized clinics and short-term exposure to hospital-based patients cannot offer a well-rounded clinical education representative of the most common neurologic presentations and may discourage residents to choose outpatient or clinic-based services as a component of their career practice.[15,16]

In this article, we describe the current status of neurology education for students and residents and revisit the flaws that may affect the quality of education while providing potential solutions/strategies for improvement.

LEARNING OBJECTIVES

By the time the proposed clerkship model of Osler was widely accepted, only a few guidelines were available for the standardization of clerkship experience. In 1930, the AAMC initiated efforts to standardize clinical education by defining learning objectives.[17] Nationally endorsed neurology clerkship learning objectives, however, did not become available until 2000 when curriculum guidelines for neurology instruction were first published.[18,19] These learning objectives were endorsed by the AAN, the Association of University Professors of Neurology (AUPN) and the American Neurological Association (ANA).[17] These learning objectives were inspired by the broader educational goals for undergraduate neurology training and also provided a basis for assessment.[17] An updated curriculum became available in 2019 to address evolving needs in medical education.[20]

The core clinical objectives of the neurology clerkship recommended by the AAN are categorized under 2 major categories of procedural skills and analytical skills, some of which are highlighted later in discussion.[19,20]

The procedural skills include:

- Obtaining a complete and reliable patient history
- Performing a reliable neurologic examination
- Delivering a clear, concise, and thorough history and examination (both oral and written presentations)
- Performing a lumbar puncture, under direct supervision or on a simulation model.[19,20]

The core analytical skills include:

- Recognition of important symptoms associated with neurologic diseases
- Distinguishing normal from abnormal findings on a neurologic examination
- Localizing the affected site in the nervous system
- Formulating differential diagnoses
- Explaining indications and interpretation of common tests used for the diagnosis of neurologic diseases
- Understanding the underlying principles of a systematic approach to the management of common neurologic diseases and potential emergencies
- Awareness of appropriate neurologic consultation request
- Review, interpretation, and application of medical literature for a specific issue related to patient care.[19,20]

Since the quality of education is usually assessed based on the competence of trainees, the learning objectives are also competency-based. The Accreditation Council for Graduate Medical Education (ACGME) competencies framework is commonly used for this purpose. It has defined six items as core competencies: patient care, medical knowledge, professionalism, interpersonal and communication skills, practice-based learning and improvement, and systems-based practice.[21] The learning objectives for residents are usually defined by postgraduate year and in the form of competency-based milestones which include:

- Patient Care: History; neurologic exam; formulation; diagnosis and management of neurologic disorders (outpatient and inpatient setting) and emergencies;

determination of death by neurologic criteria; performing and interpreting lumbar puncture; interpretation of neuroimaging, electroencephalogram (EEG), and Nerve Conduction Study/Electromyography (NCS/EMG); psychiatric and functional aspects of neurology

- Medical knowledge: Localization; diagnostic investigation
- Professionalism: Professional behavior and ethical principles; accountability/conscientiousness; wellbeing
- Interpersonal and communication skills: patient- and family-centered communication; barrier and bias mitigation; interprofessional and team communication; communication within health care systems
- Practice-based learning and improvement: evidence-based and informed practice; reflective practice and commitment to personal growth
- Systems-based practice: Patient safety; quality improvement; system navigation for patient-centered care; physician role in health care system.[22]

NEUROLOGY CLERKSHIP DIRECTORS/PROGRAM DIRECTORS

CDs and PDs have a significant responsibility and influence on the education of medical students and residents, respectively. They are responsible for the quality of clerkship or residency programs. With the progression of the education system and the introduction of new education methods, the responsibilities of directors have evolved during recent decades. Directors are clinician-educators who have the roles of both manager and leader in clinical education.[23] They should have the competencies that are required for every medical educator. Based on the ACGME framework, 6 core competencies can be defined for educators:

- Learner-centeredness (parallel to the patient care core competency), which results in tailoring the education program to meet the learner's level and need
- Content knowledge
- Professionalism and role modeling
- Interpersonal and communication skills
- Practice-based learning and improvement, which refers to the ability to increase the effectiveness and capacity by continuous learning
- Systems-based practice, which is having the knowledge of the educational microsystem and macrosystem, and using the resources to guide learners for optimal learning.[24–26]

Four specialized competencies are also required for an educator:

- Design and implementation of a sustainable program
- Evaluation of the program with a scholarly approach
- Leadership, which refers to the ability to create a shared vision of major goals, anticipating future changes, creating a stable system that is flexible, sustainable, and accountable
- Mentorship, which entails advocating and providing support for a mentee, and creating an atmosphere in which students and team members can grow and succeed.[24]

Besides competencies, the Alliance for Clinical Education (ACE) has outlined more specific responsibilities and expectations for CDs:

- Administrative responsibilities, including budget management, programmatic evaluation, recruitment of clinical training sites and ensuring comparable

experiences among these sites, oversight of the clerkship coordinator, ensuring departmental appointments for nonpaid faculty
- Curriculum development, documentation, and evaluation of the education process and outcome, evaluation of patient care learning environments, implementation of school-wide educational initiatives/priorities (eg, determine gaps in learning health systems science)
- Student education and assessment to ensure all students are gaining required clinical experience and meeting the course objectives
- Faculty development and assessment to provide a diverse educational experience for students and prepare the recruited faculty.[23]

NEUROLOGY CURRICULUM

Conventionally, a clerkship starts with observing and assisting the attending or resident physician who provides patient-centered teaching. Students fulfill the learning objectives by observation and supervised hands-on experience. Common objectives include learning the neurologic examination, applying previously acquired neuroanatomical knowledge to localize the lesion while encountering and gaining confidence with the approach to evaluating patients with common neurologic conditions.[11,27] Some curricula also offer a brief exposure to neurology subspecialties such as neuro-ophthalmology, neuromuscular medicine or movement disorders.[11] According to the standards issued by the Liaison Committee on Medical Education (LCME), the faculty is responsible for the design and implementation of the curriculum:

"The faculty of a medical school, through the faculty committee responsible for the medical curriculum, ensure that the medical curriculum uses formally adopted medical education program objectives to guide the selection of curriculum content, and to review and revise the curriculum."[28]

Based on the LCME guidelines, an AAN CNCD workgroup defined standards for neurology clerkships.[29,30] Symptom complexes were identified to guide required clinical encounter experiences, and this was subsequently updated to include the following recommended clinical encounters:

- Transient or paroxysmal alteration of neurologic function
- Acute or chronic change in mental status
- Weakness or alteration in the motor system
- Headache or focal pain
- Numbness or paresthesia, associated with peripheral nerve, nerve root, spinal cord or brain disorder
- Neurologic emergencies.[30]

These encounters can be presented in various formats, including live or simulated patients, written or discussion-based cases, or web-based modules.

The study of Tanner and colleagues on the performance of students in an ambulatory clinic demonstrated the student-perceived educational value of outpatient practice. The perception of students on the effectiveness of the clinic learning experience increased with each additional patient that was interviewed, presented, or documented.[31] The study also showed increased preceptor productivity for generated charges and relative value units per session for preceptors working with a student in clinic compared to those without a student. However, the student survey showed that the majority of assigned preceptors (53 out of 62) were less effective teachers and this correlated with clinic sessions in which there was less student engagement and responsibility. These findings highlight the need for faculty development focused on the importance of trainee engagement in patient care experiences and the benefits for all stakeholders involved.[31]

To facilitate efficiency, the updated policy on Evaluation and Management documentation by the Centers for Medicare & Medicaid Services allows the teaching physician to verify student documentation rather than redocument the work.[32] Administrators are also encouraged to provide educators with 2 clinic rooms to allow the necessary active and independent patient evaluation for trainees. When space is limited to a single clinic room, tactics to support student engagement while maintaining efficiency include allowing the student to ask the initial interview questions for a brief, designated portion of the visit while the faculty member documents and subsequently complete the interview for identified gaps. The student can also be asked to instruct the patient on components of the exam that can be observed by the supervisor and don't necessarily require repetition, such as extra-ocular movement, coordination, and gait testing. This is also a valuable opportunity to directly observe history taking and examination skills, provide real-time feedback, observe for the incorporation of lessons provided in subsequent patient encounters, and offer meaningful comments on performance evaluations.

A similar approach can be used to assess resident exam skills. The residency curriculum should also cover a wide range of neurological conditions. The diversity of cases that residents encounter during outpatient training is directly impacted by the planning of the program and clinic directors. An imbalanced case mix can result in an inconsistent training experience.[14] The most common diseases that residents encounter in clinics include headaches, cerebrovascular diseases (including stroke), neuropathies, chronic pain, epilepsies, psychiatric disorders, dementia, and movement disorders.[33,34]

NEWER APPROACHES TO LEARNING
Early Clinical Exposure for Students

Early medical exposure is a method that includes exposure of medical students to patients as early as the first year of medical college.[35] Different methods have attempted to push clinical exposure forward, such as longitudinal courses, preclerkships, and "Neuro Day" experience.[27,36] Early passive or active observation can increase the level of confidence and performance of the student.[35] In addition, early clinical exposure is a great opportunity for students to explore their interests in various specialties.

The traditional clerkship model is based on rotations involving time-limited blocks through specialty hospitals and clinics. Longitudinal Integrated Clerkship (LIC) is a newer approach that was formally defined in 2007 after the formation of the International Consortium of Longitudinal Integrated Clerkships (CLIC).[37] The implementation of a LIC can be different among medical schools and it has multiple variations. In general, this is a multidisciplinary educational approach for which the students are continuously involved in clinical correlation throughout the medical school journey. The LIC allows the students to actively participate in patient care that is not limited to a distinct discipline or episode of care. Therefore, the LIC embodies a single integrated clerkship that includes multiple disciplines and cohorts of patients from all core specialties.[37] The advocates of this method believe that the extended immersion and responsible participation in patient care facilitate the identity development of future doctors.[38]

In the traditional clerkship system, most neurology clerkships are 4 weeks in duration. Three large-scale AAN surveys (2005, 2012, 2017) of US neurology CDs reported a 4-week duration for neurology clerkships in 74–85% of the responding institutions.[11,12] These surveys reported a shift of clerkships from the fourth year to the third year, with the majority of clerkships now occurring during the third year.[11,12] This change has also shifted the timing of the United States Medical Licensing Examination (USMLE) Step 1 in many medical schools. This trend of early exposure to core clerkships is beneficial as it provides students with a more well-rounded approach to patient care. It also allows an earlier opportunity to discover and explore areas of interest for their future career. Strategic timing of core clerkships in this way can also result in better integration of the basic and clinical sciences, and facilitate the transition from preclinical to clinical training.[39]

Cross-Disciplinary Courses

An example of a cross-disciplinary course for neurology training is the combination of neurology and psychiatry. Neurology and psychiatry are interdependent specialties. With the advance in technology and the introduction of more complex subspecialties such as behavioral neurology, the need for the collaboration between these two disciplines is now more than before.[40] In neurology training, residents rarely have the opportunity to address concurrent neurologic and psychiatric problems of a patient under the supervision of experts in both disciplines.[41]

In a survey of 330 adult neurologists and 101 pediatric neurologists who were recently certified by the American Board of Psychiatry and Neurology (ABPN), Juul and colleagues[42] demonstrated that recently graduated neurologists were not prepared for psychiatric issues encountered in their patients. The experience of outpatient psychiatry during residency was reported in 53.5% of pediatric neurologists and only in 20% of adult neurologists. The most common suggestions to improve psychiatry training included an increase in outpatient exposure in psychiatry, combined clinics, and closer collaboration of program directors of the 2 disciplines.[42] A 2017 survey of neurology PDs by London and colleagues[43] showed that one-third of programs had a specific psychiatry curriculum for residents.[43] They reported that there was a strong interest in supplementing the current psychiatry rotation with an online curriculum. In collaboration with Massachusetts General Hospital in Boston, Chemali and colleagues[44] successfully implemented a combined neurology-psychiatry residency course in a low- to middle-income country (Somaliland). Despite several political and logistical problems in a country affected by civil war, they successfully developed this dual residency program.[44]

Another example of a cross-disciplinary program is the combined neurology-physical medicine and rehabilitation (N-PM&R) clerkship course which was described by Curtis and colleagues[45] They implemented this 4-week mandatory clerkship for fourth-year medical students. The new integrated N-PM&R course showed to be effective in addressing knowledge and skill gaps, boosting medical students' self-perceived confidence, and establishing an interdisciplinary approach to the management of common complaints.[45]

Balancing Case Mix

Designing a balanced outpatient case mix can be beneficial, especially for residents.[14] For instance, Stahl and colleagues[14] used a patient reassignment algorithm to ensure consistent training among residents in primary care outpatient settings. They used different models of reassignment, including the reassignment of patients for all residents with a given preceptor, reassignment of patients for all residents within a group of preceptors, and reassignment across the clinic.[14] The systematically reorganized patient panels improved the range of educational experiences for trainees. The major drawback was the loss of patient-preceptor continuity, which was especially seen with the reassignment of patients across the clinic.[14]

Residents as educators/near-peer teaching

Learning through role modeling happens on both conscious and unconscious levels. Trainees learn by examples and educators deeply affect trainees, even when they are not actively teaching.[46] Fostering the development of healthy role models is crucial for any educational system, and in medical education, this can be achieved by near-peer teaching. Near-peer teaching helps senior residents practice their role as educators and learn how to function as role models, while junior residents practice independent decision-making with appropriate supervision.[46]

A similar effect has been reported for near-peer teaching in medical students. A study by Knobloch and colleagues[47] has shown that a small-group near-peer format can help students to overcome challenges during the transition to clerkships. This method increased the self-efficacy of junior students and helped them to be more prepared for their clinical experience.[47] A recent interdisciplinary study by Taylor and colleagues[48] reported a significant improvement in neuroanatomy knowledge among second-year psychology students who were taught by third-year medical students. Near-peer teaching promotes learning in teachers, and because of the approachability of peers, provides a higher sense of safety in learners.[47]

Assigning senior students to teach junior students has shown successful results in clinical clerkships. In a study by Meller and colleagues,[49] an evaluation of 9 workshop groups, solely led by near-peer teachers, demonstrated higher ratings of near-peers compared to the faculty in terms of the perceived overall value of the workshop. The facilitators also achieved high absolute scores regarding overall value and effectiveness. The participants stated that they "really enjoyed having student facilitators for teaching" and reported "wonderful work with solid feedback." In another study by Keser and colleagues,[50] third-year neurology residents participated in small group teaching workshops to improve the quality of the neurology clerkship. The survey of 371 students (63% response rate) showed that teaching workshops and residents' involvement in the clerkship program significantly increased the quality of the students' experience, as well as teaching the effectiveness of the residents.

Active learning

Active learning is a process that aims to involve a higher level of knowledge acquisition. Instead of simple comprehension, student engagement is maximized by self-directed learning, application of the knowledge, and analysis of the topic. It includes a wide range of activities, including:[51,52]

- Preclass reading, which helps trainees prepare through reading materials prior to a teaching/clinic session
- Problem-based learning and problem-solving sessions, which are a common part of clinical care
- Team-based learning that can be used for a large group of students and includes group discussion and case-based material
- Simulation-based learning, hands-on workshops or demonstrations
- Flipped classroom, which entails being exposed to the teaching material before the face-to-face session, and dedicating the class time to student-centered activities and higher-order discussion

Although providing students with active learning experiences can be challenging due to the potential lack of resources, it can improve the learning process by increasing mindful vigilance and building upon preexisting learned knowledge.[52,53] In recent years, a few programs have tried to incorporate active learning as a part of outpatient training. Balwan and colleagues[54] demonstrated that team-based learning can result in the active engagement of trainees and increased satisfaction of both trainees and faculty. They found a 22% higher average score as a result of team-based learning compared to individual learning. Stone and colleagues[55] evaluated the effect of outpatient bedside skills modeling during the neurology clerkship, including the neurologic history taking and clinical examination. The students who were involved in a scheduled bedside skills experience as part of the pilot program reported a significant increase in observation of both a comprehensive history and neurologic exam compared with those students who went through the standard rotation without a scheduled experience. In a recent study, Will and colleagues[55] implemented a new ambulatory curriculum for obstetrics and gynecology residents with a flipped classroom format, which contained short modules and premodule assignments.[56] A majority of residents (92%) rated the curriculum as satisfactory or very satisfactory. The flipped classroom approach was found to be beneficial by reviewing basic concepts that were reinforced immediately by patient interaction.

Electronic Learning, Online Education, and Virtual Modules

Electronic learning (E-learning) can be used for both "distance learning," or "blended learning," where it accompanies conventional face-to-face sessions.[57] After the emergence of the COVID-19 pandemic, many institutions were forced to expand their infrastructure for online services. Telehealth in the outpatient realm was rapidly established and faculty and trainees alike quickly adapted. A recent publication from the AAN UES was dedicated to the development of a virtual curriculum to supplement the in-person experience for the core neurology clerkship and included advice on teleprecepting.[58]

Although online education cannot replace clinical hands-on experience, it provides a good platform for complementary education for students. In a recent survey of CDs and curriculum deans in the US and Canada to investigate headache medicine education, the most desired educational materials were case-based learning modules and online lectures.[59] As a clinical learning experience, online education can help students to productively use their time and learn clinical skills such as problem-solving, critical thinking, and approach to clinical cases.[60] Although virtual learning is not an alternative to clinical practice with an actual patient and does not replace traditional bedside evaluation and learning, the knowledge, and skills acquired through online formats can be subsequently incorporated and assessed at the bedside.

Three-dimension (3D) visualization by immersive technologies such as augmented reality (AR), and virtual reality (VR) are powerful tools for the simulation of complex concepts. These modules have gained more popularity in the education of students in the last decades; however, their use in medical education has been limited to teaching anatomy, surgery, and pathology.[61] Immersive technologies are relatively new and their potential applications in neurology training are yet to be explored. AR technology is now more accessible via new smartphones and VR-based learning is developing rapidly.

In neurology, immersive technologies have a great potential for teaching complex structures of neuroanatomy.[62] A randomized controlled study by Ekstrand and colleagues[63] with 66 medical students showed that 94% of students either agreed or strongly agreed that VR-based learning methods should be used in their curriculum. AR-based neuroanatomy learning with smartphones has shown a similar positive effect by increasing student's achievement, decreasing cognitive load, and providing real-time interaction with the environment.[64] AR and VR have proved to be beneficial in simulation-based training by increasing students' procedural skill and confidence level, and thus, filling the gap between preclinical and clinical environments.[62,65]

ASSESSMENT

Evaluation of a clerkship or residency program and trainees' performance is a multi-faceted process that should cover both knowledge and skills. Many schools incorporate the Competency-Based Medical Education (CBME) model in the design of their assessment tasks, such as the ACGME core competencies as described before.[66] However, like any other evaluation tool, designing a competency-based assessment requires basic factors such as content validity, reliability, feasibility, and acceptability.[67]

Currently, a large portion of a clerkship grade is derived from clinical performance evaluations completed by attendings and residents. Other components include the National Board of Medical Examiners (NBME) shelf exam, Objective Structured Clinical Examinations (OSCE), written essays, oral examinations, and multiple-choice questions.[12] There are substantial variations among medical schools in how much these components contribute to the final grade.[68]

Although a major percentage of the clerkship grade is based on clinical performance evaluations, they are subject to significant assessor bias that produces concerns regarding the reliability of the assessment.[66] The leniency or stringency of different examiners, known as the "hawk-dove effect," can be a major problem, especially in the absence of a standard evaluation method and adjustment of grades.[69] There have been attempts to standardize clerkship assessment. For instance, a formalized faculty assessment tool used by approximately 40 different neurology faculty showed potential for the evaluation of students' bedside skills.[70] Workplace-based assessment tools can be designed to facilitate the evaluation of ambulatory skills and are useful as feedback mechanisms.

The assessment of residents is based on the ACGME competency framework and the Next Accreditation System (NAS).[71] The Neurology Clinical Evaluation Exercise (NEX) was developed by the American Board of Psychiatry and Neurology (ABPN) to assess competency-based milestones, as described before.[72] Schuh and colleagues[73] reported poor interrater reliability between local faculty and ABPN examiners. Despite the possible bias among local faculty for the evaluation of their own residents, it still does not negate the validity of competency assessment since there was still an agreement between two series of assessors on essential issues of overall pass/fail performance 75% of the time.[73]

Formative assessments of students including the use of standardized patients (SPs) on ambulatory skills have been used widely by institutions. The use of SPs allows educators to provide exposure to the same diagnosis for all students, which is not possible in a clinical setting.[74] An SP can be coached to address a wide range of medical students with different skill levels, and this approach can be an adequate tool for the education and assessment of the trainees.[74] Comparison of the performance of medical students on the neurologic examination with and without a structured SP session has shown a significantly higher OSCE score in the group with the additional SP session.[75] Moreover, using SPs for the assessment of medical students has demonstrated good inter-rater reliability and consistency.[76] SPs are flexible and available educational tools that make it possible to assess the most important skills among a large number of examinees.

SUMMARY

Incorporating learners in the clinic can be challenging due to space and time limitations, the pressure of financial productivity, and clinic efficiency. However, to effectively train our future physicians to care for patients with an increasing burden of neurologic disease, we must provide exposure to common neurologic conditions and optimize their training in the clinic setting. We, as educators, must continue to emphasize the importance of experiential learning through "bedside" teaching in both the inpatient and outpatient settings and encourage faculty development on approaches to efficiently work with trainees and increase productivity, while providing necessary apprenticeship. Students and residents, when guided appropriately can also potentially improve the patient experience.[77,78] Faculty who effectively incorporate learners into their clinic, engage them through opportunities to interview, present, document, and provide patient education. These faculty often include the patient in the discussion and offer invaluable teaching pearls.

Educating our future physicians is incredibly rewarding and it enhances personal and professional satisfaction. It is also a social responsibility and requires collaboration among educators, departmental administrators, and institutional leaders. This support for the educational mission is essential to provide the necessary resources for a healthy working environment conducive to both the teacher and learner.

CLINICS CARE POINTS

- The World Health Organization has identified neurological disorders as an increasing public health problem and has highlighted the importance of teaching neurology at the undergraduate, postgraduate, and continuing education levels.
- Neurology educators play a vital role in providing content expertise through the delivery of clear, clinically applicable concepts to create a positive learning experience for trainees.
- Educating our future physicians is incredibly rewarding and it enhances personal and professional satisfaction. It is also a social responsibility and requires collaboration among educators, departmental administrators, and institutional leaders. Support for the educational mission is essential to provide the necessary resources for a healthy working environment conducive to both the teacher and learner.

ACKNOWLEDGMENTS

Shayan Abdollah Zadegan, MD. Research Assistant, Department of Neurology. UTHealth Houston, McGovern Medical School

DISCLOSURE

Dr E. Furr Stimming has served on the speakers' bureau for Sunovion Pharmaceuticals and as a consultant or on an advisory board for Teva Pharmaceuticals and Norvartis. She has received publishing royalties from McGraw Hill. Her institution has received research funding from Cures within Reach, CHDI, HDSA, Neurocrine Biosciences/ HSG, Prilenia, Roche/Genetech, UniQure, Vaccinex. She has no conflicts nor has she received any funding related to this article. Dr M. Soni has nothing to disclose.

REFERENCES

1. Feigin VL, Vos T, Nichols E, et al. The global burden of neurological disorders: translating evidence into policy. Lancet Neurol 2020;19(3):255–65.
2. Sandrone S, Berthaud JV, Chuquilin M, et al. Neurologic and neuroscience education: Mitigating neurophobia to mentor health care providers. Neurology 2019; 92(4):174–9.

3. Dall TM, Storm MV, Chakrabarti R, et al. Supply and demand analysis of the current and future US neurology workforce. Neurology 2013;81(5):470–8.

4. World Health Organization. Neurological disorders : public health challenges. World Health Organization; 2006.

5. Pappert EJ. Training opportunities for the nineteenth-century American neurologist: preludes to the modern neurology residency. Neurology 1995;45(9):1771–6.

6. Panda PK, Sharawat IK. Undergraduate neurology training in the inpatient and outpatient setting: How do they differ? Eur J Neurol 2021;28(7):e44–5.

7. Worley P, Esterman A, Prideaux D. Cohort study of examination performance of undergraduate medical students learning in community settings. BMJ 2004; 328(7433):207–9.

8. Dornan T. Osler, Flexner, apprenticeship and 'the new medical education. J R Soc Med 2005;98(3):91–5.

9. Sokol DK. William Osler and the jubjub of ethics; or how to teach medical ethics in the 21st century. J R Soc Med 2007;100(12):544–6.

10. Osler W. The fixed period. Aequanimitas : with other addresses to medical students, nurses and practitioners of medicine. H. K. Lewis and Company; 1906. p. 389–412.

11. Safdieh JE, Quick AD, Korb PJ, et al. A dozen years of evolution of neurology clerkships in the United States: Looking up. Neurology 2018;91(15):e1440–7.

12. Carter JL, Ali II, Isaacson RS, et al. Status of neurology medical school education: results of 2005 and 2012 clerkship director survey. Neurology 2014; 83(19):1761–6.

13. Albert DV, Yin H, Amidei C, et al. Structure of neuroscience clerkships in medical schools and matching in neuromedicine. Neurology 2015;85(2):172–6.

14. Stahl JE, Balasubramanian HJ, Gao X, et al. Balancing clinical experience in outpatient residency training. Med Decis Making 2014;34(4):464–72.

15. Gupta R, Barnes K, Bodenheimer T. Clinic first: 6 actions to transform ambulatory residency training. J Grad Med Educ 2016;8(4):500–3.

16. Luciano G, Rosenblum M, Aulakh S. Training the ambulatory internist: rebalancing residency education. Med Educ 2014;48(5):535–6.

17. Burke MJ, Brodkey AC. Trends in undergraduate medical education: clinical clerkship learning objectives. Acad Psychiatry 2006;30(2):158–65.

18. American Academy of Neurology. Neurology clerkship core curriculum guidelines. Available at: https://www.aan.com/globals/axon/assets/2770.pdf. Accessed May 24, 2022.

19. Gelb DJ, Gunderson CH, Henry KA, et al. The neurology clerkship core curriculum. Neurology 2002;58(6):849–52.

20. Safdieh JE, Govindarajan R, Gelb DJ, et al. Core curriculum guidelines for a required clinical neurology experience. Neurology 2019;92(13):619–26.

21. Edgar L, McLean S, Hogan SO, et al. The Milestones Guidebook. . Accreditation Council for Graduate Medical Education (ACGME). Available at: https://www.acgme.org/What-We-Do/Accreditation/Milestones/Resources. Accessed Feb 23, 2022.

22. Accreditation Council for Graduate Medical Education. Neurology milestones. Available at: https://www.acgme.org/specialties/neurology/milestones/. Accessed Feb 25, 2022,.

23. Morgenstern BZ, Roman BJB, DeWaay D, et al. Expectations of and for Clerkship Directors 2.0: A Collaborative Statement from the Alliance for Clinical Education. Teach Learn Med 2021;33(4):343–54.

24. Srinivasan M, Li ST, Meyers FJ, et al. Teaching as a Competency": competencies for medical educators. Acad Med 2011;86(10):1211–20.
25. Torralba KD, Jose D, Katz JD. Competency-based medical education for the clinician-educator: the coming of Milestones version 2. Clin Rheumatol 2020; 39(6):1719–23.
26. Heard JK, Allen RM, Clardy J. Assessing the needs of residency program directors to meet the ACGME general competencies. Acad Med 2002;77(7):750.
27. Gugger JJ, Reoma LB, Soni M, et al. Residency training: a practical guide for medical students who are planning a future in neurology. Neurology 2020; 94(15):673–7.
28. Liaison Committee on Medical Education. Functions and structure of a medical school: standards for accreditation of medical education programs leading to the MD Degree. Available at: https://lcme.org/publications/. Accessed Feb 22, 2022.
29. American Academy of Neurology CNCD Work Group on ED2/Core Curriculum. ED2 Core Curriculum Recommendations. Available at: https://www.aan.com/ tools-resources/clerkship-and-course-director-education. Accessed Feb 22, 2022.
30. Merlin LR, Horak HA, Milligan TA, et al. A competency-based longitudinal core curriculum in medical neuroscience. Neurology 2014;83(5):456–62.
31. Tanner JA, Rao KT, Salas RE, et al. Incorporating students into clinic may be associated with both improved clinical productivity and educational value. Neurol Clin Pract 2017;7(6):474–82.
32. Centers for Medicare & Medicaid Services (CMS). CMS Manual System: Pub 100-04 Medicare Claims Processing, Transmittal 4068. Available at: https:// www.cms.gov/Regulations-and-Guidance/Guidance/Transmittals/ 2018Downloads/R4068CP.pdf. Accessed May 24, 2022.
33. Awan S, Shafqat S, Kamal AK, et al. Pattern of neurological diseases in adult outpatient neurology clinics in tertiary care hospital. BMC Res Notes 2017; 10(1):545.
34. Akpalu A, Adjei P, Nkromah K, et al. Neurological disorders encountered at an out-patient clinic in Ghana's largest medical center: a 16-year review. eNeurologicalSci 2021;24:100361.
35. Tayade MC, Latti RG. Effectiveness of early clinical exposure in medical education: Settings and scientific theories - Review. J Educ Health Promot 2021;10:117.
36. Frey J, Neeley B, Umer A, et al. Training in neurology: neuro day: an innovative curriculum connecting medical students with patients. Neurology 2021;96(10): e1482–6.
37. Worley P, Couper I, Strasser R, et al. A typology of longitudinal integrated clerkships. Med Educ 2016;50(9):922–32.
38. Brown MEL, Whybrow P, Kirwan G, et al. Professional identity formation within longitudinal integrated clerkships: a scoping review. Med Educ 2021;55(8):912–24.
39. Pock A, Daniel M, Santen SA, et al. Challenges associated with moving the united states medical licensing examination (USMLE) step 1 to after the core clerkships and how to approach them. Acad Med 2019;94(6):775–80.
40. Heckers S. Project for a scientific psychiatry: neuroscience literacy. JAMA Psychiatry 2017;74(4):315.
41. Cunningham MG, Goldstein M, Katz D, et al. Coalescence of psychiatry, neurology, and neuropsychology: from theory to practice. Harv Rev Psychiatry 2006;14(3):127–40.

42. Juul D, Gutmann L, Adams HP Jr, et al. Training in neurology: feedback from graduates about the psychiatry component of residency training. Neurology 2021;96(5):233–6.

43. London ZN, Khan J, Cahill C, et al. 2017 Program director survey: feedback from your adult neurology residency leadership. Neurology 2018;91(15):e1448–54.

44. Chemali Z, Henderson DC, Fricchione G. Developing a dual residency program in psychiatry and neurology in an area of regional conflict: the university of hargeisa-massachusetts general hospital-boston medical center experience. J Neuropsychiatry Clin Neurosci Winter 2022;34(1):77–83.

45. Curtis CM, Eubanks JE, Charles SC, et al. A required, combined neurology-physical medicine and rehabilitation clerkship addresses clinical and health systems knowledge gaps for fourth-year medical students. Am J Phys Med Rehabil 2021;100(2S Suppl 1):S17–22.

46. Bega D, Krainc D. Challenges to neurology residency education in today's health care environment. Ann Neurol 2016;80(3):315–20.

47. Knobloch AC, Ledford CJW, Wilkes S, et al. The impact of near-peer teaching on medical students' transition to clerkships. Fam Med 2018;50(1):58–62.

48. Taylor CFC, Kurn OR, Glautier SP, et al. The efficacy of interdisciplinary near-peer teaching within neuroanatomical education-preliminary observations. Med Sci Educ 2021;31(2):387–93.

49. Meller SM, Chen M, Chen R, et al. Near-peer teaching in a required third-year clerkship. Yale J Biol Med 2013;86(4):583–9.

50. Keser Z, Rodriguez YA, Tremont J, et al. The role of residents in medical students' neurology education: current status and future perspectives. BMC Med Educ 2020;20(1):115.

51. Sandrone S, Berthaud JV, Carlson C, et al. Active learning in psychiatry education: current practices and future perspectives. Front Psychiatry 2020;11:211.

52. Schiel KZ, Everard KM. Active learning versus traditional teaching methods in the family medicine clerkship. Fam Med 2021;53(5):359–61.

53. Torralba KD, Doo L. Active learning strategies to improve progression from knowledge to action. Rheum Dis Clin North Am 2020;46(1):1–19.

54. Balwan S, Fornari A, DiMarzio P, et al. Use of team-based learning pedagogy for internal medicine ambulatory resident teaching. J Grad Med Educ 2015;7(4):643–8.

55. Thompson Stone R, Tollefson T, Epstein R, et al. Education research: positive effect of scheduled faculty modeling on clerkship student bedside skills exposure and learning. Neurology 2017;88(24):e236–9.

56. Will EM, Altchek CL, Shukla HP, et al. AuduBon-bons: bite-sized learning for residents in the ambulatory obstetrics and gynecology clinic. J Grad Med Educ 2022;14(3):326–31.

57. Chhetri SK. E-learning in neurology education: principles, opportunities and challenges in combating neurophobia. J Clin Neurosci 2017;44:80–3.

58. Govindarajan R, Vu AN, Salas RME, et al. Accelerated implementation of a virtual neurology clerkship amid a global crisis. Neurology 2022;98(7):279–86.

59. Pace A, Orr SL, Rosen NL, et al. The current state of headache medicine education in the United States and Canada: An observational, survey-based study of neurology clerkship directors and curriculum deans. Headache 2021;61(6):854–62.

60. Kasai H, Shikino K, Saito G, et al. Alternative approaches for clinical clerkship during the COVID-19 pandemic: online simulated clinical practice for inpatients and outpatients-A mixed method. BMC Med Educ 2021;21(1):149.

61. Bui I, Bhattacharya A, Wong SH, et al. Role of three-dimensional visualization modalities in medical education. Front Pediatr 2021;9:760363.
62. Sandrone S, Carlson CE. Future of neurology & technology: virtual and augmented reality in neurology and neuroscience education: applications and curricular strategies. Neurology 2021. https://doi.org/10.1212/wnl.0000000000012413.
63. Ekstrand C, Jamal A, Nguyen R, et al. Immersive and interactive virtual reality to improve learning and retention of neuroanatomy in medical students: a randomized controlled study. CMAJ Open 2018;6(1):E103–9.
64. Küçük S, Kapakin S, Göktaş Y. Learning anatomy via mobile augmented reality: effects on achievement and cognitive load. Anat Sci Educ 2016;9(5):411–21.
65. Cook DA, Erwin PJ, Triola MM. Computerized virtual patients in health professions education: a systematic review and meta-analysis. Acad Med 2010;85(10):1589–602.
66. Santen SA, Ryan M, Helou MA, et al. Building reliable and generalizable clerkship competency assessments: Impact of 'hawk-dove' correction. Med Teach 2021;43(12):1374–80.
67. Norcini J, Anderson MB, Bollela V, et al. 2018 Consensus framework for good assessment. Med Teach 2018;40(11):1102–9.
68. Senecal EL, Askew K, Gorney B, et al. Anatomy of a clerkship test. Acad Emerg Med 2010;17(Suppl 2):S31–7.
69. McManus IC, Thompson M, Mollon J. Assessment of examiner leniency and stringency ('hawk-dove effect') in the MRCP(UK) clinical examination (PACES) using multi-facet Rasch modelling. BMC Med Educ 2006;6:42.
70. Thompson Stone R, Mooney C, Wexler E, et al. Formal faculty observation and assessment of bedside skills for 3rd-year neurology clerks. Neurology 2016;87(21):2266–70.
71. Nasca TJ, Philibert I, Brigham T, et al. The next GME accreditation system–rationale and benefits. N Engl J Med 2012;366(11):1051–6.
72. The American Board of Psychiatry and Neurology. Neurology clinical evaluation exercise. Available at: https://www.abpn.com/access-residency-info/residency-training-information/neurologychild-neurology/. Accessed Feb 26, 2022.
73. Schuh LA, London Z, Neel R, et al. Education research: Bias and poor interrater reliability in evaluating the neurology clinical skills examination. Neurology 2009;73(11):904–8.
74. Barrows HS. An overview of the uses of standardized patients for teaching and evaluating clinical skills. AAMC Acad Med 1993;68(6):443–51 [discussion: 451-3].
75. Safdieh JE, Lin AL, Aizer J, et al. Standardized patient outcomes trial (SPOT) in neurology. Med Educ Online 2011;16doi. https://doi.org/10.3402/meo.v16i0.5634.
76. Braksick SA, Wang Y, Hunt SL, et al. Evaluator agreement in medical student assessment across a multi-campus medical school during a standardized patient encounter. Med Sci Educ 2020;30(1):381–6.
77. van der Leeuw RM, Lombarts KM, Arah OA, et al. A systematic review of the effects of residency training on patient outcomes. BMC Med 2012;10:65.
78. Parekh N, Lebduska E, Hoffman E, et al. A longitudinal ambulatory quality improvement curriculum that aligns resident education with patient outcomes: a 3-year experience. Am J Med Qual 2020;35(3):242–51.

Moving?

Make sure your subscription moves with you!

To notify us of your new address, find your **Clinics Account Number** (located on your mailing label above your name), and contact customer service at:

Email: journalscustomerservice-usa@elsevier.com

800-654-2452 (subscribers in the U.S. & Canada)
314-447-8871 (subscribers outside of the U.S. & Canada)

Fax number: 314-447-8029

Elsevier Health Sciences Division
Subscription Customer Service
3251 Riverport Lane
Maryland Heights, MO 63043

*To ensure uninterrupted delivery of your subscription, please notify us at least 4 weeks in advance of move.

Printed and bound by CPI Group (UK) Ltd, Croydon, CR0 4YY

03/10/2024

01040474-0008